Advance Praise for Creativity

"Countless contributions have dealt with the psychological, socio-cultural, cognitive, evolutionary aspects of creativity. The neuroanatomical and physiological aspects have been explored to a limited extent: which is odd, as creativity is the product of brain's activity. Elkhonon Goldberg's book has the brain as its undisputed main character; this makes it uniquely important. The role of the brain's physiology and anatomy in the generation of creativity, with the frontal lobe and the prefrontal cortex in the privileged position, are discussed exhaustively and masterfully. Goldberg spices the discussions with his experiences as a young neuroscientist in the Soviet Union to deal with important, but lesser known, aspects of creativity. This book is written with great literary skill, making reading it really enjoyable. Goldberg is a first rate neuroscientist and a born writer."
>   —**Ernesto Carafoli, MD**, Venetian Institute of Molecular Medicine,
>   University of Padova, Italy

"Creativity, that most charismatic of human mysteries, can't be reduced into the action of a few simple brain processors. In *Creativity*, Elkhonon Goldberg, a pioneer in research into novelty and routine in the brain, and one of the greatest integrative thinkers in modern neuroscience, is subtle, judicious, relentlessly curious, fun and brutally honest about what neuroscience knows, and doesn't know, about the subject. He guides us through decades of research, to show that perhaps the most striking thing about our plastic organ of creativity, is that, while there are certain basic patterns in the creative brain, they are only starting points; the brain's circuitry, being so plastic, likely has just as many different ways of helping to produce creative states, as there are human ways of being creative. No one interested in the neuroscience of creativity can afford to miss this book."
>   —**Norman Doidge, MD**, author of *The Brain That Changes Itself*
>   and *The Brain's Way of Healing*, Toronto, Canada

"As a former copywriter and Worldwide Creative Director of a large international advertising company, my days were spent trying to control and direct the 'creative' efforts. There was no manual to refer to, we had to 'be' creative. After reading Dr. Goldberg's new book, I realize we had no understanding of what that really meant. There is so much in here I wish I could have accessed and was unsettled by the accurate description of the mental ping pong game which I have unconsciously employed throughout my career. Dr. Goldberg has obviously travelled extensively and his observations and experiences seem like a beautifully written journey in themselves until he leads one to the point where he reveals even more involving aspects of creativity in other cultures and even species. As far as this book is concerned, Dr. Goldberg clearly knows what he's doing when it comes to *Creativity*."

—**John Fawcett**, Creative Director, Balucate, Sydney, Australia

"What an inspired marriage of Creativity and Neuroscience (big C, big N), officiated by a brave scientist and original thinker. This book will spark new research, new toolkits, new conversations—and much creativity."

—**Alvaro Fernandez, MBA, MA**, CEO & Editor-in-Chief of SharpBrains, Washington, DC

"Elkhonon Goldberg's new book, *Creativity: The Human Brain in the Age of Innovation* is a very insightful study of our brains in a time of accelerating and multi-dimensional change. It is the fruit of both scholarly research and many decades of experience. He explores several key concepts: Salience, how does our brain determine what is of real importance and relevance and put it ahead of the neural line? Hyperfrontality-Hypofrontality, our brains going through intense engagement with a problem and then the 'Aha' moment comes during sleep or when taking a walk. Small-world networks, whose strong connectivity with each other leads to new and surprising insights and solutions. *Creativity* is a wonderful addition to Dr. Goldberg's body of work."

—**Bienvenido F. Nebres**, National Scientist, Professor of Mathematics, Past-President of Ateneo de Manila University, Manila, Philippines

"Elkhonon Goldberg, PhD, a leading-edge neuropsychologist and broad-ranging thinker, has provided a brilliant, synthetic account of human creativity. A sophisticated understanding of brain function is combined with insights from contemporary psychology, evolutionary biology, and cross-cultural studies to elucidate the key processes underlying innovation in the arts, sciences and all areas of human endeavor. Indeed, Goldberg says that creativity is not a unitary phenomenon, and many different neural functions and network interactions coordinate to produce and appreciate novel, meaningful thoughts and acts. How and why this all comes together, and what it means for our species and its future, are just a few of the big issues addressed in this masterful and engaging book."

—**David Silbersweig, MD**, Co-Director, Neuroscience Center and Professor of Psychiatry, Brigham and Women's Hospital, Harvard Medical School, Boston, MA

Creativity

Also by Elkhonon Goldberg

The Executive Brain: Frontal Lobes and the Civilized Mind
(Oxford University Press, December 2002)

The Wisdom Paradox: How Your Mind Can Grow Stronger
As Your Brain Grows Older
(Gotham Books, February 2006)

The New Executive Brain: Frontal Lobes in a Complex World
(Oxford University Press, August 2009)

Creativity

The Human Brain in the Age of Innovation

By

ELKHONON GOLDBERG

OXFORD
UNIVERSITY PRESS

OXFORD
UNIVERSITY PRESS

Oxford University Press is a department of the University of Oxford. It furthers
the University's objective of excellence in research, scholarship, and education
by publishing worldwide. Oxford is a registered trade mark of Oxford University
Press in the UK and certain other countries.

Published in the United States of America by Oxford University Press
198 Madison Avenue, New York, NY 10016, United States of America.

© Elkhonon Goldberg 2018

Library of Congress Cataloging-in-Publication Data
Names: Goldberg, Elkhonon, author.
Title: Creativity : the human brain in the age of innovation /
by Elkhonon Goldberg.
Description: New York, NY : Oxford University Press, [2018] |
Includes bibliographical references and index.
Identifiers: LCCN 2017008677 | ISBN 9780190466497 (alk. paper)
Subjects: | MESH: Brain—physiology | Creativity
Classification: LCC QP376 | NLM WL 300 | DDC 612.8/2—dc23
LC record available at https://lccn.loc.gov/2017008677

1 3 5 7 9 8 6 4 2
Printed by Sheridan Books, Inc., United States of America

*The book is dedicated to the anonymous creative minds
who were so far ahead of their times that nobody
noticed. Their valiant spirit is herein acknowledged.*

Contents

Preface

WHAT IS AN aging neuropsychologist doing writing a book about creativity, the province of the young and the brash? A lifelong focus of my work has been trying to understand how the brain deals with novelty and complex decision making, and the way it evolved into an interest in creativity was actually not entirely of my own doing. Over the years, whenever the conversation about cognitive novelty arose, I was quizzed about creativity—frequently by colleagues and almost invariably by the members of general educated public. I didn't have much to say, other than voicing my general skepticism that creativity could be understood as a monolithic trait, that it could be linked to a narrow set of neural structures, or that it could be understood in strictly biological terms. Occasionally, I also shared my being generally unimpressed with the laboratory "creativity" tests, which on a few occasions I had been asked to take, and found, at least from a subject's perspective, to be contrived and of dubious relevance to real-life consequential creativity. I also felt that the never-ending deliberations about the relationship between creativity and intelligence were going nowhere as long as either construct lacked a meaningful definition. But I could appreciate how naturally the discourse about novelty morphed into one about creativity. Based on my, at the time very limited, familiarity with "creativity research," I also knew that the structures implicated in dealing with cognitive novelty, which I had studied and written about extensively—the prefrontal cortex and the right hemisphere— have been often linked to creativity both in scientific literature and in tabloid sources. And it was also clear that the capacity for innovation is only part of the creativity story, the other one being the cultural context, societal relevance and salience. This called for the convergence of neuroscientific and the humanities/ social science perspectives—a convergence that has always appealed to me both intellectually and temperamentally. It also brought into the discourse the relationship between two sides of the innovation process: its generation by the creative individuals or teams, and its reception and acceptance (or rejection) by the consumer, the general public,—something akin to what Eric Kandel referred to as "the beholder's share" in his discussion of the visual arts.

The range of influential approaches to creativity research seemed to be defined by two polarities—a cultural/humanitarian perspective so eloquently represented in the writings by Mihaly Csikszentmihalyi on one end, and the neuroscientific studies where performance on the tasks of "divergent thinking" was combined with various neuroimaging, biochemical, and genetic techniques on the other end—but these two narratives were often unfolding in parallel rather than in concert. Even though it was clear that the two perspectives—neuroscientific and cultural—had to be integrated into a coherent narrative for the processes of innovation and creativity to be understood, this integration sounded like a dauntingly tall order. It was a challenge worth rising to, or at least trying to meet.

Then there was an almost aesthetic sense of symmetry waiting to be satisfied. Creativity and wisdom are often regarded as two pillars supporting the same arc bracketing the essence of the meaningful life of a productive mind. An earlier book of mine, *The Wisdom Paradox*, examined one of these pillars from a neuroscientific perspective, and the project seemed incomplete without examining the other. The idea of writing a book about cognitive novelty had been on my mind for some time, and as my thoughts about the future book evolved, the subject of creativity was increasingly in the picture. The book you are about to read is the product of this evolution, where the novelty and creativity themes are closely intertwined. While working on the book, I made an earnest effort to acquaint myself with some of the "creativity research" literature, but also quite intentionally maintained a certain distance from it and was guided mostly by my own understanding of how the brain works and how it doesn't, in the hope that this balance may foster original insights.

As was the case with my previous books, this book is also a bit of a Trojan horse (one of my favorite animals, second only to my dogs), providing a vehicle for addressing a wider range of topics related to the brain and the mind, which transcend the more specific novelty/creativity focus. In writing this book, I aimed for it to be of interest both to my scientist and clinician colleagues and to the educated general public. This has inevitably led to the interweaving of more general and more technical narratives, hopefully with a reasonable balance between the two.

I am writing this Preface with the rest of the book having already been written. Finishing a book is usually fraught for me with emotional ambivalence. There is a sense of fulfilment but also of a loss; it is the end of a deeply personal journey. At least this is how it felt with my previous books, but this book is turning out to be different as it begins to animate my sense of the directions of my own future work. Perhaps because the whole quest for understanding creativity and innovation by converging the biological and cultural perspectives is a relatively new enterprise, it is ripe with new possibilities, new ideas, and provocative hypotheses potentially capable of propelling original and innovative (pun intended) research in a number of uncharted directions. A few such ideas and new directions are outlined in the book you are about to read. In addition to aiming to shed light on the nature of human (and not only human) creativity, these ideas aim to advance our understanding of how knowledge is represented in the brain; of the evolutionary roots of language; of the trendy but not sufficiently understood "working memory"; of how the two halves of the brain are both different and together in humans and other species; and of the nature of human intelligence. They also aim to refine, or perhaps even change our understanding of certain neurological disorders; to make the case for the need of creativity, and more generally cognitive neuroscience, research in diverse cultural contexts and not just in the Western societies; and even to introduce a few ideas potentially useful in artificial intelligence designs. While some of these ideas and hypotheses may prove to be wrong or wrongheaded (a risk anyone aspiring to being creative must be prepared to take), others will not. I hope that the members of the general public among the book's readers will find these ideas intriguing, and the scientists will find them worthy of pursuing in their future work. Such scientists will surely include me.

Elkhonon Goldberg
New York City, 2017

Acknowledgments

SEVERAL INDIVIDUALS HELPED make this book possible in a variety of ways. My agents, Michelle Tessler and Michael Carlisle, provided invaluable encouragement at the early stages of the project. My editor, Craig Panner, has been the source of unfailingly cogent guidance, benevolent but firm, throughout the work on the book. Assistant editor Emily Samulski has provided superb assistance at every stage of the project. Richard Gallini provided the artwork with patience and precision. Daniel Feldman assisted with literature searches and chapter notes. Anton Shapovalov designed the small-world and random network images for the book. Ida Bagus Yogi Iswara Bawa recorded the video of the Sanghyang Jaran dance on the island of Bali. Dmitri Bougakov, Bienvenido Nebres, Harry Ballan, Igor Glavatski, and Luz Casimiro-Querubin have provided invaluable feedback on various aspects of the manuscript. My late bullmastiff, Brit, and my new English mastiff puppy, Brutus, have been my junior partners at various stages of writing the book, with unconditional devotion and cheerful disposition. My sincere gratitude goes to all of them. This is my fourth book with Oxford University Press, and the association has been highly rewarding and gratifying, for which I am thankful.

Creativity

I

The Age of Novelty

IN ANCIENT EGYPT, life had not changed much from the age of the Great
Pyramid of Giza to the age of Ramesses the Great—a span of approximately
1,300 years. This is roughly the same span as that between the fall of the Roman
Empire through Europe's descent into the Dark Middle Ages and to the dawn of
the Industrial Revolution, a span of immense transition. And in our time, much
of the knowledge acquired in graduate school ten years ago is obsolete today. If
Ray Kurzweil's Law of Accelerating Returns is to be believed, the rate of growth
of information technology, and by extension knowledge accumulation in general, is exponential (Figure 1.1).[1] In a similar vein, "Moore's law" and other estimates predict that the rate of scientific and technological process will progress at
an increasingly neck-breaking rate.[2] We are confronted with novelty at an ever
accelerating rate, both as individuals and as a society. This quantitative progression leads to a profound qualitative change. As recently as two generations ago,
a cognitive skill set acquired in one's youth could see one through a lifetime. But
today an octogenarian nimbly operating an Apple iPhone or a Samsung tablet
clearly is not relying on something learned in her youth. This societal paradigm
shift is so pervasive that we often fail to notice it, but it is here.

In this context, understanding how the human brain deals with novelty
becomes an issue of paramount importance. Granted, most of us do not share an
intrinsic interest in science or technology, but even as consumers of technology,
we will inhabit a world where tomorrow will be unrecognizably different from
today, and our brains will be increasingly challenged by novelty whether we like
it or not.

In an informationally stagnant society where change previously occurred at a
glacial rate, relatively few individuals were engaged in creative processes; the lives
of the vast majority of society were driven by routines that, once acquired, could
be followed without much change through their life span. But in a society where
knowledge and skills become obsolete even before they become routine, virtually

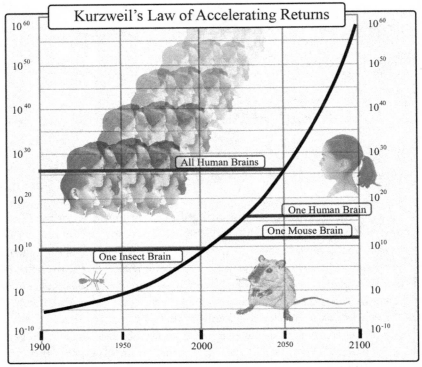

FIGURE 1.1 Kurzweil's Law of Accelerating Returns. On X axis—year. On Y axis—calculations per second per $1,000.

every member of society becomes part of the creative process: if not generating the unique ideas, then grasping and incorporating them in their lives, these new ideas, concepts, and skills. Does this trend now require a different deployment of our neural resources, of our brain power by the members of a novelty-driven society? Will it affect the way our brain changes as we age? I will argue that the answer to these questions is probably "Yes."

Punctuated Equilibrium in History

The history of our civilization is marked by a progressive accumulation of information, ideas, and technologies. But this process has been neither simple nor straightforward. According to Niles Eldredge and Stephen Gould's "punctuated equilibrium" theory of evolution, biological evolution is not a smooth or gradual process, but is rather driven by bursts of change interspersed by periods of relative stasis.[3] In his book *The Great and Holy War*, the historian Philip Jenkins proposes that this is also true for the cultural evolution.[4] Indeed, beginning with the mysterious explosion of artistic expression somewhere on the boundary of biological evolution and culture 30,000 years ago, the accumulation of knowledge and ideas proceeded in fits and starts. The period of 2700–2500 BCE in Ancient Egypt was a period of great ferment—the age of Imhotep, the first great polymath in recorded history, and of the Great Pyramids. It was followed by many centuries of relative cultural stasis dominated by tradition and imitation. The same was true for ancient Mesopotamia, regarded by many as the cradle of the Western civilization, where the cultural ferment in the third millennium BCE was followed by a long succession of imitation societies. In ancient Greece, the cultural bursts of the Minoan and later Mycenaean civilizations of the second millennium BCE were succeeded by the Greek Dark Ages, followed by a long period of relative stasis before the eighth century BCE resurgence, culminating in the creative splendor of the Classical period in the fifth century BCE, the Athenian Golden Age. The cultural sophistication of Emperor Augustus' Pax Romana in the beginning of the first millennium AD was followed by Europe's Dark Ages, until the High Middle Ages and finally the Renaissance infused the Continent with a new burst of creative energy. The Industrial Revolution on the cusp of the eighteenth and nineteenth centuries was another such burst of radical innovation. The cumulative effect of these cultural spikes has resulted in the unprecedented accumulation of knowledge. Contrary to the meaning of the popular expression, the "Renaissance man" (or woman) was probably the first human in history no longer able to have a grasp of all, or even most of, the essential knowledge of the time. The dizzying rate at which information is accumulated and knowledge expands is exhilarating and inspiring, but it comes at a price. That price is the fragmentation of knowledge, whose extreme case is sometimes referred to as "Balkanization." Balkanization is described in Wikipedia as "a geopolitical term, originally used to describe the process of fragmentation or division of a region or state into smaller regions or states that are often hostile or non-cooperative with one another.... The term is also used to describe other forms of disintegration.... It is considered pejorative by some"—for instance, by me. I imagine it bedevils most disciplines; it certainly bedevils mine—neuropsychology and neuroscience. Later in the book, we will encounter several examples of its retarding effects on neuropsychology and neuroscience, as well as attempts that have been made to overcome its ill effects.

Many Kinds of Revolution

In his sweeping tour de force *Sapiens: A Brief History of Humankind*, the historian Yoval Noah Harari proposes several "inflection points" in our species' ascendancy.[5] The first one was the Cognitive Revolution, with the emergence of language capable of formulating speculative propositions as its hallmark, about 70,000 years ago. The second one was the Agricultural Revolution, with the departure from the hunter-gatherer lifestyle, the domestication of plants and animals, and the emergence of permanent settlements as its hallmark, about 30,000 years ago. This was also the age of the "cultural revolution" (not to be confused with the social upheaval unleashed by Mao Zedong in China millennia later and known under the same name). The third inflection point was the Scientific Revolution, with the systematic accumulation of empirical knowledge, the age of maritime expansion and discovery of America by the Europeans, and the rise of capitalism as its hallmark, about 500 years ago. This inflection point ushered in something absent from the human *zeitgeist* up to that point: "the admission of ignorance." According to Harari, up to that time, society operated on the implicit assumption that everything worth knowing had already been discovered, and that individual ignorance could be remedied by consulting some older texts—in an informationally static society, you turned to the past to receive guidance for the future. It was only about 500 years ago that this fundamental premise changed in favor of the admission of societal ignorance and the ongoing quest for new knowledge. The fourth inflection point was the Industrial Revolution, with the rise of market economy and the rise of machines as its hallmark, about 200 years ago.

The chronology of these inflection points is approximate and imprecise. Yet even with this caveat, the examination of the time intervals separating them is highly instructive: 40,000 years between the Cognitive and Agricultural revolutions; perhaps less than 30,000 years between the Agricultural and Scientific revolutions; 300 years between the Scientific and Industrial revolutions; and 200 years between the Industrial and Digital revolutions (Figure 1.2).

The rate of change has not been merely speeding up, it has been speeding up by orders of magnitude—from tens of millennia to hundred-year intervals. And if we extrapolate into the future, the order of magnitude of this change is likely to be compressed even further. By all accounts, we are in the beginning of another great creative cultural burst driven by the digital revolution and by the prospect of a nearly complete fusion of the physical and virtual worlds, of biology and artifice, the *"fusion revolution."*

In an environment characterized by such a rate of change, a major redeployment of neural resources may be necessary in any individual brain, a major change in the way the human brain processes information. The basic cognitive habits, and perhaps even the underlying brain machinery itself operating in a relatively static environment, may be very different from the habits necessary to operate in an ever-changing environment. If this is true, then the implications of such changes for society are profound.

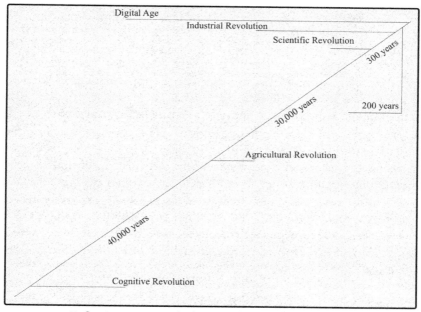

FIGURE 1.2 Inflection points in the history of civilization. Rate of development of human society through history, after Yoval Harari.

Culture and Cognitive Styles

Cultural dependence of cognitive styles has been increasingly on my mind, prompted by the observations made in a very different "compartment" of my life. My typical working day is often a juxtaposition of very disparate activities—like writing this book in the morning and wearing my clinical hat in the afternoon, or vice versa. This juggling of diverse activities—clinical, research, teaching, industry consulting, and writing—has been at times a mixed blessing, possibly detracting from any one of them, but on the whole I have enjoyed it over the years and felt that the beneficial effects of mutual enrichment outweighed those of crowding. My clinical work is in itself a study in diversity: New York City being the modern-day Tower of Babel, I get to see patients of every social stratum from every corner of the world. It so happened that while I was writing this book and over a short period of time, I was asked to see several patients from various developing countries of Asia and Africa. They were all simple older people with zero formal education, complete products of the traditional "old country" societies who, even while living in the United States, had had little contact with the larger world. By the nature of the cases, the patients stood to gain something from the diagnosis of genuine cognitive impairment—financial awards or various accommodations—and I was asked to conduct neuropsychological evaluations to assess their cognition. In such cases, the possibility of "malingering" or "symptom magnification" is never out of the question, and part of the neuropsychological evaluation involves the determination of whether such untoward behaviors in fact are taking place. Special tests even exist to help determine whether the patient is malingering or failing to exert sufficient "good-faith effort" required by the cognitive tasks s/he is asked to perform. I am not a great fan of these tests and have been on the record referring to them as "ersatz neuropsychology," but use them anyway when I am required to.

Without exception, all the patients of this particular run performed abysmally on the neuropsychological tests—including the "malingering" ones—in a way which was vastly out of proportion to the known or suspected maladies that brought them to my office and could not be explained by them. Yet they were neither demented, depressed, nor anxious in a way that could interfere with their performance; nor were they oppositional or resistant to the testing. They were genial older people who were compliantly doing everything I was asking them to do . . . except that they were not. The obvious "by the book" conclusion a neuropsychologist is expected to draw in such situations is that the patient was malingering or sabotaging the evaluation by failing to exert the requisite effort; but as a seasoned clinician with more than forty years of experience, I was convinced that they were neither malingerers nor saboteurs. At the same time, it was clear that despite my numerous admonitions, they were not exerting the mental effort necessary to solve the little, moderately challenging tasks I was giving them. I was quite certain that the tasks were well within their cognitive capacity, but they would require a bit of mental effort. And I was increasingly under the impression that the stumbling block was not that the patients didn't *want* to mentally exert themselves but that they simply *didn't know how to*—*they did not have the habit of mental effort*. The whole proposition of exerting mental effort seemed as foreign to them as attempting cartwheels would be to me. When I shared this observation with Bienvenido Nebres, a leading scientist and educator in the Philippines, he described a similar phenomenon in some parts of his country, "where there has not been a tradition of schooling and parents cannot understand why their children have to go to school every day." Such observations lead to an interesting distinction between *cognitive skills* and *cognitive habits*. Different cultural milieus engender not just different *cognitive skills,* but also different *cognitive habits*.

Cultural differences in cognition have been studied for decades, and it has been known, to a substantial degree owing to the work of my mentor Alexander Luria, that major differences exist between the ways hypothetical logical and conceptual tasks (syllogisms, classifications, and so on) are approached by the members of literate "modern" societies and those of illiterate traditional ones.[6] But here I felt that I had stumbled onto something more fundamental and profound: that the whole enterprise of "mental effort," and even more broadly what can be termed "cognitive habits," may be culture-dependent in a general sense. A person with no experience of mental effort all of a sudden faced with a situation requiring one, is like someone who grew up in a gravity-free environment and suddenly transported into one governed by the laws of gravity, not realizing that objects must be held up in order for them not to fall on the ground. Far-fetched as this idea may be, it did not surprise my friend Michael Cole, a distinguished cross-cultural psychologist at University of California, San Diego. When I shared my patients' experiences, not to mention my own surprise, with him, he immediately remarked that separation of abstract thought from practical action is a cultural phenomenon.

If the very habit of cognitive effort and perhaps other basic cognitive habits is a function of the society's informational demands, then the increase of these demands in a rapidly changing environment may have profound effects on the brain itself. The changes in the rate of knowledge accumulation will change the neural demands, not just for those who create human culture, but also for those who consume it, which means for everyone. This means that the demands on the brain may be very different during cultural "bursts" compared to the periods of cultural stasis.

Major technological changes were intertwined with societal and political changes during earlier surges of cultural ferment, and we are witnessing it again today, often in ways no one anticipated; such as the "Arab Spring," whose unfolding, for better or worse, a few years ago across North Africa and the Middle East would not have been possible without the Internet and social media; nor would the worldwide recruitment of disgruntled malcontents by ISIS. And just as the Western powers were bombing ISIS to no great effect, the hackers' community known as "Anonymous" declared its own war on ISIS through a masked spokesman on social media. Who knows, in a world where an unconventional organization was able to come into existence because of the Internet and social media, attacking it in cyberspace may prove to be more effective than with the means of conventional warfare. Meanwhile, Donald Trump's unrestrained but probably effective use of Twitter may have played a role in his unexpected win of the 2016 presidential elections in the United States. Life is stranger than futuristic fiction!

How Realities Fuse

Among the technology-driven societal changes, I find one particularly intriguing and potentially profound: the fusion of physical and virtual realities. Pedestrians bumping into one another on Manhattan sidewalks because the virtual goings-on on the screens of their mobile devices evidently take precedence over the physical events on the street around them have become so ubiquitous that we don't usually perceive them as portending a seismic societal shift; and it is safe to assume that the bumbling pedestrians know the difference between the real and the virtual, even though they often do look alarmingly disoriented when they tear themselves momentarily from their mobile devices to make a brief and reluctant contact with the old-fashioned physical world. The boundary between physical and virtual reality is increasingly blurred intentionally and rationally in various training regimens designed to enhance real-life skills in education, medicine, and particularly in the military. But here, too, unintended, or at least unanticipated, consequences abound. In an editorial in *The New York Times* titled "A Band of Tweeters," John Spenser, a U.S. Army major and West Point scholar, compared his Iraq battlefield observations in 2003 and 2008. Following an engagement with the enemy in 2003, soldiers would talk about what happened; but in 2008, each was "sitting silently in front of computer screens, posting about their day on Myspace and Facebook." Where in 2003 strong bonds were developing between soldiers serving in the same unit, it seemed that in 2008 each of them was more immersed into his personal "virtual" world than in their shared physical world.[7]

Far more striking is an event that actually happened in South Korea, when parents allowed their real, flesh-and-blood biological child to starve to death because they, the parents, were immersed in raising a virtual child in a video game. It seems that in the minds of the South Korean couple permitting this to happen a few years ago, an actual blurring of the boundaries between the physical and virtual realities may have taken place. I truly believe that within the next few generations—and possibly even one generation—such blurring will become near complete. Outlandish as this prediction may sound, I will stand by it, particularly since I won't be around to eat the crow should it fail to materialize. And as a reflection of the point that technological progress is for the most part morally agnostic, we find the prefiguration of this fusion in one of the ugliest phenomena of our time—the rise of ISIS, referred to by Fareed Zakaria as an evil "messaging machine." This was captured in a repentant letter written by a teenage would-be ISIS recruit: "By assimilating into the Internet world instead of the real world, I became absorbed in a 'virtual' struggle while disconnecting from what was real: my family, my life and my future."[8] I can believe that, for a teenager, the crossing of the boundary separating the virtual world of "heroic" posturing from the oh-so-physical world of unspeakable cruelty may occur before he realizes what is actually happening to him. The vast consequences of such fusion of physical and virtual elements into one "synthetic" world are impossible for someone old-fashionably rooted in the physical reality, like myself, to imagine, but it is going to happen—very likely within the span of a single generation, the "fusion generation."

This fusion will not just change the world our not-so-distant descendants will live in, the synthetic world will *become* their world—the one to which the epithet "brave new" will apply like to no other era in human civilization. Imagine the dose of novelty that will befall these "fusioners" to digest! This futuristic change will be arguably more profound than moving to a different planet, yet in an odd way it will validate the eighteenth-century philosophical musings by Immanuel Kant, seconded a century later by Hermann Helmholtz and Ernst Mach—a thought that first crossed my mind and amused me to no end about a decade and a half ago, at the very crack of the twenty-first century. In his *Critique of Pure Reason* (*Kritik der reinen Vernunft*), Kant argued that all we experience is the "phenomenal world" conveyed by our senses, and that the actual physical source of these experiences—the "noumenal world"—populated by "thing[s] in itself" (*Dinge[n]-an-sich*) is never available to us directly and ultimately doesn't matter—a position that may have sounded counter-intuitive and even bizarre to his contemporaries as well as to ours, but is likely to have the ring of self-evident truth to the "fusion" and "post-fusion" generations.⁹ Yet the emergence of the "synthetic world" will arguably be the most profound and fundamental change in the cultural history of our species—one that the hackneyed expression "paradigm shift" does not do justice to, even remotely. Along with this shift in our species' cultural history is likely to come a biological shift in the way our brain functions under these radically different conditions. The exact consequences of this change are unpredictable, but they are certain to be profound, and some of them are prophesied by the noted British neuroscientist and my good friend Susan Greenfield in her novel *2121*. As implied in the novel's title, its protagonists are "post-fusioners" living their lives in a thoroughly fused synthetic world.¹⁰

The Human Brain in the New Age

Not only will the digital revolution change the workings of the normal brain, but it will also change the way brain disease manifests itself. Temporal lobe epilepsy (TLE) may turn out to be a case in point. TLE is among the most fascinating neurological disorders, which, contrary to a commonly held popular belief, does not "come and go" with stretches of complete normality between seizures. A patient with seizure disorder is often affected by the disease all the time even between seizures, and profound personality changes are known to occur in TLE. Among such changes, "hyper-religiosity" is particularly intriguing. A person previously indifferent to religious themes and practicing a secular lifestyle may develop a keen interest in religion, sometimes in the extreme, and start practicing religion fervently. A number of important religious and quasi-religious personalities were known or suspected to have had seizures (even though we cannot be sure what kind)—Mohammed, Martin Luther, Joan of Arc, and Pope Pius IX among them.[11] But the notion that TLE is necessarily associated with hyper-religiosity is challenged by the fact that a number of historic personalities known or suspected to have had seizures were religious only in the breach or outright blasphemous—Alexander of Macedon who proclaimed *himself* god; Julius Caesar who came to regard his hereditary position of High Priest (*Pontifex Maximus*) a career dead-end and quit it promptly, only to become a very secular dictator; or Peter the Great of Russia, whose favorite pastime during the early stages of his reign was to humiliate clergy by cutting off their beards and dressing them up in bizarre costumes.

What are the mechanisms of hyper-religiosity in TLE? Its association with a neuroanatomically specific site of dysfunction—the temporal lobes—has even led to speculations that religiosity is hardwired in the human brain, a rich terrain for tabloid speculations indeed. But I believe that the hyper-religiosity in TLE is a cultural phenomenon. Indeed, how else would one be expected to interpret hearing voices, gut-wrenching visceral premonitions, and emotional surges of dread or elation—all common experiences in a temporal-lobe seizure—in a society infused with religious motifs (and even most advanced societies were infused with such motifs as recently as a generation ago, and many still are)? A religious explanation and subsequently "finding religion" would be the most likely one in such a society. But I predict that, unless a definitive cure for it will have been found, the future-generation "fusioners" afflicted by TLE in the "synthetic" society will be much more likely to interpret such experiences in virtual reality terms than in religious terms.

The rapidly accelerating "novelty curve" will have a profound impact on our minds and brains by forcing every one of us to be a consumer of innovation to an unprecedented degree, and understanding the impact this constant exposure to novelty will have on the "consumer brain" is a challenge facing neuroscience. But then there is the other side of the coin, the *creation* of novelty. How is the novel idea created? In the age of innovation, understanding how the human brain processes novelty becomes an issue of paramount importance for more than one reason. As a society, we have a dual motivation for striving to uncover the brain mechanisms of confronting novelty: to understand both how it is consumed and how it is created. It is precisely this dual motivation that was the impetus for writing this book.

Novelty is inexorably linked to creativity, that most precious yet most mysterious gift of the human mind that drives progress. Understanding the brain machinery of novelty is a crucial step toward understanding human creativity.

We will examine the relationship between generating novel content and creativity in the human brain, and will present a new understanding of how different cognitive functions and brain structures come together for the creative act to happen. We will speculate how *dynamic network connectivity,* recently discovered by Yale neuroscientists, drives the process; and we will discover how, when it comes short, a process we call *directed wandering* takes over and produces that ineffable spark, the creative moment.

No single structure exists in the brain solely in charge of novelty-seeking, let alone of creativity. Rather, these complex functions arise from the interplay between many brain structures. The relationship of some of these structures to novelty and creativity is more direct and more transparent than that of the others; but ultimately they all play a role. In the forthcoming chapters, we will examine these numerous moving parts of the brain and their complementary roles in the complex machinery of innovation and creativity.

2

The Neuromythology of Creativity

From Neuroorphans to Neurofads

Unraveling the brain mechanisms of dealing with novelty is one of the most important stepping stones to understanding complex cognition; as a cognitive neuroscientist I find it fundamental. But it is not the kind of question likely to excite the general public's imagination. When I decided to write a book about cognitive novelty and proposed that the title of the book should be anchored by the word "novelty," my editor—undoubtedly more experienced than myself in ways of capturing the readers' interest, and wishing my book to succeed—objected. "How many people want to be novel?" he asked rhetorically, the implicit answer being "few to none." In contrast, "creativity" has a very personal allure. Presumably, everyone wants to be creative, or at least (or more importantly?) to be perceived as a creative individual. And the very opaqueness of this construct allows any number of self-serving interpretations. Over the last few decades, the brain mechanisms of creativity have been of considerable interest both to cognitive scientists and to the general population, and the boundary between these narratives—those of neuroscience and of pop-science—are sometimes blurred. The brain structures most commonly linked to creativity are the prefrontal cortex and the right hemisphere.

I will argue through much of the book that both structures are indeed closely linked to creativity as well as to dealing with novelty. But I will argue as stridently that neither of them—nor any other brain structure in particular, for that matter—can be thought of as the exclusive "seat" of creativity; and that the whole idea that a complex function like creativity can be linked to a narrow subset of brain regions is both misguided and naïve. I will also argue that, relatively less excitement-generating though it may be, the inquiry into the brain mechanisms of processing novelty may be a productive, perhaps even critical, stepping stone toward understanding creativity, as well as being important (perhaps even more so) in its own right.

One of the most exhaustive reviews of the "creativity" literature has been conducted by neuroscientist Arne Dietrich. German by birth, Dietrich was educated in the United States and works today at the American University in Beirut, Lebanon. This arguably unorthodox career trajectory suggests a restless spirit and an inquisitive mind, and Dietrich's work on creativity deserves close attention. Having meticulously selected and reviewed more than 60 research papers using a rigorous selection algorithm, Dietrich concluded that the findings were appallingly devoid of consistency, and this lack of consistency extended to the putative roles of the frontal lobes and the cerebral hemispheres in the creative process. Yes, the frontal lobes were activated in some of the neuroimaging studies of the creative process, but they were deactivated in others (we will aim to make sense of this bimodality later in the book). And yes, the right hemisphere was particularly active in some of the studies, but so was the left hemisphere in others (as the forthcoming chapters will hopefully show, this finding makes a lot of sense if one considers the roles of the two hemispheres in cognitive novelty versus cognitive routines).[1]

So it appears that both the frontal lobes and the right hemisphere play a role in creativity, but so do the other brain regions, including the left hemisphere. In the chapters that follow, we will attempt to apportion the roles played by these diverse structures in the creative process. Among other topics, we will examine the relationship between creativity and novelty seeking, the latter being a necessary but far from sufficient prerequisite of creativity. We will argue that while the claim of an exclusive role of the frontal lobes and the right hemisphere in creativity is a far-fetched oversimplification, the claim of their role in processing novelty is not. And we will see how conflating these two related but not identical constructs—creativity and novelty—may have contributed to the "frontal lobes and the right hemisphere" neuromythology of creativity.

"Bad and Useless"

Ironically, the brain structures most commonly implicated by neuroscientists in processing novelty, and invoked by popular science as being central to the creative process, had been in the doghouse of psychology and neuroscience until relatively recently. The prefrontal cortex and the right hemisphere are crucial for dealing with novelty, and while not holding a monopoly on just novelty, they are also relevant to that which is creativity. Yet for many years, one of them was dismissed as "useless" (the frontal lobes) and the other one as "evil" (the right hemisphere).

There are princesses and Cinderellas in life and also in science, and just as in most human pursuits, science has had plenty of false starts and misconceptions.

Frontal lobes were the "orphaned lobes," a Cinderella of neurology of sorts. For years it was believed that they didn't serve any useful purpose and were sitting there to support some poorly understood but expendable function. It was even thought that various brain disorders could be "cured" by severing the connections between the frontal lobes and the rest of the brain. This now-discredited belief was the basis for the infamous frontal lobotomy whose inventor, the Portuguese neurologist Antonio Egas Moniz, first performed it in 1935 and later received the Nobel Prize in Medicine in 1949, arguably one of the most misplaced in the history of the award.

A stiletto-like instrument called "leucotome" was inserted through a hole drilled in the patient's skull, and a lesion severing the connections between the frontal lobes and the rest of the brain was made. Since the modern neuroimaging technologies, such as computerized tomography (CT) scan or magnetic resonance imaging (MRI), were still decades away, the lesion was inflicted literally "in the dark." By the time this truly barbaric procedure was on the wane in the 1960s, an untold number of patients had been rendered zombie-like, the symptoms of mental illness removed together with most symptoms of mental life.[*]

Inspired by this "innovation," the psychiatrist Walter Freeman began to practice frontal lobotomy on an industrial scale in the United States beginning in 1936. He "simplified" it in a way that did not require drilling through the skull and could be performed by inserting an icepick-like device into the brain through an eye-socket. For this truly awful procedure, casually referred to in its heyday as the "icepick" lobotomy, no training in neurosurgery was deemed necessary, and it was performed by psychiatrists in numerous psychiatric hospitals across the United States. With jolly levity, the good Dr. Freeman referred to it as "my jiffy lobotomy" and performed it as an outpatient procedure with his patients seated in a dental chair installed in his private office in Washington, D.C. He also traveled around the country in a specially equipped van, which he cutely referred to as the "lobotomobile," and dispensed lobotomy generously and casually in numerous psychiatric hospitals across the land. The results were for the most part disastrous—many of his patients suffered cerebral hemorrhage, and some died. Those who survived could be seen wandering aimlessly and absently in the hallways of state psychiatric hospitals even in the 1980s (I have seen my share of them while consulting at one such hospital)—lobotomized twenty or thirty years prior and never regaining a semblance of human personality.[2]

---

[*] In a feat of what some would call poetic justice, Muniz was shot by a paranoid patient and spent the rest of his life confined to a wheelchair. Ironically, the offending patient had not undergone frontal lobotomy; had he had one, he probably would have lacked the mental facility necessary to do the vile deed.

If the frontal lobe was one "Cinderella" of neurology, then the right hemisphere was the other Cinderella. If the prefrontal cortex was regarded for decades as "useless," then the right hemisphere was dismissed as "subdominant" and, well, also useless. In that spirit, the old-school neurosurgical mantra had been that the left hemisphere (whose primacy in controlling language clearly established its importance) had to be approached with great care, whereas the right hemisphere could be operated on with relative impunity, without fearing significant side effects. In a similar vein, electroconvulsive therapy (ECT) or "shock therapy" used to treat depression but known for its side effects was applied to the right hemisphere with far less hesitation than to the left hemisphere. The notion of the right hemisphere's relative unimportance has been so entrenched among some old-school neurosurgeons that, a few years ago, a young neurosurgeon on the faculty of a prestigious East Coast medical school arranged an invitation for me to give a talk in her department ("Grand Rounds" in the common medical parlance) to disabuse her more senior colleagues of the notion that the right hemisphere is dispensable and can be manipulated with impunity.

The old-school neuroscientists should have known better, and the more recent studies have demonstrated how important the right hemisphere and the frontal lobes really are. People with one hemisphere surgically removed to treat intractable epilepsy in childhood have a higher IQ in adulthood if they had lost the left hemisphere than the right hemisphere; so in some sense the right hemisphere is the "smarter" of the two.[3] And people with severe damage of the frontal lobes become catastrophically disorganized even though their specific cognitive skills—reading, writing, and such—remain intact.[4]

Why did it take neuroscientists so long to fully grasp the role of these structures in cognition? Because traditional neuropsychology and cognitive science focused on isolated, usually "crystallized" mental skills that corresponded to the lay taxonomy encoded in our everyday language and thus invited the illusion of being self-explanatory: movement, perception, language, even memory. As it turns out, the contributions of the frontal lobes and the right hemisphere to the mental orchestra mostly lie elsewhere. For many centuries of human history, the present was basically shaped by the past, since the curve of new knowledge accumulation, the "novelty curve," was relatively sluggish. In that environment, referring to the left hemisphere as the "dominant" one was not unreasonable. But in the brave age of novelty, the neural priorities have changed, and the two orphan structures, the frontal lobes and the right hemisphere, assume a new and dominant role.

Deconstructing Innovation and Creativity

Innovation and creativity are complex and multifaceted constructs with cognitive, biological, and social components, which elude unequivocal definitions.

Any attempt to understand creativity and its neural underpinnings will benefit from identifying its many ingredients and examining each of them first. The more multi-componential a mental process is, the more moving parts collaborate in supporting it, the less feasible is the idea of locating it to a particular part of the brain.

Here are a few of these moving parts, each involving its own neural networks and at times at loggerheads with one another. (And there are probably additional ones, not mentioned here.)

Salience: The ability to pose central problems and to ask important questions. Creativity requires more than mental virtuosity. It also implies relevance. Had Albert Einstein expended his exceptional gift of visual imagery on a lifelong quest of perfecting the art of pleasure-garden landscaping, he would have been remembered within the narrow niche of professional landscapers, but he would have hardly been rated as one of history's greatest minds.

Novelty: An interest in, and the ability to find solutions for, problems not tackled before. This is self-explanatory. An individual perfectly satisfied with making use of already available knowledge or practicing fully developed art forms is not likely to embark on a creative pursuit. Attraction to novelty is a central prerequisite of creativity. So is intellectual nonconformity, the ability to distance oneself from the established scientific theories and concepts, or artistic forms.

Ability to relate old knowledge to new problems: The opposite of the above, this is the ability to recognize familiar patterns in seemingly new and unique problems. Isaac Newton acknowledged in a letter to a colleague that "if I have seen further it is by standing on the shoulders of Giants." A friend of mine, Allan Snyder, a professor at University of Sydney, likes to say that "anything that is totally new is probably wrong." This casually deflating pronouncement contains a good grain of truth. Many highly innovative scientific concepts and artistic forms are in fact evolved and modified earlier concepts and forms. A visitor to the Picasso Museum in Barcelona's Barri Gotic, where the works of the great painter are exhibited in a meticulously chronological order, may be surprised to discover that the founder of Cubism started as an accomplished painter in the tradition of realism. A continuity of ideas intricately intertwined with discontinuity is common in science as well.

Generativity and mental flexibility: The ability to generate multiple and diverse approaches to a problem is essential to the creative process in science. A scientist would be exceptionally lucky to hit upon the solution of a daunting problem from the first go. It is usually necessary to attack the problem from multiple—and different—angles. The ability to experiment with multiple forms is also central to the creative process in the arts. Pablo Picasso was a painter, sculptor, ceramicist, print maker, and stage designer; these diverse art forms mutually enriching each other.

Drive and doggedness: In a sense, the opposite of the previous, an ability to deploy sustained effort toward tackling a problem. This is about the relationship between "inspiration" and "perspiration." While examples of "lazy geniuses" exist (Claude Debussy is sometimes mentioned as one), most instances of great scientific discoveries or artistic creations are product of hard work extending over years. Capacity for sustained effort, commitment to the chosen subject, and resilience to failure are the *sine qua non* of most successful creative careers, except for the very lucky few.

Mental wandering: The mysterious capacity for the productive and seemingly effortless pursuit of ideas wherever they take you. Individual accounts by a number of exceptionally creative individuals from various fields of human endeavor, from music to science, allude to seemingly effortless mental states, whereby a solution to a problem or a melodic contour appears all of a sudden, as if from nowhere. What are the neural mechanisms of this phenomenon, and what is its relationship to other mental processes? Do periods of "mental wandering" have to be preceded by, and interspersed with, periods of conscious, systematic, and directed mental effort in order to be productive? Much more will be said on this subject in Chapter 7.

Mental focus: The opposite of mental wandering, this is an ability to systematically pursue a logical train of thought. While this is a less "mysterious" aspect of the creative process, it is an indispensable part of any scientific discovery, one which works synergistically with "mental wandering."

Iconoclastic frame of mind: This is self-explanatory. In order to forge ahead of society, a creative individual must be driven by a sense of dissatisfaction with the intellectual, scientific, or artistic status quo. The creative individual must also possess the strength of character and faith in one's work to persevere despite rejection and disapproval. Before they were embraced by society, paintings by Vincent van Gogh and music by Igor Stravinsky were rejected by critics. This was the fate of many other great artists and scientists.

Resonance with central societal and cultural themes: The opposite of the previous quality, this may sound counter-intuitive. A creative individual, and certainly a genius, is ahead of society, but his/her work must be recognized by society as important and valid in order to survive, or else it will be lost to history and culture. This notion contains a paradox: in order to be recognized, a creative individual must be ahead of society, but not too far ahead. If, through some implausible combination of factors, differential equations had been invented by a Cro-Magnon genius, the invention would have fallen on deaf societal ears, ignored and forgotten. I find the thought of the creative outliers too far ahead of their contemporaries to make an impact so poignant that I decided to dedicate this book to them.

Social grace: Certain supremely creative individuals were known to history for their social suaveness and adaptability, and others for a notorious lack thereof. Leonardo was an example of the former and Caravaggio of the latter. While probably extraneous to the creative process itself, the social attributes of the creative individual are likely to play an important, sometimes definitive role in his or her access to the resources necessary to support the creative process, and to the fate of the creative product itself. In certain instances, these attributes may even spell the difference between immortality and oblivion.

A favorable cultural milieu: Historically, certain societies and epochs were richer in discovery and innovation than others. The Athenian "Golden Age" and Florentine Renaissance are usually invoked as such societies, but there were others. The relationship between a creative individual and his/her social and cultural milieu deserves a closer examination.

Multiple Creativities

It should be clear from the foregoing that creativity is a very complex construct consisting of many moving, often conflicting, parts. It should also be clear that the multiple prerequisites and ingredients of creativity are unlikely to be very strongly correlated. This means that the search for a single key to creative process is likely to be futile, and that there are many forms the paths to creativity may take and many different profiles of "a creative individual." It might even mean that these multiple traits, profiles, and prerequisites may contain certain contradictions.

We often talk about creativity as if it were a unitary attribute, such that a person may have or not have; or may have it in degrees—to be highly creative, modestly creative, or not creative at all. But this approach, taken to its logical extreme, would imply that a highly creative mathematician would also be a highly creative choreographer; and a highly creative novelist would be a highly creative architect. Does one really believe this to be the case? Yes, certain types of talent seem to be highly correlated: good mathematicians are often also good amateur musicians. But just as, or perhaps more, often, such "domain-specific" talents are not correlated at all.

Any specific creative process is not an abstract enterprise; it occurs within a particular area of human endeavor, building on a particular body of knowledge, experience, and skills unique to that content area. Considering all this, how reasonable is it to think of creativity as a unitary gift? Just as there are "multiple intelligences" not always strongly correlated, there are almost certainly "multiple creativities" drawing on different neuronal ensembles. If this is so, then the very way the "creativity question" is often posed may be fundamentally misguided. The way this question is posed often assumes that creativity is a monolithic trait; but this assumption is almost certainly false. That there are multiple, and most likely very different, creative paths even within a single field of human endeavor, becomes clear when the lives and working styles of great mathematicians are examined.

Mathematics is sometimes referred to as "the queen of the sciences." Far from being mere numbers manipulation, so-called pure (theoretical as distinct from applied) mathematics in particular requires an exceptional feat of imagination, an ability to conjure up highly abstract "objects" devoid of explicit parallels with any experientially obvious physical reality. It has been suggested that the mental processes of a groundbreaking mathematician represent creativity in its purest form. Consider two of the arguably greatest and most creative mathematicians of all times: Evariste Galois (1811–1832) and Carl Friedrich Gauss (1777–1855). Each of them made seminal contributions to multiple areas of mathematics, including algebra, geometry, number theory, group theory, and others. Yet their personalities and working styles couldn't have been more different.

Galois was a quintessential rebel deeply enmeshed in the political turmoil of post-Napoleonic France, whose short and volatile life was bent on political and physical confrontation. He died from an abdominal gunshot wound in a duel at the age of twenty, yet in his short life he made seminal discoveries in multiple areas of mathematics: algebra, group theory, and polynomial equations among them. Many of his mathematical insights were hastily summarized in a letter to Auguste Chevaliere the night before the duel.[5] In contrast, Gauss, a politically conservative father of six, blessed with a long and orderly life, was known for a meticulous and deliberative reworking of his ideas for years or possibly decades before publishing them. So meticulous was his working style that it has been suggested that he unnecessarily delayed the publication of important results by decades.[6]

Are we to assume that the creative processes in these two great mathematicians unfolded in similar ways, that they followed the same trajectory? Highly unlikely, particularly if one takes into account the striking differences in their personalities and circumstances: Galois' short and volatile life of a young revolutionary versus Gauss' orderly and outwardly uneventful life extending well into old age. In my own education, I came to believe that one can better grasp the substance of an idea if one is also informed about its author's personality and circumstances. This must be equally true in any attempt to reconstruct the creative process giving birth to a consequential idea. It is highly unlikely that the diametrically opposite personalities of Gauss and Galois followed the same creative path toward the pantheon of mathematics.

Similar contrasts abound in a very different arena of creative expression: music. Wolfgang Amadeus Mozart (1756–1791) and Ludwig van Beethoven (1770–1827) are another case in point. Mozart wrote his last three symphonies—the Thirty-ninth, Fortieth, and Forty-first—in a span of a few weeks.[7] By contrast, Beethoven worked slowly—it took him six years to compose his Ninth Symphony, according to some opinions his greatest.[8] Even though he lived a much longer life, Beethoven's oeuvre was considerably sparser than Mozart's. One would surmise that the creative processes were very different in these two great composers. My musicologist-turned-lawyer friend Harry Ballan remarked that Beethoven's symphonies are "architectural," guided by a plan, while Mozart's symphonies are "spontaneous," probably devoid of a thought driven by a plan. This is suggestive of very different creative processes.

Clearly, different types of creative processes unfold at vastly different time scales, and this may be true even within the same—broadly considered—area of human endeavor. So both across and within various areas of creative pursuits, striking individual differences abound, forcing one to reject the notion of creativity as a unitary monolithic process. Instead, the inescapable conclusion is that the creative endeavors that are similar on the surface may in fact engage vastly different cognitive tools and processes and rely on multiple different neural structures.

None of the time scales implicit in these real-life, consequential creative processes has much in common with the time scales of the laboratory tests commonly used to study creativity, such as the Torrance Tests of Creative Thinking, tests of "divergent reasoning," and similar techniques designed to measure "creativity" in the lab[9] —which is one of the many reasons why the relationship of these techniques to the real-life consequential creativity must be questioned. Different time scales are not likely to be merely stretched or compressed versions of one another; they are likely to have very different cognitive compositions.

Given the multiplicity of the cognitive, metacognitive, and social ingredients of the creative process, their multiple forms and mutual contradictions, how reasonable or realistic is it to expect that a single magic "creativity" center exists in the brain? Not so much! Instead, multiple brain regions and structures operate in concert, and sometimes in contradiction, in a highly interconnected way to support the creative process. Furthermore, this cooperation (or tension) may take very different forms and involve different constellations of interacting brain structures in different creative individuals, even if their creative work takes place in the same broad field of endeavor.

In the next chapters, we will examine various cognitive processes that work in concert to support the creative process, as well as their neural machinery.

3

The Conservative Brain

How We Know What We Know

In the previous chapter, we discussed how the frontal lobes and the right hemisphere used to be dismissed by the old-school neuropsychologists as inconsequential. What then, was the neural real estate of interest to them? Said "real estate" was really pretty sparse—certain parts of the left hemisphere. But even there, the old-school science got it wrong, or at least not entirely right (no pun intended). It is true that in an adult individual the left hemisphere supports language—this has been understood for many years—but it does much more than that. And in order to understand how language came to inhabit the left hemisphere, some other, more fundamental, functions of the left hemisphere must be first recognized and analyzed.

The brain does not spin novel knowledge or creative ideas out of thin air. Much, and perhaps even most, of what we do is shaped to some degree by previously acquired information, and that includes even most groundbreaking innovation and most daring feats of creativity. The relationship between the old and the new is fluid and intimate. The very impulse to embark on a creative quest usually finds its origin in the sense that existing established knowledge or theories are incapable of providing a solution for the problems at hand; or that existing esthetics and artistic forms fall short of resonating with the sensibilities of the time or the individual's needs for self-expression. Furthermore, innovation is not necessarily a wholesale rejection of the previously accumulated knowledge, ideas, and beliefs. More often than not, the old morphs into the new in subtle and fluid ways.

This is also true for the brain mechanisms of innovation and creativity. The brain is one big network. Even though distinct sub-networks exist that are dedicated to specific tasks, they are not entirely separate; they are closely interconnected and strongly overlap. In order to understand the brain mechanisms of innovation and creativity, we must also understand the brain mechanisms of representing established knowledge, the knowledge that is the point of departure for any creative process. In this chapter, we will examine how knowledge is represented in the brain.

How *is* knowledge represented in the brain? Before tackling the sublime, let's discuss the seemingly banal, since the underlying brain machinery is fundamentally the same. Just think about it: we constantly encounter objects in our environment that are, strictly speaking, new to us and unique, yet we have no trouble relating to them as if they were familiar. On vacation in an exotic country, you are walking through the market and see a jacket of unusual color made of a fabric you have never seen before; or a lamp of unusual shape. Technically, you have never encountered these objects before, but you know right away what they are. You may even buy them using unfamiliar currency, which you nonetheless immediately recognize as money. And by the way, have you ever thought about how it is possible that in an exotic restaurant while on vacation in an exotic country you are instantly able to handle exotically shaped knives, spoons, and forks, despite the fact that you had never encountered such silverware before?

We don't even need to travel far to accomplish this seemingly oxymoronic feat every day and every hour of our lives. We bump into total strangers on the street and know that they are humans and not dogs, and we also know that the unfamiliar dogs being walked by the strangers are dogs and not humans. Have you ever stopped and thought about how this happens—encountering a totally unfamiliar thing and knowing instantly what it is? The process is so ubiquitous, so effortless, and so natural—like eating or drinking—that the odds are you never paused to appreciate it.

The process that enables us to accomplish this feat, and in which the left hemisphere excels, is called "pattern recognition." As we encounter unique but similar objects, a mental representation is formed in our brain that captures the essential shared properties of these objects, while disregarding the superfluous attributes. A mental representation of a "pen" will capture its obligatory elongated shape with a sharp end and a rounder end, but it will disregard the color. A mental representation of a "plate" will capture its round shape, relative flatness, and a concavity in the middle, but it will disregard the decorative design around the edge. These are patterns. So when we encounter a new object belonging to the same category of things, we recognize them for what they are because they resonate with, and activate, one of the patterns previously stored in our brains.

How is a pattern represented in the brain? Neurobiologically speaking, a pattern is a network of strongly interconnected neurons. When a part of the network is activated by incoming sensory input—let's say, a visual image of an object in your environment—the rest of the network is also activated. This activation of the whole network, by just its part, is the mechanism of pattern recognition, by which the brain recognizes a new object as a member of a familiar category: a table, a chair, or whatever it may be.

Complex ideas are represented in the brain in a fundamentally similar way. Just as we experience the everyday physical world through the prism of previously formed patterns, so, too, a scientist, an artist, an entrepreneur, a politician, or a corporate leader approaches his or her challenges through the prism of previously formed concepts, artistic forms, or institutions. When a mathematician looks at a formula and recognizes it as a linear equation and not a quadratic equation, the process of recognition also occurs through an activation of a network that represents the essential shared properties of linear equations. When an art critic looks at a painting and recognizes it as a product of the Flemish School and not of the Dutch School, this, too, occurs because the image of the painting activated a sufficient number of neurons of the network encoding the essential shared properties of Flemish masters for the whole network to become activated. And when a physician examines a patient and promptly diagnoses the disease, this is also possible because, based on the physician's previous experience, a neural network had been formed in his or her head representing the essential properties of the disorder. The neural nets representing essential attributes of whole classes of similar objects (here we use the word "object" broadly) are sometimes called *attractors*, since each of them "attracts" a multitude of specific inputs. The term was borrowed from mathematics but now is commonly used in computational neuroscience. Such neural "attraction" is the mechanism of the subjective experience of recognition. The left hemisphere is particularly adept at storing attractors of all kinds, whether verbal in nature or not.[1]

Now suppose a patient presents with a collection of symptoms not encountered by the doctor before; or a physicist encounters a process that cannot be described by any known type of equation; or an artist has an idea, a creative stirring that does not lend itself to being expressed through any established artistic tradition; or—more prosaically—a simple object was not recognized as anything familiar. The act of recognition failed to happen because the impact on the brain by the object at hand failed to activate any of the previously formed attractor networks.

The brain has encountered a novel challenge. A subjective feeling of being confronted by novelty is mostly the result of the left hemisphere's failure to find a solution, by failure of the incoming information to resonate with any of the previously formed attractor networks. What happens in the brain next will be the subject of chapters 6 and 7. But the important point we have made so far is that embarking on the search for a novel solution is usually preceded by the failure of known solutions to crack the problem at hand.

Mapping the World in the Brain
Agnosias and the Left Hemisphere

Much as we take pattern recognition for granted, this process may be broken following certain forms of brain damage. Such brain damage results in a class of disorders called "associative agnosias"—when the patient loses the ability to recognize meaningful objects for what they are, or "apraxias"—when the patient loses the ability to perform previously well-rehearsed motor skills. In a way, these patients are like people who have never encountered such objects before. An ancient Egyptian or Roman presented with a cellphone would have been able to describe its features—flat, rectangular, smooth surface, a certain color—but would have had no idea what it was, not because of brain damage, but because an appropriate mental representation, a pattern, had never been formed in his head. Nor would he know how to wind a wristwatch, manipulate a steering wheel, or ride a bicycle—for a similar reason.

It is interesting to note that several forms of associative agnosia and apraxia exist. They may be caused by various diseases—stroke, dementia, or brain trauma—but they all share the same neuroanatomical property: the left hemisphere must be affected for the ability to recognize unique things as members of generic categories to be lost.[2] The latter observation has led to the conclusion that the left hemisphere must play a particularly important role in storing and maintaining the patterns representing classes of familiar objects and actions. Clearly, the existence of such patterns is essential to our ability to navigate and manage our environment. Were these patterns to be erased from our brains or degraded, we would have to relearn the meaning of every specific object, as well as the movements necessary to manipulate it. Life would be beyond unmanageable, it would be unlivable. But this is precisely what happens to certain patients when the left hemisphere is affected by disease.

Suppose I show such a patient a pen (a quaint example in the age of texting!) and ask him to describe it. "It is a thin long thing with a sharp end. It is round and shiny," comes the response, along with the correct description of the pen's color. So far, so good, but when I ask the patient to name the object, the response is, "It's a knife." Is it perchance the case that the patient forgot the meaning of words? But no, when I ask the patient to describe the function of the object and to demonstrate it through a pantomime, my patient says "cutting food" and engages in make-believe cutting movements. It appears that the patient truly sees the pen as a knife, despite the fact that all the visual features of the object were identified correctly.

We have just encountered *visual object agnosia*—a form of associative agnosia. While relatively rare in its pure form, this condition has been studied by a number of neurologists and neuropsychologists. A patient described by Alexander Luria looked at the picture of a pair of glasses and ventured the following guess: ". . . a circle, then another circle, and some sort of crossbar . . . it may be a bicycle." Henry Hecaen and Martin Albert described a patient who perceived a pen and a cigar as "cylindrical objects or variable sticks" and a bicycle as "a pole with two wheels, one in front one in the back," while being unable to identify them.[3] What makes visual object agnosia so remarkable is that the patient can correctly identify the visual attributes of an object or a picture and may even be able to draw it correctly, but he does not know what it is. Nor is it a naming deficit, because the way patient names the object concurs with the way he describes or pantomimes its function. The patient behaves like a person who has never encountered the object before, even though he most certainly has. It is as if the mental representations of categories of things, which normally enable us to recognize specific objects as members of such categories (pens as pens and bicycles as bicycles), have been erased from the patient's brain, or at least severely degraded. And this is indeed what happens. Hans-Lucas Teuber described such patients' perception as being "stripped of its meaning."

But now comes the moment of revelation. I allow the patient to take the object in his hand and examine it by touch, and he immediately recognizes it as a pen. Or I retract and expose the writing tip of the pen several times by pressing on the blunt end that emits the characteristic clicking sound; hearing the characteristic sound will also cause the patient to recognize the object as a pen. Now we know that the mental representation of the "pen" category has not been erased completely, but only its *visual* aspect, since as soon as other sensory modalities—proprioceptive or auditory—were brought into play, the patient could easily recognize the object. The lesion responsible for the peculiar disorder called *visual object agnosia* is found in the left hemisphere; more specifically, in its occipito-temporal region.

If we move a little up and forward in the brain's cortex—but still remain within the left hemisphere—we encounter an area in the parietal lobe whose damage may result in a similar disorder, but affecting the ability to recognize objects by *touch* through the tactile and proprioceptive channels. This disorder is called pure *astereognosia*. Suppose we place a pen in the patient's hand, with his eyes closed. The patient's response may go as follows: "This is a long a skinny thing, of cylindrical shape and with a smooth surface . . . some kind of stick." Yet the moment the patient opens his eyes, he knows exactly what the object is, and says "pen." As in the previous example, the patient is able to give a pretty good account of the pen's shape and surface, yet unable to integrate these sensory details into a coherent percept, as if he had never encountered such objects—except in this case, the deficit affects, and is limited to, the tactile and proprioceptive sense.

Damage to yet another area of the left hemisphere, this one in the temporal lobe, will result in a similar disorder, but the *auditory* modality will be affected. A patient afflicted with such a condition, known as *associative auditory agnosia*, will have a hard time identifying the sources of various environmental sounds. He may hear the clicking sound of a pen without realizing what it is. He may hear the sounds of a heavy downpour outside yet will walk out of the house without an umbrella, unless he also sees the rain through the window. Or quite the opposite, he may hear the drumbeat sounds of a marching band outside and leave the house with an umbrella, assuming that there is a downpour outside. In a typical test of associative auditory agnosia, the patient will hear the recordings of various environmental sounds and will be asked to point to the picture of objects or living creatures that are the sources of the recorded sounds. The patient will find the task utterly confusing, pointing to the picture of a car while hearing the sound of a barking dog, or to the picture of a dog while hearing the sound of a roaring automobile engine.

And then there is *apraxia*, a deficit of motor planning and execution of overlearned skilled movements. Apraxia may take several forms known by different names. In *ideational apraxia*, the patient is unable to perform the movements appropriate for the overlearned motor skill (e.g., will hold a pen the way you hold a toothbrush or vice versa). In *ideomotor apraxia*, the patient may be able to perform an overlearned motor task automatically but be unable to do so in a pretend situation in the absence of the appropriate object (e.g., to make believe that she is combing her hair in the absence of a comb or brush her teeth in the absence of a toothbrush). In *kinetic apraxia,* the smooth transition between the components of a complex skilled movement, like tying a tie or shoelaces, is impaired.

Any of these odd disorders may be caused by bilateral brain damage, but if the damage is unilateral, it is likely to be in the left hemisphere.[4] This suggests that the patterns that allow us to recognize and manipulate unique exemplars as if they were familiar and spare us the nightmare of relearning the function of every single object in our environment from scratch somehow "reside" mostly in the left hemisphere.

The Question of Brain Design

How are such patterns represented in the left hemisphere? Imagine yourself the designer (we won't presume to say "creator"—too many unintended connotations) of an artificial brain trying to figure out how to represent the outside world. You may consider two very different design principles. According to the first principle, all the attributes of an object—its size, shape, color, the sound, and the odor it emits—are "bundled" in one concise brain region. According to the second principle, the representation is distributed, with different attributes of the object inhabiting different parts of the brain. Since the actual brain was a product of evolution and not of some inspired "intelligent design" and "the wisdom of evolution" is a rather tenuous notion, we will not debate the relative strengths and weaknesses of such alternative blueprints.

The neuroanatomy of associative agnosias offers a window into the way the physical world is represented in a healthy brain, and it appears that the second principle prevails. Why? Because in none of the associative agnosias does the totality of information about the object become erased or severely degraded, but only part of it—that portion that is linked to a particular sense: visual, tactile, or auditory. The territories of different associative agnosias are quite dispersed in the cortex of the left hemisphere. Therefore, one can conclude that the normal processes whose breakdown results in agnosias are also highly distributed in the brain (see Figure 3.1). Most things have multiple attributes—visual, auditory,

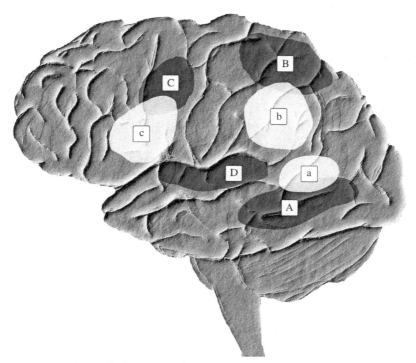

FIGURE 3.1 **Cortical territories of associative agnosias, apraxias, and anomias.**
(A) Visual object agnosia; (B) Pure astereognosis (C) Apraxia; (D) Auditory associative agnosia.
(a) Anomia for object words and colors; (b) Anomia for relational terms; (c) Anomia for action words.

tactile—and these attributes are coded in different parts of the left hemisphere, this resulting in highly distributed mental representations.

So, based on the studies of brain damage effects, we can say that it is mostly the left hemisphere that serves as the repository of our accumulated prior experience with the world. It captures this experience in a generalized way as patterns through which we interpret the incoming new information.

Agnosias and the Right Hemisphere

The effects of brain damage offer a glimpse into the function of the right hemisphere as well, and a very different picture emerges. Damage to the right hemisphere may result in *apperceptive agnosias*, when the patient loses the ability to recognize a thing or a living being as its own self in an ever-changing environment.[4] Just think about it. You see a thing—a household utensil or an article of clothing—on numerous occasions, and there is no doubt in your mind that it is the same object. That is despite the fact that the actual sensory input is never quite the same: you never observe the same object at exactly the same distance, the same angle, or under exactly the same lighting. Nor do you always touch that object with exactly the same force and with the same grip (not even mentioning the unpleasant fact that your hand may be sweaty on occasion but hopefully not all the time). Nor is the sensory input from the face or the voice of the same individual exactly the same whenever you talk to her, and for similar reasons. The brain somehow has the ability to cut through the sensory "noise" and recognize things as their own selves, despite that fact that their sensory impressions on your brain never are exactly the same. This ability, sometimes referred to as *perceptual constancy*, appears to be particularly closely linked to the right hemisphere, since damage to the right hemisphere is particularly likely to disrupt it.

Apperceptive agnosia may take several forms. For a social species such as ours, the ability to recognize a unique object under constantly changing sensory conditions is particularly important when it comes to human faces—to know that Anne is Anne, who is different from Mary, and not just a generic face of a middle-aged Caucasian female. When the ability for facial recognition is lost, a particularly dramatic form of apperceptive agnosia sets in, called *prosopagnosia* (roughly translated from Greek as "lacking the knowledge of faces"), and it is usually caused by damage to the fusiform cortex found in the right occipito-temporal region of the brain. Presented with photos of several people taken from different angles, the patient will find it difficult to decide that photos represent the same face as opposed to different faces. In more severe cases, this ability may be disrupted even with actual people. Imagine yourself walking into an office or a classroom, finding yourself surrounded with people you have known before, yet not recognizing them and not knowing who is who. An inconvenience to say the least! The late neurologist and author Oliver Sacks, who diagnosed himself with a mild form of this disorder, described it in his famous book *The Man Who Mistook His Wife for a Hat.*[5]

"You Aren't You!"

A peculiar, related, disorder is known under the name of *Capgras* (after its discoverer French psychiatrist Joseph Capgras) *syndrome*, sometimes referred to as the "reduplication syndrome."[6] A patient with Capgras syndrome will recognize a familiar face but will refuse to accept it at face value, so to speak. He will look at a familiar person and say, "Yes, you surely look like my neighbor John but you are really not John, you are John's double." Capgras syndrome is often explained by postulating a dissociation between the perception of a person and the affective experience associated with the face. This explanation may well be accurate, but a simpler and more parsimonious explanation is that Capgras syndrome is a manifestation of impaired perceptual constancy. Technically speaking, a person never looks exactly the same to an observer, and if the perceptual constancy mechanisms are weakened, the experience of someone "not looking the same" will be magnified. Depending on your point of view, you can think of Capgras syndrome as a form of prosopagnosia, as the deficit of facial recognition; or as its inverse, an enhanced appreciation of minute differences between faces. Either way, facial recognition is clearly affected, and again the right hemisphere must be affected by brain damage for this peculiar disorder to arise.

Taken together, these clinical observations point to a striking division of labor between the two hemispheres. The left hemisphere is mostly in charge of identifying things as members of previously learned broad categories (like recognizing various objects for what they are). In contrast, the right hemisphere is mostly in charge of identifying things as their own unique selves (like human faces). Both cognitive skills are essential for navigating the complex and everchanging world around us, and the breakdown of either of them dissolves this world into perceptual chaos, but in very different ways.

How Language Found Its Home
Words and Patterns

If you are a careful reader, which you undoubtedly are, you may be puzzled by how little resemblance this chapter's content bears to a typical account of the "dominant" left hemisphere that you have encountered in numerous books and articles. Where is language? What is the relationship between the left hemisphere's role in pattern recognition and its role in language? What is the connection between the two narratives? Not to worry, language is very much in the picture, and it may well be that it owes its affiliation with the left hemisphere, and even its very existence, to the pattern recognition mechanisms described earlier in this chapter. How come?

Language is such an exquisitely powerful cognitive tool because of its several attributes. It is a tool of communication. It is a tool for generating a practically infinite number of statements (more about this in Chapter 4). And language is also a tool for representing the world around us. This is a fundamental aspect of language without which there would have been nothing to communicate and no content to generate. Yes, I agree with Noam Chomsky emphatically and unreservedly that generativity and the grammatical structure may be the single most distinguishing characteristics of language (more about this, too, in Chapter 4), but without the representational content, generativity is merely a set of vacuous formalisms.[7]

We represent the world around us, as well as our intents, plans, and suppositions, through words, which represent various objects, actions, and relationships, as well as abstract concepts. It is common to distinguish between concrete words (a table, a chair, to sit, to walk) and abstract ones (independence, wisdom, to equivocate, to deduce). Each word is more than an utterance, it represents a concept, and even the most concrete words are high-order abstractions. We don't invent a separate word for every chair or every table, for every act of walking or sitting. The mere fact that we use the same word, "chair," to refer to a huge number of specific objects that are individual chairs reflects a high level of abstraction inherent in this humble, pedestrian word. Even though we use such words to refer to specific objects, they really refer to abstractions. During the early stages of the emergence of language at the dawn of our species, in order for a lexicon, that collection of the building blocks of any language, to develop, our distant ancestors must have already possessed the ability to abstract patterns from the ever-changing, bewildering in its diversity, world around us, so that the same word could be related to a number of specific objects. Without the ability to extract patterns from the environment as a prerequisite, early lexicons could not have been formed as an effective cognitive tool, since every specific object would have had to be represented by a different word, and that would have introduced confusion rather than order into our early ancestors' already befuddling world.

Indeed, the capacity for abstraction as a necessary prerequisite for the earliest words in a "protolanguage" has been noted by a number of evolutionary psychologists. The ability to extract patterns capturing the shared properties of large numbers of specific objects from the surrounding environment is present to varying degrees in any creature capable of learning, and it reaches a considerable level of abstraction in apes. According to the evolutionary psychologist Richard Byrne, the refinement of this ability occurred approximately 16 million years ago in the common ancestor of the great apes and humans, and it served as an "essential precursor of the later language development in the hominid line."[8] (Curiously, in the individual development of a child in the modern world, the relationship between perception and language is often reversed; and in the course of acquiring language, the child learns how to organize and pattern the surrounding physical world, thus shortcutting the individual cognitive developmental process by internalizing the previously accumulated knowledge of the species codified in language.)

How did language end up in the left hemisphere? For starters, consider this paradox. Language is a fundamentally new cognitive asset that separates us from other species, even from those closest to us, like the chimpanzee or the bonobo. But the emergence of language was not accompanied by the emergence of a separate, totally new neural structure; it is not as if a new lobe emerged in the human brain that had been absent in other primates. Granted, the human brain is different from that of other primates in many respects, but the fundamental macroarchitecture is very similar. Language somehow attached itself to the neural real estate already existing in other primates. But how?

Numerous theories exist that aim to explain the link between language and the left hemisphere. One possible explanation was offered by Norman Geschwind, arguably the most important behavioral neurologist of his generation, and his associates. They discovered that the brain region called the *planum temporale* is larger in the left than in the right hemisphere. Shortly thereafter, another area, called the *pars opercularis* (known also as *frontal operculum*), was found to be larger in the left than in the right hemisphere; and so was the adjacent *pars triangularis*.[9]

These areas are important for the recognition and production of speech, and this, assuming that "bigger is better," could explain why the left hemisphere is more adept at supporting language. But these regions are larger also in the left hemisphere of the great apes, which, with all due appreciation of their cognitive skills, do not have language, at least not in its conventional narrow definition. This, in turn, means that any possible link between language and the large left planum temporale and frontal operculum is a product of functional "repurposing" of certain features of the brain structure whose original development was a response to very different evolutionary pressures or possibly even a product of random processes. The emergence of new functions in evolution is a process that is neither orderly nor parsimonious. It is very often a hodge-podge of multiple separate adaptations whereby many old structures are "coopted" to support new functional ends in a way that an "intelligent designer" would consider pretty odd. This, in turn, means that many evolutionary adaptations are the products of many processes working together. Parsimony could be reasonably expected of an "intelligent designer" hired by Google to come up with an artificial brain, but it is out of place in trying to grasp the fits and starts of the evolutionary process. Together with other factors (such as the asymmetries of the planum temporale and frontal operculum), the cortical organization of pattern recognition must have played a role in shaping the cortical representation of language. Just as the *existence of pattern recognition* very likely played a role in enabling the emergence of language, the *neuroanatomy of pattern recognition* must have played a role in shaping the neuroanatomy of language.

More on Brain Design

Let's place ourselves again in the position of an imaginary designer. For the lexicon (the meaning and use of words), two radically different designs are possible: (1) to bundle it all together and put it in one particular part of the brain; or (2) to have it dispersed throughout the brain. Just as the studies of agnosias tell us how evolution resolved this dilemma for perception, so, too, the studies of language disorders, *aphasias,* shed light on how the cortical representation of a lexicon is organized.

The second design wins again. Cortical representation of the lexicon is distributed, and it is distributed in a way that parallels the cortical representation of the physical world. In an adult native speaker, the ability to understand and correctly use object words (nouns), action words (verbs), and the words denoting spatial and other relations (prepositions) is disrupted following damage to different regions of the left hemisphere far separated from one another. Damage to a posterior region of the temporal lobe on the boundary of occipital lobe in the left hemisphere disrupts the production and understanding of object words (nouns). In contrast, damage to an area in the left posterior frontal lobe disrupts the production and understanding of action words (verbs). Both types of damage may result in a phenomenon called *paraphasia*, when the intended word is replaced by either an incorrect word or by a neologism, a word-sounding non-word (neologisms are not unique to neurological patients; many words commonly used by all of us, like "guesstimate" and "frenemies" started out as neologisms and then became accepted as real words). But the types of paraphasias caused by the two focal lesions discussed before are different and telling: when damage affects the left posterior temporal lobe region, the patient often uses intact action words (verbs) to make up for the lost access to object words (nouns): "a looker" instead of "glasses" or "a writer" instead of "a pen." When damage affects the left posterior frontal regions, the opposite may happen: the patient may say "I glass" instead of "I look" when asked what he does with the glasses.[10]

Neuroimaging studies are consistent with these earlier clinical observations. In an elegant experiment using positron emission tomography (PET), Alex Martin and his colleagues asked their neurologically healthy subjects to look at the pictures of animals and tools and to name them. Under both conditions, "language areas" lit up in the brain, but there were also differences: animal-naming triggered the activation of left visual cortex of the occipital lobe where information about their visual appearance is stored, and tool-naming triggered the activation of left premotor cortex, also involved in the actual execution of action.[11] The results of studies using repetitive transcranial magnetic stimulation (rTMS) point in the same direction: suppression of the left anterior midfrontal gyrus (where control over actions resides) interfered with verb (action words which refer to what we do with things), but not noun, production.[12]

It is important to clarify what the lesion and neuroimaging studies show, and what they do not show. They show that certain cortical regions are particularly important for representing various aspects of the physical world and others for representing various parts of the lexicon. They do not show that the cortical representation of specific types of objects or lexical items (words) is restricted to specific, narrowly defined cortical territories. Quite the contrary: these representations are widely distributed in the cortex, and their exact cortical topography is probably subject to considerable variability, reflecting the individual differences in experiences. But certain regions are more strongly involved in these distributed representations than others.

The next observation is critical for understanding how language landed in the left hemisphere. It turns out that the two distributed representations—of the physical world and of the language describing it—are closely linked: nouns involve the areas found next to the visual representation of the physical world (interestingly, in primates, like us, visual modality is the dominant one); verbs involve areas next to the motor cortex that controls movements; and prepositions involve areas found next to the cortex representing the attributes of the physical world that we learn about through the tactile and proprioceptive channels (see Figure 3.1).

What Came First?

The two cortical representations, one of the physical world, the other of language, are both distributed and are attached to each other like a pair of twins joined at the hip. This twin-like arrangement between perception and language makes too much computational sense to be merely coincidental. It is much more likely that language inhabited the left hemisphere because the generic representation of the physical world had already been established in the left hemisphere. In the evolutionary "search" for the cortical real estate for the new cognitive asset—language—the territory adjacent to, and perhaps even overlapping with, the cortical territory of that which it denotes makes for the most computationally economical allocation of cortical space. After all, the lexicon represents the world in generic terms, and so do the distributed patterns whose breakdown results in associative agnosias.

Now we encounter an interesting "chicken-and-egg" question: Did the cortical mapping of pattern recognition determine the cortical mapping of the lexicon, or did the cortical mapping of the lexicon determine the cortical mapping of pattern recognition? In fact, the latter possibility has been entertained by a number of cognitive scientists under the name of the "snowball effect" of language on perception. According to this point of view, categorical perception ended up in the left hemisphere because it is driven by language and language's affiliation with the left hemisphere.[13] This point of view is appealing, and it makes a certain sense, since the notion that language is the defining function of the left hemisphere is so entrenched. There is one good and one bad thing about this point of view. The good thing is that, unlike many psychological theories, it is falsifiable. The bad thing about it is that it is probably wrong.

Let's start with the falsifiable part and think logically. Suppose that pattern recognition ended up in the left hemisphere because language is in the left hemisphere. That would mean that the division of labor between the two hemispheres encountered by us earlier—categorical perception linked to the left hemisphere and perception of uniqueness to the right hemisphere—must be present only in humans, since only humans possess language. Conversely, should it turn out that such a division of labor between the hemispheres is present in other species; this would imply that at the very least, its emergence predated the emergence of language in evolution. This would in turn imply that the fact that language also landed in the left hemisphere is either coincidental with the left hemisphere's being the seat of pattern recognition, or more likely is secondary to it. Furthermore, the wider the array of species characterized by such a division of labor between the hemispheres—categorical on the left, unique on the right—and the farther these species are removed from our own in evolution, the less wind will be left in the rearguard argument that some kind of mysterious "proto-language" played a role in shaping this division.

Evidence abounds that the division of labor, whereby the left hemisphere excels at generic pattern ("categorical") recognition and the right hemisphere at recognition based on unique features, is ubiquitous across species, not all of them primates or even mammalians.[14] Take pigeons, for instance. When trained to recognize pictures of humans, they process such stimuli categorically if they are presented to the right eye (and consequently to the left hemisphere, since the pathways are crossed) and in terms of unique features if presented to the left eye (and consequently to the right hemisphere).[15] Pigeons are also better with their right than left eye (left hemisphere, rather than the right hemisphere) in learning general patterns; and they exhibit a distinct lateralization of bottom-up (sensory input-driven) processing to the right hemisphere and top-down (previously formed pattern-driven) processing to the left hemisphere.[16]

In several mammalian species (monkeys, dogs, sea lions, mice, and gerbils), the left hemisphere is better at recognizing calls conveying certain information to other members of the same species and recognized by all of them, a process that is clearly categorical even though nonverbal. In contrast, the right hemisphere is better than the left at recognizing vocalizations specific to unique exemplars of its own species (conspecific) in sheep[17] and in rhesus monkeys. And our best friends, dogs, employ mostly the right hemisphere in recognizing unique human faces.[18] Likewise, lateralized brain damage in monkeys results in effects very similar to the human agnosias described earlier in this chapter. For example, Japanese macaque and rhesus monkeys are better able to recognize species-specific (conspecific) vocalizations with their right ear, and damage to the monkey's left but not right temporal lobe has a particularly severe disrupting effect on this ability.[19] All these observations imply that pattern recognition exists already in other species, and so does the division of labor between categorical pattern recognition and recognition of uniqueness. The capacity for pattern recognition and its affiliation with the left hemisphere is a pervasive feature of brain organization across numerous species, predating the advent of language by millions of years.

For all these reasons, it is not too far-fetched to conclude that the cortical organization of pattern recognition plays an important role in shaping the cortical organization of language, particularly of the lexicon, and steers it toward the left hemisphere. This is how we resolve the "chicken-and-egg" conundrum and tie together the two narratives—one linking the left hemisphere to pattern recognition and the other one linking it to language. By so doing, I propose a new understanding of how language ended up in the left hemisphere: the left hemisphere's link to language was both preceded by in evolution, and to a large extent caused by, the left hemisphere's link to perceptual generic pattern recognition. (See, it is possible to introduce new ideas without rejecting the old ones. A case in point about the intimate and fluid relationship between the old and the new.)

Studies of hemispheric specialization in other species have a relatively long history, and it has been known for some time that perception is lateralized already in primates and therefore has to be independent of language.[20] More recent studies confirmed the basic similarity in the ways perception is organized across different primate species[21] (much more on the subject in Chapter 8). Why, then, did this knowledge fail to make much of a dent in the ways most cognitive neuroscientists and neuropsychologists continue to think about hemispheric specialization today? Is it the entrenched assumption of our species' exclusivity, or the bedeviling effects of balkanization (the fragmentation of a field of knowledge discussed earlier), or both?

"Isomorphic Gradients"

The broad lesson that brain lesion effects teach us is that the way perceptual and linguistic categories are represented in the cortex is not modular—they are not represented as a collection of "grandmother cells" or even of "grandmother regions"—but in a way which is continuous and distributed. I gravitated to this conclusion as an undergraduate at the University of Moscow in the 1960s, probably by way of a contrarian reaction to being taught a rather modular, localizationist view of the brain. To capture this idea, I came up with the concept of "cognitive gradients," which are continuous mappings of cognitive space into neocortical space, and wrote a paper with a youthfully ambitious title, "The Gradiental Approach to Neocortical Functional Organization," in which I went as far as proposing a "neuroanatomical-functional isomorphism." The idea was so drastically at odds with the dominant modular dogma of the time that publishing the paper proved to be difficult, and having been rejected by several journals where I felt it would have made the most impact, it was finally published twenty years later in a journal (and then as a book chapter) where its impact was predictably rather modest.[22]

For what it was worth, my early intuition about the gradiental nature of functional cortical organization and the "functional-neuroanatomical isomorphism" was based on low-tech observations of brain lesion effects, which are by their very nature coarse and devoid of either neuroanatomical or cognitive precision. It took another twenty years for it to be confirmed, elaborated, and detailed with the method of functional neuroimaging called "representational similarity analysis." This was accomplished in an important study by a team of neuroscientists from the Helen Wills Neuroscience Institute at the University of California, Berkeley, led by Alexander Huth.[23]

Using functional magnetic resonance imaging (fMRI), the researchers recorded the brain activity of healthy subjects while they were watching movies. Why movies? Because movies contain a great variety of objects and activities representative of everyday human experience. From these recordings, the cortical activation patterns corresponding to 1,705 specific object and action categories were extracted, and the relationship between these cortical activation patterns

was compared with the relationship between the corresponding semantic categories as specified in WordNet, an English-language database devised by George
Armitage Miller, one of the most important American psychologists and a
founding father of cognitive psychology as a discipline.[24] What they found was
that the semantic categories were mapped into the cortical space along "smooth
gradients." This mapping suggested a virtually isomorphic relationship between
the semantic space and the cortical space, similar across the five subjects who
participated in the study. In a follow-up fMRI study, the Berkeley neuroscientists constructed a cortical map of the semantic system based on the patterns of
cortical activation while subjects were listening to long narrative stories. Again,
the gradiental pattern of semantic categories mapping into the cerebral cortex
was revealed.[25]

Dementia with a Silver Lining?

Dementia is by any reckoning a bad thing to have, and it comes in many forms.
Most members of the general public have heard about Alzheimer's disease and
the memory impairment associated with it. But Alzheimer's disease is far from
the only form of dementia, and memory is not the only cognitive function that
may be affected. Frontotemporal dementia (FTD, known in the past as Pick's
disease) targets the frontal lobes (particularly its orbitofrontal subdivisions)
and the temporal lobe (particularly its anterior portion). Depending on which
of these two regions is mostly affected, this results in impaired judgment, poor
impulse control, and loss of social inhibitions; or in language impairment; or
both. FTD tends to affect patients at an earlier age than Alzheimer's disease,
is often characterized by a more rapid decline, and when the frontal lobes are
affected, "anosognosia," the patient's unawareness of the deficit, is often present.
Whenever you hear of an aging individual beginning to exhibit impulsive, inane,
socially inappropriate, and out-of-character behaviors, the possibility of FTD
must be considered. In my earlier book *The New Executive Brain,* I talked about
a surgeon who, having performed a technically competent surgery, carved his ini-
tials on the patient's abdomen, later explaining that his surgery was such a "masterpiece" that he had to sign it. When he was predictably criminally charged, his
attorneys successfully argued that he suffered from Pick's disease. And some time
ago, a female patient whom I ended up diagnosing with FTD, insisted on dancing in my office with my (much younger) clinical practice associate.

But sometimes FTD comes with a peculiar silver lining. It has been reported
that despite the generally devastating impact of this dementia, patients occasionally exhibit artistic creativity that had not been present before the disease onset.
Bruce Miller and colleagues studied five patients who became visual artists at

early stages of FTD. In four out of five of them, language and social skills were severely impaired, but visuospatial skills were spared. Neuropathology or SPECT (single photon emission computerized tomography) suggested a spared dorsolateral prefrontal cortex but an impaired anterior temporal lobe, most likely particularly affecting the left hemisphere.[26]

What is the mechanism of this late-life bittersweet gift? The answer may lie in the experiments by the Australian neuroscientist Allan Snyder. Allan proposed that the generally useful role of the patterns inhabiting the left hemisphere comes at a price. Yes, patterns allow us to perceive the world in categorical terms, with all the adaptive benefits discussed earlier in this chapter, but they also force us to perceive the world in certain preconceived, predictable ways. This phenomenon, somewhat akin to Gestalt phenomena first described by the early-twentieth century German psychologists Kurt Koffka, Wolfgang Koehler, Max Wertheimer, and Kurt Lewin, causes us to perceive the outside world as we expect it to be, rather than as it actually is. By "liberating" perception from the impact exerted by the previously formed patterns, it may be possible to make it more precise, sensitive to nuance, and open to new possibilities. Allan aimed to accomplish this by applying low-frequency transcranial magnetic stimulation (TMS) to the left temporal cortical regions of his healthy subjects, and by so doing, temporarily inhibiting the part of the brain where the patterns normally reside. Also, since the relationship between the two hemispheres is to a large extent one of mutual inhibition via the corpus callosum and the commissures, the inhibition of the left hemisphere probably enhanced the activation of the right hemisphere. The result was a dramatic improvement in the precision and nuanced detail of the subjects' drawings. Based on these findings, Allan claimed that there is an artistic "savant" hidden in all of us, that it "resides" in the right hemisphere and can be "liberated" by removing the constraining impact of the left hemisphere.[27]

We don't have to focus on savants, however. Instead, we will examine how these fascinating findings help us understand the late-life "creativity" in some FTD patients. Evidence exists that brain atrophy in FTD is asymmetrical: the orbitofrontal and temporal-lobe structures in the left hemisphere are affected more than in the right hemisphere. The causes behind this asymmetry are unclear, but they may reflect an aberration of asymmetrical gene expression in the neocortex.[28] If this is true, then the enhanced creativity effect caused by Allan Snyder in his neurologically intact subjects by temporarily suppressing certain regions of the left hemisphere with TMS could have been mimicked in FTD patients by the lateralized pattern of their brain atrophy—but irreversibly and at an unacceptably high price.

Similar effects were reported in three patients with "semantic dementia," a condition affecting language and closely related to frontotemporal dementia. At a certain stage of the disease process, the patients began to exhibit newfound feats of verbal creativity: writing poetry, engaging in innovative wordplay, and even writing a lifestyle guidebook. In all three of them, cortical atrophy was particularly prominent in the mesial temporal structures of the language-dominant (usually left) hemisphere.[29]

Obviously, any creativity arising in FTD patients as a result of their condition will be sooner or later overridden and negated by the catastrophic effects of disease progression. But frontotemporal dementia's dubious "silver lining" may provide an interesting window into the role of the right hemisphere in the creative process, once it has been "liberated" from the conservative influence of the left hemisphere. More on the subject will be found in chapters 6 and 7.

4

The Mermaid and the Lego® Master
(and the Cave Lion-Man)

How Is a New Idea Born?

Cognitive neuroscience is preoccupied today with working memory, mirror neurons, and a host of other very worthy, somewhat worthy, and less worthy subjects. Considerable interest has been directed at the question of how ideas are selected. Yet, before they are *selected*, ideas have to be *generated*, or else there will be nothing to select from. Oddly, the question of how new ideas emerge is not frequently asked directly. It is time that we do so. And in order to address the question cogently, not only must the brain be discussed, but also culture and the structure of knowledge must be brought into the narrative.

Solutions of novel problems and the creation of novel content do not occur in a vacuum. New knowledge is built upon the old knowledge, yet it is new. How is the new knowledge derived from the old? Even during the most conservative times in history, society changes, albeit often slowly. Scientific ideas evolve, and so do artistic forms. True, they are rooted in the past, but they are also novel. What is the relationship between the old and the new in the creative process? How does novelty arise from the past without being its mere replication?

Most creative giants "stand on the shoulders of giants" who came before. Virtually without exception, consequentially creative individuals had acquired the mastery of their respective fields as they had already existed, before they were able to advance them further. This is reflected in the "ten year rule"—which is how long it takes, on the average (but with plenty of exceptions), for a member of a creative profession or a scientist to practice one's field before he or she is able to make a truly innovative, consequential contribution (at least this is how it has been so far; whether the "ten-year rule" survives the rapid increase in the rate of knowledge accumulation remains to be seen).[1] The notion of a total naïf's coming up with a feat of genius "out of nowhere" may have a certain romantic appeal, but this is not how things happen in the real world. It may be tempting to invoke savants as examples of such "out of the blue" artistic or mathematical feats, but most individuals recognized as truly important contributors to human culture are not savants.

As we already saw in Chapter 2, a visitor to the Picasso Museum in Barcelona's Barri Gotic will discover that the founder of Cubism started as an accomplished painter in the tradition of realism. A cultural historian will point out El Greco's and Goya's influences in Picasso's paintings. Likewise, an historian of science will tell you that Darwin's theory of natural selection was influenced by Malthus' musings about population growth, and Einstein's special relativity theory was influenced by Planck's quantum mechanics. Revolutionary as the famous $E = mc^2$ formula was, the concepts of mass and energy had existed before. And even the art of the flamboyant twentieth century iconoclast Salvador Dali strikes a distant resonance with the paintings of the fifteenth-century Hieronymus Bosch, whose whimsical, fantastic images prefigured surrealism. Any individual creative act can only be understood in the cultural context in which it occurs, a point so eloquently made by Mihaly Csikszentmihalyi in his landmark book *Creativity: The Psychology of Discovery and Invention.*[2]

Contrary to popular lore, a creative process is not a solitary process, even when the creative individual is temperamentally a loner and subjectively feels that it is a solitary endeavor. It is embedded in, and propelled by, the cultural milieu in which it occurs. Yet such an endeavor is not a mere replica of the past. The greatness of Picasso, Darwin, and Einstein lies in their creative gift of innovation, not in the mere mastery of their respective fields as they existed before.

Conjuring Up the Future

How does the brain conjure up future out of the past? Even though this is a whole-brain enterprise involving multiple brain structures, the brain structure that plays a particularly important role in this process is the dorsolateral and frontopolar prefrontal cortex, that famously "useless" part of the brain whose connections to the rest of the organism were severed in lobotomy, as we learned in Chapter 2.

The prefrontal cortex arose quite late in evolution, possibly in response to the pressures to superimpose order and organization upon the increasingly complex cognitive demands of the organism. While most other parts of the cortex are invested with relatively specific functions, the prefrontal cortex is in charge of "metacognition." It steps in to organize and coordinate those specific functions into complex, meaningful, and purposeful behaviors. It is important for setting goals, planning, making decisions, predicting the outcome of one's own and other people's actions, and impulse control. In performing these tasks, the prefrontal cortex seems to have access to the specific information stored elsewhere in the brain, particularly in the posterior (parietal, temporal and occipital) association cortex. In my earlier books *The Executive Brain* and *The New Executive Brain*, I draw the analogy between the emergence of the prefrontal cortex late in evolution, and the development of search engines, "the digital frontal lobes." Both the biological and digital "frontal lobes" arise in response to the increased complexity of the system and the need to overcome the potential for, respectively, biological informational chaos, or "digital anarchy." Both the frontal lobes and the digital search engines are "capable of constraining the system's degrees of freedom in any specific goal-directed situation while preserving these degrees of freedom in principle."[3]

Different parts of the prefrontal cortex make different contributions to these complex "metacognitive" processes. Although their roles overlap, the orbitofrontal cortex is particularly important for deciding what is "salient" for the organism's well-being: the lateral prefrontal cortex for organizing behavior directed toward the outside world, and the frontopolar cortex for integrating the functions of the first two regions (see Figure 4.1). Although the prefrontal cortex is the youngest part of the brain in evolution, it is also far more developed in humans than in any other species, including the great apes. Likewise, the prefrontal cortex is

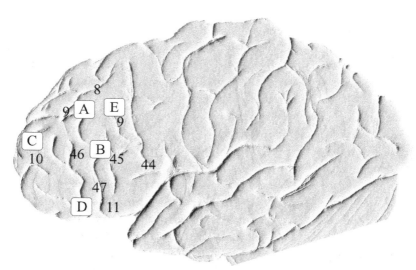

FIGURE 4.1 **Major prefrontal subdivisions.** (A) Dorsolateral; (B) Ventrolateral; (C) Frontopolar; (D) Ventromedial/orbitofrontal; (E) Anterior cingulate. Numbers correspond to Brodmann's areas (a standard taxonomy of cortical regions).

also among the last parts of the brain to mature during the lifespan—it is fully developed only by the age of one's early to middle thirties.

Brain Manipulation (But Not What You Think)

The lateral prefrontal cortex, in particular, has the ability to manipulate the mental representations stored in the brain like Lego® pieces: to assemble them into new configurations through a deliberative, goal-driven process. The actual "Lego® pieces"—the information manipulated by the prefrontal cortex—may be stored in other parts of the brain, to a large extent in the parietal, temporal, and occipital lobes—and the prefrontal cortex acts like the player accessing the pieces from various compartments according to the mental blueprint he or she has devised.

This process allows us to form new mental representations out of the fragments of old, previously formed ones; and these new mental representations do not have to correspond to anything we have experienced in real life so far (or ever will). *Generativity*, the ability to juxtapose old elements into new configurations, is essential to many human activities and functions. If there is anything at all that distinguishes the human brain from the brains of other species, however advanced, it is probably the capacity for generativity, mediated by the prefrontal cortex. In some sense, these newly assembled mental representations are predictions; they are models of the future—as we expect it to become or as we intend to make it so, a point made with almost poetic eloquence by Joaquin Fuster.[4]

Another distinguished neuroscientist, David Ingvar, coined the extravagant-sounding phrase "memories of the future" to refer to these predictive neural models of things to come.[5] It has been said—rightly or wrongly—that the prefrontal cortex, the brain structure central to assembling the "memories of the future" from the fragments of "memories of the past," is what makes us humans. Not a great fan of an exceptionalist, anthropocentric view of anything, I gravitate toward a more gradualist view of the development of traits in evolution. Then again, not being a primatologist, I have to go in making my admittedly dilettante observations by what I have—dogs. My late bullmastiff Brit was able to develop a very modest model of the future of sorts but it extended only a few minutes into the future. Upon seeing me take the leash, ready to take him for a walk, Brit would rush to his corner of the apartment to gobble up his food in anticipation of being separated from it; but he began to exhibit this behavior only in the canine ripe middle age: it took eight or nine years of his life for this rudimentary "memory of the future" to develop. My new English mastiff puppy Brutus, 11 months old at the time of this writing, still shows not even a hint of such predictive behavior. It appears that in a canine, even the rudimentary "memories of the future" are very slow to form, and they lack the ability to extend far into the future.

Language Generativity and the Frontal Lobes

There is one territory where my gradualist assumptions break down, or at least it can be argued so—language. Many theories about the evolutionary prerequisites of language development have been proposed, but they often forget Noam Chomsky's admonition that what distinguishes true language from other communication systems is its generativity.[6] Human language can generate a practically infinite number of statements that do not necessarily have to reflect empirical reality, and it can refer to things that do not exist or are not even possible—like "the negatively aged triple-headed purple unicorns are flying from the Mars to the Saturn on a solar-energy-fueled magic carpet at the caterpillar speed back in time" (I just made it up). This generativity is a unique attribute of the prefrontal cortex, and its emergence late in evolution enabled the development of genuine language, the ultimate Lego®. Human language also has the capacity for recursion, which makes it possible to generate linguistic structures where complete statements are embedded into larger statements, like the Russian *matryoshka* dolls: "The negatively aged triple-headed purple unicorns, expecting to meet up with positively aged headless striped multicorns, are flying from the Mars to the Saturn on a solar-energy-fueled magic carpet, which has been masterfully crafted by winged mastodons on the Moon, at the caterpillar speed back in time." Construction of a recursion, and particularly of multiple recursions (here we go—a recursion, can't get away from them!), is essentially a hierarchical process, and assembling cognitive hierarchies is also under the control of the prefrontal cortex. It is doubtful that an organism without a strongly developed prefrontal cortex would have been able to generate recursive linguistic structures.[7] Chomsky argued that recursion—the capacity for hierarchical organization—is a universal characteristic of all languages. Even though this assumption in its absolute form has since been challenged, a challenge that itself has been challenged (another recursion!), recursion is undoubtedly a property of most languages.[8]

Assembling the New from the Old

The ability to combine the elements of old ideas into new configurations is essential for generating new ideas and new concepts, which in turn is essential to creativity. This is how the figments of human imagination like mermaids (half-human–half-fish denizens of fairy tales and legends) and unicorns came into being, and this is how many important scientific ideas, technological inventions, and artistic creations have been born. As we already know, new ideas, solutions, and art forms are not created in a vacuum. To a very large extent, they arise as novel configurations of the elements of previously formed ideas, solutions, and art forms. The prefrontal cortex is uniquely equipped to configure and assemble bits of previously acquired knowledge and ideas in novel ways. One does not need the prefrontal cortex to evoke a mental image of a human or a fish; they are grounded in experience. But one needs the prefrontal cortex to construct a mental image of a mermaid or a unicorn, the figments of human imagination not grounded in experience. Flippant as this may sound, one can think of consequential scientific ideas and artistic concepts also as the mermaids and unicorns of our human imagination.

In his book *Sapiens: A Brief History of Humankind*, Yuval Noah Harari[9] muses about the nature of the "cognitive revolution" that presumably took place sometime around 70,000 years ago and resulted in an avalanche of inventions: boats, oil lamps, bows and arrows, needles—which finally really signaled the emergence of the "modern human." What was at the root of this revolution? Harari and many others believe that it was a mutation affecting the *Homo sapiens* brain and conferring on this species (us) the dominion—not always benevolent—over from the animal kingdom and even over the other hominid species inhabiting various parts of Eurasia at the time—Neanderthals, Denisovans, *Homo erectus,* and a few others. How, exactly, did the hypothetical mutation change the human brain? We don't know for sure, and any attempt to answer this question remains a speculation, but a plausible answer to this question is offered by the famous ivory figurine of a "lion-man" or "lioness-woman," also mentioned in Harari's book, with a human body and a lion's head (presumably that of the cave-lion inhabiting Europe at the time) (Figure 4.2).

One of the earliest examples of prehistoric representational art, the "lion-man" was found in the Hohlenstein-Stadel Cave in Germany and is 30,000–40,000 years old. The creation of this mermaid's distant ancestor most likely required a reasonably well-developed prefrontal cortex, just as the development of language meeting the Chomskian definition did, since both require Lego®-like generativity. As we already argued, one does not need this ability to conjure up an image of a human, a fish, or a lion, since these representations are rooted in reality and thus in one's actual experience. But the image of the mermaid is not based on actual experience, nor is the image of the lion-man, since such creatures don't exist in the physical world. These images had to be truly created by combining elements of the old into a *de novo* configuration that did not correspond to anything encountered before. Whatever other properties this mysterious mutation may have conferred on the human brain, its effect on the frontal

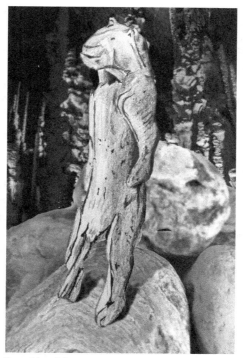

FIGURE 4.2 The Cave Lion-Man.

lobes had to be part of the story—or possibly even the whole story. Some paleo-anthropologists believe that what doomed the Neanderthals was their inability to adapt to the changing environment. For many generations throughout millennia, they existed on the same diet and practiced the same hunting methods. The capacity for change, the mental flexibility conferred by the developed frontal lobes, was absent.[10] Another archaic human, *Homo erectus*, who inhabited East Asia for almost two million years, continued to make, according to Harari, the same type of tools all these millennia without much modification.

Harari proposes that the far-reaching manifestation of the Cognitive Revolution was the *Homo sapiens*' ability to create cognitive fictions (or "social constructs," or "imagined realities"), constructs that do not immediately correspond to any physical, directly experienced reality. In their highest expressions, the concepts like "law," "state," "corporation," and "religion" are examples of such constructs. Complex and intangible from a sensory standpoint as they are, these constructs all begin with a "lion-man" or a "mermaid," where the figment of one's imagination is only one step removed from the tangible physical world. Then the process, shared across individuals and generations, is iterated at increasingly high levels of abstraction and becomes increasingly removed from the tangible physical reality.*

So if there ever was a crucial mutation affecting the brain and turning the archaic *Homo sapiens* into the modern *Homo sapiens sapiens*, it most likely involved the prefrontal cortex, endowing it with its Lego®-like prowess in assembling various components of one's mental representations at will, and increasingly liberated from the constraints of the physical reality. In an uncanny way, this reverses the direction of causation. If more limited cognition is restricted to the mental representations reflecting the physical world, then in the cognition empowered by the prefrontal cortex and related structures, the arbitrarily assembled mental representations, or "imagined reality," drive behavior, ultimately changing the physical reality according to these cognitive fictions.

Both the individual act of innovation of modest consequences and the forging of "social fictions" with their seismic effects on society hinge on the organism's ability to combine old elements into new configuration, and this in turn requires the highly developed prefrontal cortex. While other mammalian species may have relatively developed frontal lobes, their development peaked precipitously in *Homo sapiens sapiens*, this enabling the Cognitive Revolution and modern language.

Mechanics Behind the Metaphor—the Macro View

Of course, the frontal lobes as the Lego® master and the generative process of innovation as rearrangement of Lego pieces is merely a metaphor. It may convey the general idea of new solutions arising from old experience, but it tells us nothing about how these processes actually arise in the brain. Are we ready to move beyond the metaphor and have a glimpse into the neural machinery of innovation? We are ready to try. Do we have a comprehensive understanding of this machinery? We do not, at least not yet, but we are beginning to ask probing questions. These questions can be asked at different levels: at the macro level of whole brain structures and their interactions; and at the micro level of intricate neural circuits.

---

* The cultural evolution of religious beliefs illustrates the point. In its earliest, animist forms, the supernatural practically mimicked the natural: a separate deity (or "spirit," or whatever) was posited for every type of thing—a tree, a creek, a stone. Over multiple iterations, more abstract constructs increasingly removed from concrete physical reality gradually evolved, culminating in ideas such as monotheism (yet still with a multitude of prophets, saints, apostles, and angels lurking in the background, the vestigial remnants of earlier abstractions). The iterative and hierarchical evolution of "social fictions" is very similar to the generative nature of language (even though these two kinds of processes occur on vastly different time scales), and a well-developed prefrontal cortex is essential for both.

"Canonical" Networks

How does the prefrontal cortex interact with other brain structures in the course of a complex cognitive task? By its very nature, this interaction cannot be understood by looking at separate brain structures; one needs to look at networks. The shift from the research into the functions of separate brain regions to that of constellations of interactive brain structures (i.e., networks) has been one of the major developments in cognitive neuroscience of the last few decades. Today, three networks are often invoked in brain research: the central executive network (CEN), the default mode network (DMN), and the salience network (SN). These networks are schematically represented in Figure 4.3.

The central executive and default mode networks have been particularly extensively studied, and the assumption is often made of a sharp discontinuity among them. They are "anticorrelated"—when one is active, the other one is inactive. Each network consists of a relatively small number of macroscopic "hubs"—areas known to have bilateral connections with a particularly large number of brain structures and regions.[11]

An intelligent neurobiological naïf, an engineer, or a mathematician, may be perturbed by the frequently encountered inclination in today's cognitive neuroscience to invoke these two networks (CEN and DMN) as the explanation of too broad a range of cognitive processes. He may also question the realism of reducing all possible interactions afforded by the rich matrix of myelinated pathways in the brain to just a few networks, as well as of the assumption that the two major ones among them cannot operate in parallel. Indeed, a number of additional, often overlapping networks have been introduced, including the attention network, language network, and frontoparietal control network (FPN). The latter two are presumed to be unique to humans, and the FPN in particular to reflect the pattern of evolutionary expansion of the cortex, especially pronounced in the frontal and parietal regions.[12]

And before we knew it, old temptations reasserted themselves in a new guise: the yearning for a finite (and preferably not too long) list of neatly defined modules. Sometime in the 1970s and 1980s, neuropsychologists were infatuated with the notion that the cortex was a collection of "modules," discrete entities with rigid boundaries and fixed functions. It was the last "hurrah" of the peculiar state of affairs whereby cognitive science was mostly unconnected to neuroscience, and as the fusion of the two disciplines progressed toward the end of the twentieth century (to a large extent due to the advent of functional neuroimaging), the notion of "cortical modularity" was abandoned in favor of a nimbler understanding of cortical organization. Today, even though instead of brain regions, the new modules are defined as "networks," their proliferation bears an uncanny resemblance to the heyday of the old-school modularity a few decades ago, and it represents the same epistemological esthetics (which never

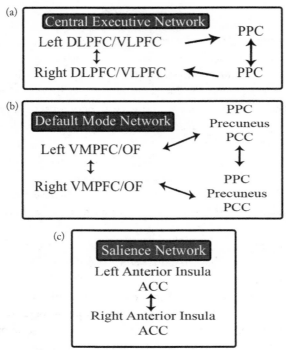

FIGURE 4.3 **Major large-scale networks.** (a) Central executive network (CEN) involves the dorsolateral and ventrolateral prefrontal cortex (DLPFC and VLPFC) and posterior parietal cortex (PPC). (b) Default mode network (DMN) involves the ventro-medial (VMPFC)/orbitofrontal (OF)cortex, posterior parietal cortex (PPC), precuneus, and posterior cingulate cortex (PCC). (c) Salience network (SN) involves the anterior insula and anterior cingulate cortex (ACC).

particularly appealed to me). As the number of the proposed networks grows, they begin to look increasingly like the classic functional systems, assembled in an ad hoc fashion in response to the cognitive demands at hand, rediscovered with the tools of functional neuroimaging.[13] And the fact that in different studies the neuroanatomy of each of these networks is often outlined somewhat differently also suggests that the attempts to force all the observations into a small number of "canonical" networks is a questionable exercise whose outcome is not to be taken literally. Instead of unique canonical networks, it is probably more heuristically useful to think in terms of "network categories," while realizing that there are potentially as many networks as the topology of long pathways in the brain permits. It would not be particularly surprising if the ascendancy of this new brand of modularity were to follow a trajectory similar to that of the old one, and like the "modularity" of brain regions, the "modularity" of brain networks will be tempered in due time in favor of a more nuanced understanding.[14]

But even if probably too coarse, the macro network taxonomy is "true enough" for many aspects of the current state of neuroscientific affairs, and it carries a certain explanatory value. It is useful to think of these networks as major highway systems that can accommodate a wide range of traffic patterns and specific subsystems. Each of the three commonly invoked networks will be dealt with more closely later in the book.

Central Executive Network (CEN)

The CEN, also known as cognitive control network (CCN), is a complex constellation of brain regions working together when we strain, consciously and persistently, to solve a challenging cognitive task. This is why this network is often referred to as "task-positive." The exact description of CEN's components may vary from study to study, probably as a reflection of the differences in the specific cognitive tasks involved, but the lateral prefrontal cortex (whose dorsal and ventral subdivisions are often lumped together and collectively referred to as the "dorsolateral prefrontal cortex" or DLPFC) and posterior parietal cortex (PPC) are invariably its main components.[11]

The temporal dynamics within CEN shed light on the relationship between the prefrontal cortex and posterior association cortex, where complex knowledge is represented in cognitively challenging tasks. When scientists examined the order in which different components of the network became active, it became clear that the activation within the network is driven by the prefrontal cortex.[15] Prefrontal cortex becomes active first, and the activation of the other CEN components, the regions found in the parietal and sometimes temporal lobes, follows.

The CEN may not be unique to humans. Using near-infrared spectroscopy (NIRS) and surface field potentials (SFPs), Joaquin Fuster and his colleagues described a network anatomically very similar to CEN in the rhesus macaque monkeys performing a working-memory task. The network, involving the lateral prefrontal and posterior parietal regions, was characterized by a complex pattern of synchronizations and desynchronizations in time, frequency, and brain space, this highlighting the point that identifying the highway is only the first step in understanding the neural traffic patterns, and a more detailed analysis of these patterns is in order.[16]

Default Mode Network (DMN)

The DMN is a network that becomes activated when no externally imposed task drives the workings of the person's cognitive processes, and the brain is left to its own devices. It is sometimes referred to as "task-negative," but this really is a misnomer, since the brain is not idle: rather, instead of being driven by an externally imposed task, it is engaged in internally selected and internally directed ones.[17]

More will be said about DMN in Chapter 5, but here we will just compare the two networks—CEN and DMN—in terms of their neuroanatomical components. Both networks are centered around two macroscopic hubs: the prefrontal cortex and the posterior parietal cortex. These two areas are so-called heteromodal association cortices, and their unique role in most complex cognition, their extensive connectivity, and their propensity to work in concert have been recognized for a long time.[18] Seen in that light, the discovery of the two large-scale networks has been a functional neuroimaging reconfirmation of, and elaboration on, a well-known basic feature of functional cortical organization.

But while both CEN and DMN incorporate the prefrontal cortex and posterior heteromodal association cortices, different subdivisions thereof are involved in the two networks; this is what makes their discovery particularly interesting. The most clear-cut difference between CEN and DMN is evident in the prefrontal cortex. Whereas in CEN, the dorsal and ventral lateral aspects of the frontal lobe are active, in DMN, it is the orbital and ventromedial aspects.

The posterior components of CEN and DMN appear to overlap but are somewhat different nonetheless. Both involve the heteromodal association cortex of the posterior lateral parietal lobe, but more extensively in CEN than in DMN. In contrast, DMN involves the posterior cingulate cortex and precuneus (an area found on the mesial aspect of the posterior parietal lobe), which CEN does not.

Based on what we know about these brain structures, CEN appears to be turned toward the information about the outside world, and DMN toward the internally generated inputs. Note that the lateral aspect of the prefrontal cortex (CEN) is somewhat larger in the right than the left hemisphere, and the opposite is true for the orbitofrontal and cingulate (DMN) cortices.[19] To the extent that "bigger is better" (a coarse but often surprisingly valid motto when it comes to the relationship between structure and function in the brain) this asymmetry may contain a hint about the relative roles of the two hemispheres in CEN vs. DMN.

Salience Network (SN)

The SN provides an interface between CEN and DMN. It was described more recently and has been less extensively studied. It consists of the anterior insula and anterior cingulate cortex and appears to become active—particularly the right insula—when switching between DMN and CEN occurs. In the experiments that led to the discovery of SN, switching was unidirectional, from DMN to CEN but not the other way around, and the switch was triggered by an abrupt change in the sensory input—an abrupt shift in musical "movements" (themes) or the appearance of an infrequent ("oddball") stimulus. Because of the unidirectional nature of the switch, it could be argued that the switch was really precipitated by the detection of novelty rather than of "salience" in the sense of "significance" (more about the multiple uses of the term "salience" and the potential for confusion because of this in Chapter 5). As we will find out in Chapter 6, the right hemisphere is critical for dealing with novelty, which helps make sense of the asymmetrical (right more than left) insula involvement in the switching process.[20]

Another noteworthy feature of the switching process is that it entails not just the activation of CEN, but also the concurrent dampening of DMN (remember, the two networks are "anticorrelated"—when one is active the other one is inactive). This implies an inhibitory relationship between the two networks. How does this happen? Interestingly, the two prefrontal regions that drive the two networks exhibit opposite functional properties across a wide range of contexts. Dorsolateral lesions produce symptoms similar to depression—it is for this reason that the dorsolateral prefrontal syndrome used to be known as "pseudodepression" in the old neurological literature. In contrast, orbitofrontal lesions often result in the shallow euphoria and jocularity known as *Witzelsucht*. Likewise, in depression, dorsolateral cortex is often hypoactive, and orbitofrontal cortex is hyperactive.[21] Taken together, these data suggest that a reciprocally inhibitory relationship exists between these two prefrontal regions.

The central nervous system thrives on reciprocal inhibitory mechanisms. Could it be that the opposite, "anticorrelated" relationship between CEN and DMN is a consequence of the mutually inhibitory relationship between the two prefrontal regions that "drive" them? Indeed, the lateral (ventral and dorsal) prefrontal cortex and medial prefrontal cortex work in opposite regimes: when one is active, the other one is not. On the other hand, it has been argued that the effective mutually inhibitory, anticorrelated relationship between the two large-scale networks does not require the presence of overtly inhibitory long-distance pathways and may be a consequence of global network dynamics.[22] Thus the issue remains unsettled.

Either way, SN may be the relay through which the effective mutual inhibition takes place. Indeed, the anterior insula is interconnected with vast cortical areas, particularly with multiple regions of the prefrontal cortex, including the orbitofrontal and ventrolateral regions. This makes it a likely relay of inhibitory relationships between the drivers of CEN and DMN—the lateral and orbital prefrontal regions, respectively. According to this scenario, SN is more of a "switch" than a "switching hand": once novelty is ascertained in the right hemisphere, the extroverted lateral prefrontal cortex inhibits the introverted ventromedial/orbitofrontal cortex. As a result, CEN is activated, and DMN is dampened.

The supposition of an "anticorrelated" mutually inhibitory relationship between the lateral and mesial/orbital prefrontal cortices leads to another interesting conclusion: that each of the two prefrontal regions in question tends to gravitate toward relatively extreme, and opposite, activation levels, eschewing the middle grounds: at any given moment in time, one of them is in a state of high arousal, and the other one in a state of low arousal. The propensity to bypass neutral activation levels in favor of relatively extreme ones invokes the concept of "bistability" as a major characteristic of the workings of the lateral and mesial prefrontal cortex. More about this in Chapter 7.

The Working Memory Conundrum
How It All Began

The large-scale networks provide an aerial view of how the prefrontal cortex interacts with the rest of the brain. But we are still in the metaphor-land, and crucial questions remain unanswered. What does it mean for the prefrontal cortex to "engage" the posterior parietal cortex (PPC) and other cortical structures where knowledge is represented? Does it extend a little neural "hand" and move the neural circuits around? Probably not, but then what exactly does happen? We still don't have the answers to these questions, but significant progress has been made—to a large extent owing to the work of four remarkable neuroscientists: C. F. Jacobsen, Joaquin Fuster, Patricia Goldman-Rakic, and Amy Arnsten.

C. F. Jacobsen, working in the 1930s at Yale University, was the first to demonstrate that experimental bilateral lesions in the frontal lobes disrupted a monkey's performance on the delayed response and delayed alternating response task, where the monkey had to "remember" in which of the two locations the bait had been found previously and go to either the same or the opposite location. Jacobsen described this impairment as "out of sight, out of mind" behavior, and he was the first to link the frontal lobes to a certain kind of memory.[23] Joaquin Fuster's work confirmed and further clarified the role of the frontal lobes in delayed response. He demonstrated that the cryogenic depression (freezing) of the frontal lobes interfered with delayed response, and was also able to identify neurons in the frontal lobes of the *Macaca mulatta* monkeys that increased firing during the delay between cue presentation and response.[24] As a result of this work, a particular form of memory was identified, linked to the frontal lobes and referred to in contemporary literature as "working memory."[25] Many years later, Patricia Goldman-Rakic, one of the pioneers of working-memory research, was very fond of the "out of sight, out of mind" phrase, both as a way of conveying the essence of frontal-lobe lesion effects, and as a way of teasing her acquaintances in social situations.

Is the lesioned monkey's "out of sight, out of mind" behavior the result of genuine memory loss, or is it the result of the lost ability to treat the memory as important or relevant; in other words, loss of its designation as a "salient" one? The answer to this question is not clear, at least not to me. After all, the monkey doesn't care about the scientist's research agenda; all it cares about is getting the bait. Although the "out of sight, out of mind" behavior is commonly interpreted as a form of forgetting, the alternative "loss of salience" explanation is possible, and it merits further investigation. The difference between the two possibilities is far more than merely semantic, and bringing salience into the narrative may result in the change of our understanding of "working memory." The fact that the neurotransmitter dopamine plays a critical role both in supporting frontal-lobe function *and* in tagging information as salient (none of which was known in the days of Jacobsen's experiments) lends credence to the latter possibility (more about this in Chapter 5).

Working Memory and Long-Term Memory

Patricia Goldman-Rakic built on Jacobsen's work and was among the first to propose that the unique attribute of the prefrontal cortex was its ability to "work with mental representations" of things, even when these things were no longer present in the animal's physical environment; and that the pyramidal cells of layer III in DLPFC are central to these processes.

Goldman-Rakic laid the foundation for understanding the underlying mechanisms by demonstrating that, in the monkey, the regions of the temporal lobe processing object identity (part of the "what" pathway) and the regions of the parietal lobe processing object location (part of the "where" pathway) send separate projections to the distinct areas of the DLPFC and are therefore represented there; and that similar representations exist in the frontal lobes for the auditory signal and its location. She also demonstrated that the projections between the regions of the frontal lobes and those of the posterior parietal and temporal cortex are bidirectional, allowing back-and-forth reentrant communication between the frontal lobes and posterior cortex; and that this connectivity is hard-wired and innate.[26] The description of circuits provided by Goldman-Rakic for the classic animal models of working memory was remarkable for its clarity and mechanistic precision. More broadly, a variety of posterior cortical and subcortical regions may be engaged in such reentrant reverberating-loop interaction with the prefrontal cortex, depending on the specific features of the task at hand.[27]

But many questions remained unanswered. These questions become particularly intriguing if we assume—as most neuroscientists today do—that Goldman-Rakic's findings about "what" and "where" representations in the monkey's frontal lobes are a special case of a more general relationship between the frontal lobes and the association cortex of the parietal and temporal lobes, and that a similar relationship exists in the human brain.

Some of these questions must address an important difference between the experimental paradigms commonly used in animal "working memory" research; and the way working memory is used in real life by humans and most likely also by other developed species. In a typical experiment, the monkey has to keep "online" relatively recently presented sensory information about the location of the bait; the task does not require access to long-term memory content. In contrast, in humans, real-life access to long-term memory content is very much part of the processes involving working memory. As I am writing this very chapter, I am juggling several "theme lines" in mind and deciding how to organize them as I go: the Lego and mermaid metaphors, the history of "working memory" discovery, the properties of layer III pyramidal neurons, the content of previous chapters lest I repeat myself, the plan for subsequent chapters lest I jump the gun, detours into paleoanthropology, and so on. I am straining to organize all these themes in a coherent and logical fashion (you are the judge of my success or failure) and must keep them in my head "online" all at once along the way. The process is seriously taxing my working memory; I can feel it almost viscerally as I am typing these very words. But unlike in Jacobsen's monkey experiments, none of the information I am "working" with derives from recent sensory inputs. It derives from my long-term memory store, which contains knowledge acquired by me a long time ago and represented in diverse cortical regions of my aging brain, most of it probably outside my prefrontal cortex.

Long-term memory comes into play not only in real-life use of working memory, but also in experimental paradigms designed to study it in humans. Take, for example, the "N-back task." First introduced by Wayne Kirchner more than half a century ago, it has undergone a recent revival as the workhorse of working-memory research (Figure 4.4).[28]

The idea behind the N-back task is both simple and elegant. Imagine a conveyer with various items moving behind a wall separating it from the observer. There is a window in the wall, so that at any given time, the observer sees only one object. The observer is instructed to report whether the item appearing in the widow is the same as, or different from, the one that appeared one step before (N = 1), two steps before (N = 2), three steps before (N = 3), and so on. The task requires the observer to constantly update which two items must be compared, and not just passively keep certain information in memory. If the items are meaningless squiggles never encountered by the observer before, then the experiment is somewhat akin to the animal "working memory" experiment in that it is driven by recent sensory inputs. But if the items are letters, or words, or drawings of common objects, then the content of the subject's long-term store is brought into the process.

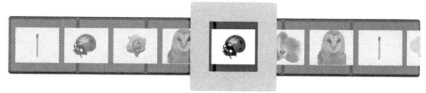

FIGURE 4.4 The N-Back Task. Is the image in the window the same as, or different from, the one *n* steps before?

One doesn't even have to be human for one's behavior to be guided by the content of long-term store as opposed to recently encountered sensory inputs. While my dogs' ability to form "memories of the future" seems limited at best, their ability to use long-term store is more substantial—an interesting distinction most likely related to the degree of frontal-lobe involvement in these processes. My late bullmastiff Brit was a picky eater and often ignored for hours the food laid out for him in "his" corner of our apartment—that is, until he saw me reach for the leash, the implication being that we were about to go out and he would be separated from his assets. The moment that happened, he would run to "his" corner from wherever in the apartment he happened to be, gobble up his food, drink his water, and only then approach me to get his leash put on. As I mentioned earlier, the predictive aspect of this behavior took years to develop, and Brit began to exhibit it only toward the end of his life (he died at 12 years old, and I still miss him), but there was another component to his behavior—long-term memory. Most likely, Brit's behavior was guided by the knowledge of the location of his food and water bowls, which had remained the same for years and was the content of his long-term memory store, and not by the recent memories of my putting food there, which he usually did not even witness (unless, of course, him being a dog, Brit's behavior was guided by olfaction that informed about the location of food through real-time sensory inputs). My new English mastiff Brutus exhibits an even more unequivocal behavior. When I bring him home from the "dog hotel" where he has been boarded during my two-week absence, he immediately runs to the corner of the apartment where his food and water are usually arranged, even though there is nothing there—the place had been emptied, thoroughly cleaned and deodorized before my departure. His behavior exhibits good "working memory," but it is guided by the content of long-term store and not by recent or current sensory input. At the age of 11 months, Brutus's behavior reveals a rather dramatic dissociation: virtually total absence of predictive, future-oriented behavior and at the same time a reasonably well-developed ability to utilize long-term memory store representing the past in his behavior. This is probably a reflection of frontal-lobe development in canines—modest but non-negligible, almost comparable to that of the rhesus monkey in terms of its size relative to the total cortex.[29]

Long-Term Knowledge and the Frontal Lobes

So understanding the nature of the interaction between the prefrontal cortex and the long-term knowledge store, presumed to be distributed throughout the neocortex, is of fundamental importance. Without it, the commonly used expressions like "bringing information online" and "mental scratch pad" will remain heuristic metaphors—useful and evocative but lacking precise meaning or mechanistic clarity.

Obviously, the brain of an undistinguished human being, let alone that of an ambitious intellectual, concerns itself with orders-of-magnitude more complex matters than the basic information about simple objects and their location in space, like my Brit's and Brutus's food bowl's location in the apartment. If the mental machinery of a contemporary thinker forging new ideas while "standing on the shoulders of giants" depends on the interaction between these two highly evolved cortical regions—the prefrontal cortex and posterior heteromodal association cortex, where presumably much of our general knowledge is stored and which are the main components of the "task-positive" central executive and "self-tasked" default mode networks—then what kind of information is being exchanged between them, and how? To the extent that some information reduction takes place, what is its nature, and how is it conveyed? For all such information to be permanently "copied" from the posterior cortex, where it is originally stored, to the prefrontal cortex without some sort of compression would probably amount to an evolutionary extravagance, a resource-consuming redundancy that, on balance, would be maladaptive. Furthermore, it would probably be a computational oxymoron, since a permanent exact copy may require that the informational volume of the source (vast areas of the posterior cortex) exceed the informational capacity of the recipient (lateral prefrontal cortex). This would run afoul of Gödel's incompleteness and Tarski's undefinability theorems, two of the most important formulations of twentieth century mathematics, both of which dictate that a system cannot fully represent itself or another system of equal or greater complexity.[30]

Here are a few questions that must be addressed to clarify the relationship between the prefrontal cortex and long-term memory store distributed throughout the brain and involving to a large extent the posterior neocortex:

- We know that a reentrant back-and-forth relationship between the prefrontal and posterior cortices exists in the course of a working-memory task,[31] but exactly what information is being exchanged?

- Does the content of long-term memory store, brought "online" by the prefrontal cortex in the course of a cognitive task, remain exclusively where it had been previously stored in the posterior cortex, albeit in an activated state; or is it somehow "copied" temporarily to the prefrontal cortex?
- If the latter is the case, then is all the task-relevant information contained in the posterior cortex "copied" in the frontal lobes, or is there some data compression?
- If the latter is the case, what is the nature of such compression? Is it "lossless," to use the lingo of data-compression technology, implying that no salient information is lost; or is it "lossy," characterized by some degree of information loss?
- If the latter is the case, then what information is lost and what information is retained?
- Whatever the informational content conveyed from the posterior association cortex to the prefrontal cortex, what is the neural "mechanics" mediating the process?

Phantoms in the Brain—the Micro View
Dynamic Network Connectivity

Answers to all these questions remain shrouded in mystery, at least for now, but some relatively recent findings may provide an important piece of the puzzle. Amy Arnsten and her colleagues at Yale University discovered a previously unknown type of interaction within neural networks that is unique to the prefrontal cortex—dynamic network connectivity (DNC). DNC involves changing connectivity within a neural circuit without changing the structural architecture of the network. The changes are rapid, ephemeral, and reversible, and they occur at the molecular rather than the synaptic level (which is why the structural architecture of the network is not altered). This makes DNC very different from the more extensively studied long-term information storage (LTS) which is orders-of-magnitude slower and involves the production of new synapses, altering connectivity within the network in a stable, structurally robust way.[32]

According to Arnsten and her colleagues, DNC mostly involves pyramidal cells of layer III (one of the six neuronal layers of which human cerebral cortex is composed) in the DLPFC. These neurons, whose triangular bodies gave rise to their name, had already been linked to complex cognition more than a century ago by the man who discovered them, the great Spanish neuroanatomist Santiago Ramon y Cajal. With their very long axons, a long apical dendrite, and multiple basal dendrites, they are uniquely suited for integrating information from multiple sources and for forming complex networks. Pyramidal cells are found in many parts of the brain, but they are especially prominent in the prefrontal cortex where their connectivity is particularly rich. The exceptional ability of prefrontal pyramidal neurons to integrate diverse and complex information is reflected in the complexity and density of their branching. This is especially true for layer III, the "external" layer, which is in charge of connecting the prefrontal cortex with much of the rest of the brain. In humans, a prefrontal layer III pyramidal cell has up to 23 times more dendritic spines (the microscopic protrusions making contact with other neurons) than does a pyramidal cell of the visual cortex. The density and richness of the prefrontal pyramidal cell connectivity have increased steadily throughout the primate evolution, reaching their peak in the human brain. A human prefrontal pyramidal cell has, on the average, almost twice as many basal dendritic spines as its macaque counterpart, and almost four times more than its marmoset one.[33]

These structural attributes are ripe with functional consequences that allow us to relate neural networks to complex cognition in a number of new and interesting ways, some of which will be discussed here. It is for this reason that I believe the discovery of DNC by Amy Arnsten and her team of Yale neuroscientists to be among the most important recent advances in neuroscience, and that it may prove to be key in cracking some of the previously intractable central conundrums of our field. What follows is a set of interrelated hypotheses, a speculative account that should be treated as such, while keeping in mind that a hypothesis remains just that, until it either finds support or is negated; but equally so, that most important breakthroughs begin with a hypothesis, a speculation.

Introducing "FROPs"

At least hypothetically, one can imagine a mechanism such that, when a stable, synaptically mediated network representing certain knowledge in long-term store is activated in the posterior association cortex, a temporary "copy" of that particular network (or several networks) is replicated in the frontal lobes in the DNC form via a mechanism that we still don't understand. We will refer to this process as *frontal resonance*, and to the hypothetical ephemeral copy as a *frontal phantom*, or FROP for short. Because at any given time, only a small subset of all the neural networks existing in the posterior cortex is "fropped" to the frontal lobes, the previously mentioned informational capacity conundrum is circumvented. Let's also assume that in order for the frontal resonance to occur, the prefrontal cortex (particularly DLPFC) must be in a "task-positive," active state. Such a state of frontal activation is sometimes referred to as "hyperfrontality," and it will be discussed in more detail in Chapter 7.

Our hypothesis does not specify how detailed the "frops" are, whether they capture all or only part of the information contained in the posterior cortical network that is being copied; whether it is an exact copy or a "stripped-down" one. Under the "stripped-down" scenario, the prefrontal representation of an extensive posterior network is not, strictly speaking, a copy; but it may help keep the original posterior neural network active for as long as the prefrontal "stripped-down" representation exists in a DNC-mediated form.

The frontal resonance "fropping" scenario may strike a rigorous, conservatively minded neuroscientist as a far-fetched fantasy bordering on the frivolous, until one recognizes its similarity to the scenario that is widely accepted to describe the "keeping online" mechanisms of working memory in animal experiments. The difference is that, instead of simple sensory information of limited informational content, we are extending this scenario to apply to orders-of-magnitude more complex and diverse information contained in the long-term memory store accumulated over years and decades. But this modified scenario requires a mechanism of representing such complex, diverse, and constantly changing information in the prefrontal cortex, albeit temporarily, for relatively brief periods of time. The ability of DNC to mediate such representations is a consequence of its rich combinatorial properties, which in turn are the consequence of pyramidal neurons' exquisitely rich connectivity. And the emergence of DNC in evolution has endowed working memory with the capacity to manipulate the complex content of long-term store and not just relatively simple sensory information.

Amy Arnsten was a student and a close associate of Patricia Goldman-Rakic, and a strong continuity exists in their work. (Being myself a student and former close associate of a great scientist, Alexander Luria, I know that a spectacular pedigree is both a distinction and a burden.) The discovery of DNC provides a way of infusing with a mechanistic content the concept of "working memory," to whose understanding Fuster and Goldman-Rakic contributed so much, but which nonetheless remained so frustratingly opaque and elusive for so long. As stated earlier, the "mental scratch pad" and "bringing information online" metaphors have been so frequently invoked to highlight the nature of working memory that they have created an illusion of understanding. But evocative as they were, these metaphors fell short of providing a mechanistic understanding of the actual brain processes involved in human working memory. The discovery of DNC by Amy Arnsten and her colleagues may prove to be a major step toward this understanding.

Pandora's Box of Consciousness Reopened

Assuming that the DNC-based frontal resonance and frontal phantoms ("FROPs") are real neural phenomena, and not the mere phantoms of my unhinged imagination, what is their relationship to the phenomenon of conscious experience?

I am tempted into this deliberation almost against my better judgment, since consciousness is the Pandora's box I usually try to stay clear of. For one thing, I have always regarded the subject's importance overrated, since the vast majority of our cognitive processes are automatic, guided by "mental autopilot" rather than by conscious awareness. Furthermore, I have felt that the infatuation with the subject of consciousness both among neuroscientists and among the general public was an epistemological cop-out, which basically represented a reluctance to completely let go of the Cartesian dualism; that consciousness was soul in disguise; and that "like many recent converts we continue to honor the old gods in secret—the god of soul in the guise of consciousness."[34] Regarding the conscious experience itself, my position has been parsimoniously minimalist to a fault: that it is nothing more and nothing less than a sufficiently large neocortical network activated for a sufficiently long period of time with a sufficient intensity. With consciousness understood in this way, the real role of "consciousness research" should be in characterizing the three critical parameters: the network's size, the duration of its remaining activated, and the intensity of this activation necessary for a neural event to become a conscious experience. A related phenomenon, that of a vague, poorly articulated, ephemeral thought, which we sometimes refer to as "intuition" or "gut feeling," can also be studied parametrically, since it can be understood in this framework as an activation of a smaller network, or one activated for a briefer period of time or at a lower level of intensity.

But I could also see how this minimalist understanding of consciousness would be regarded as woefully inadequate by many, perhaps even by most among those interested in the subject. Intuitively, consciousness implies the organism's self-referential capacity: an ability to form a representation of its own self, its own internal states. The self-representational ability has been regarded as a fundamental property of a developed nervous system by the philosophers of mind,[35] yet a mechanistic understanding of how this actually happens was lacking, and I would be the first to concede that a minimalist conceptualization of consciousness akin to the one described here fails to provide it either.

The frontal phantoms, or "FROPs"—assuming that they are real—fill this conceptual gap because they are essentially self-representational, and by being so, they may qualify as the mechanistic basis for conscious experience. Since according to our scenario the self-representational "fropping" occurs in the prefrontal cortex, the latter is placed at the core of the consciousness narrative, echoing some of the earlier assertions of the prefrontal cortex's role in consciousness and the relationship between the emergence of consciousness and frontal-lobe development in evolution.[36] At any given time, the phantom networks "copied" into the prefrontal cortex are limited in scope, and they may be rapidly supplanted by other phantom networks equally limited in scope, which agrees with the subjective experience of the narrow focus of consciousness at any given time. In contrast, the scope of neural representations potentially available for being phantom-copied to the prefrontal cortex is very broad, which agrees with the subjective sense of difference between what an individual is conscious of at any given time and what is potentially available for conscious experience—the former being very narrow, and the latter very broad. Of late, the notion of a "global workspace" as a metaphor for the focus of consciousness with fleetingly rapidly changing content has been taking hold.[37] To the extent that the metaphor is a useful one, the lateral prefrontal cortex with a rapid, kaleidoscopically fluid stream of "frontal phantoms" is that "global workplace."

The Making of a Mermaid

The discovery of DNC may also shed light on the central theme of this book: how mermaids, cave lion-men, Chomskian impossible statements, and great scientific ideas are created. The forging of all of these requires combining elements of several neural networks (each representing certain "old" information, image or concept) into a single "new" one. These different representations may have very little in common under most circumstances, and the neural networks embodying them may have little or no overlap. Herein lies a puzzle. Absent a homunculus' magic hand, how can these non-overlapping neural nets be brought together? It has been assumed that this ability is the unique purview of the prefrontal cortex. To illustrate the point, let's consider a commonly used neuropsychological test, Verbal Fluency. The subject is asked to generate as many words as possible of a particular kind in a pre-specified period of time, usually a few minutes. The task may take two distinct forms, each presumably probing the functional integrity of different parts of the cortex. In one form, the subject is asked to generate as many possible members of a particular category as they can—for instance, names of clothing items or animals. In the other form, the subject is asked to generate as many words as possible that begin with a certain letter. On the face of it, the two tasks are quite similar: both require accessing one's lexicon and pulling certain items from it. Yet many neuropsychologists believe that, despite the apparent similarity, the neural demands of these two seemingly similar tasks are different: the latter requires the participation of the frontal lobes, and the former does not. Why so? Because the lexicon is organized in the brain on the basis of semantic hierarchies and not on the basis of phonological or graphemic word forms. This means that if the task is to generate names of items belonging to the same category, the subject is accessing neural representations that are stored in the cortex close to one another, and the underlying neural nets strongly overlap. But in order to generate words that begin with a certain letter, the brain must "do violence" to the natural metric of language's cortical representations and access disparate networks located far apart from one another, with very limited overlap. Juxtaposing distant ideas, concepts, or facts in unusual and unexpected combinations is also at the heart of innovation and creativity of a more consequential kind, and the neural machinery behind them may be fundamentally similar to the one driving performance on the humble neuropsychological test described here.

How does this happen in the brain? How do elements of different, perhaps neuroanatomically disparate neural networks become integrated into cohesive new networks? What follows perhaps may not even qualify as a scientific hypothesis. I will call it a "scientific fantasy," and will indulge myself by pursuing it here at the risk of having it derided by my scholarly peers as a platitude or a lunacy, just on the chance that it may turn out to be a prophecy. At the very least, it lends itself to interesting computational neural net models as a way of confirming—or refuting—the idea's viability.

Let's consider two not mutually exclusive scenarios to account for the process. One of the scenarios involves "frontal phantom" resonance, and the other does not; but both are predicated on the exquisitely rich connectivity inherent in layer III pyramidal cells involved in DNC.

Scenario 1—"FROPs" and "double resonance": Suppose that several robust, synaptically encoded neural nets that inhabit distant, non-overlapping areas of the posterior association (parietal, temporal, or occipital cortex) are "copied" (or "fropped") into the prefrontal cortex via the DNC-mediated frontal resonance mechanism at the same or nearly the same time. These "neural copies" now find themselves in a more restricted cortical territory, a limited workspace of sorts, where they literally do overlap, albeit in an ephemeral way. That the "phantom" replicas of the neural circuits that were far apart in the posterior cortical space now literally overlap in the prefrontal cortex is crucial to the idea that we are developing here. It facilitates the formation of connections between their components that would not have been possible, or at least would have been highly improbable, before. In a way, it is like mixing different soundtracks and getting a new tune as a result (Figure 4.5).

The neural nets that inhabit vastly different areas of the cortex and do not overlap are temporarily "copied" into a constrained cortical space (the frontal lobes) together, providing that their activation was close in time. The combined temporary neural net may result in entirely novel activation patterns connecting elements that had never been previously combined. Even though most of these activation patterns do not represent any valuable new solutions of the task facing the organism, some of them may. As the double Nobel laureate Linus Pauling said, "The best way to have a good idea is to have a lot of ideas."

Various combinations of previously unrelated components of these networks are now possible. Suppose now that some of the *de novo* products of this overlap are "judged" by the brain as meeting the goal of the cognitive task at hand. We have yet to discover how this appraisal process takes place, but the prefrontal cortex is almost certainly involved, and the fact that the *de novo* networks are being formed in the prefrontal cortex will facilitate the process. The neural nets so selected are "copied" back into the posterior cortex, where they will be treated in a way similar to the way impressions coming from the external world are treated. In due time they may acquire a robust, structural, synaptically mediated form and become part of the long-term store; or they may fall

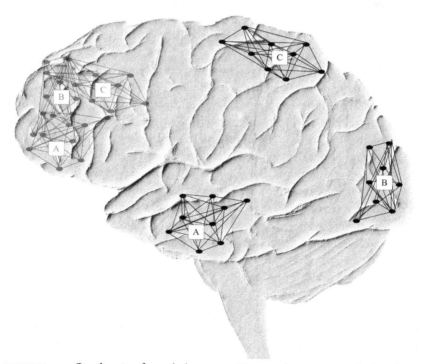

FIGURE 4.5 **Overlapping frontal phantoms.** Non-overlapping networks distributed in distant areas of the posterior cortex are temporarily "copied' in the prefrontal cortex where they overlap.

by the wayside. We will refer to this back-and-forth copying process between the prefrontal areas and the rest of the neocortex as *"double resonance."* The mediation of such resonance may well be among the main functions of the central executive ("task-positive") network.

Under what conditions are the neural nets "copied" back and forth between the prefrontal regions and the rest of the neocortex? Robust, structurally represented neural nets are being activated in our brains all the time. When I bump into a friend on the street and say "Hi, Bob," the network containing the knowledge, that the man's name is Bob and associating the name with the image of his face, became activated. Does it mean that it would be automatically "copied" to the prefrontal cortex, according to our scenario? Almost certainly not, since such a lack of selectivity would flood the prefrontal cortex with neural noise, turn it into a veritable information garbage bin, and would derail any useful decision-making process instead of facilitating it. But we have already constrained our scenario (it is too loose for me to call it "model") by positing that in order for the structural network to be "copied" via the DNC mechanism into the prefrontal cortex, the brain must be in a "task-positive" *hyperfrontal* state. A similar gating mechanism probably controls the double resonance: in order for it to occur, both the prefrontal cortex and posterior association cortices must be in a "task-positive" optimal arousal state.

Clearly, this is a very loose scenario of how new ideas are generated from the elements of old knowledge, merely a first-iteration sketch with more holes than flesh on the bones. Just to point out some of these loose ends, we don't know what information is retained and what is lost in the double-resonance process, nor do we understand its neural mechanics. Nonetheless, it may prove to be a start, a productive heuristic point of departure for future research and computational model-making, made possible by the discovery of DNC. Central to this scenario is the proposition that when structurally articulated neural circuits are activated, they are, under certain yet-to-be-identified circumstances, "copied" to the prefrontal cortex in a DNC form; and that several such "copies" end up overlapping in the same constrained regions of the prefrontal cortex at the same time, this making the assembly of the fragments of "old" networks into new ones possible.

Scenario 2—the "supernet": Because of their dendritic richness, the prefrontal pyramidal layer III cells connect to vast neural networks throughout the neocortex. Each such neuron both receives inputs from a vast network and (particularly so) sends outputs to it. Suppose now that a network of simultaneously active prefrontal pyramidal neurons is assembled via the DNC mechanism. Since each of these neurons is connected to a large number of neurons through its highly branched axon, this will result in a simultaneous activation of several vast networks elsewhere in the neocortex, which usually don't overlap, or overlap only minimally. Together they will form a temporary "supernet" enabling an interaction of cortical representations that otherwise would not have interacted. As a result, novel juxtapositions of the elements of "old" representations will be possible, this leading to the formation of new images, concepts, and ideas (Figure 4.6).[38]

These hypothetical scenarios, or a combination thereof, represent the essential components of a deliberate, conscious, goal-driven problem-solving process. Even though both are highly speculative at this point, their properties can be studied on computational models and perhaps experimentally as well. These scenarios provide a hypothetical mechanistic framework for thinking about how novelty is generated in the brain, and about the role played by the prefrontal cortex in the creative process.

The goal-oriented systematic machinery of the prefrontal cortex, which we attempted to sketch here, often goes a long way toward driving the creative process to fruition. It succeeds often but not always, and not all the way.

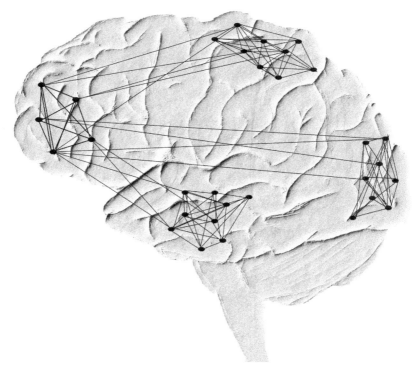

FIGURE 4.6 **Formation of a supernet.** A network temporarily formed in the prefrontal cortex co-activates posterior networks that otherwise don't interact.

When these mechanisms fall short, other brain mechanisms may have to be brought into the picture to complement the processes driven by the prefrontal cortex. We will discuss them in Chapters 6 and 7. But even when not sufficient in and of itself, the goal-directed search for solutions guided by the prefrontal cortex is necessary in most cases to prepare the grounds for that proverbial "creative spark."

5

It Is All About Salience!

The Salience Circuit

Free will is about making choices. Picking the right battles is as important as winning them. The choice of novel pursuits is as important as their outcome. Unlike college tests or cognitive tests used by psychologists, most real-life conundrums do not come with precisely formulated questions. It is up to the person to home in on what is *salient*, what should be the central theme of scientific or artistic endeavor. *Salience* is an ambiguous term, and this ambiguity is reflected in its definitions. In *The Cambridge Dictionaries Online, salience* is defined as "the fact of being important to or connected with what is happening or being discussed." In *The Oxford Advanced Learner's Dictionary,* it is defined as something "most noticeable or important."[1]

So salience may mean either importance or noticeability. As the word "salience" has become a bit of a buzzword, it is used in different disciplines and by different authors to mean different things. Because this word is commonly used by neuroscientists and will figure prominently in the book, we need to start by explaining how we will use it here. *Salience* is used by some authors to mean sensory prominence: a very loud sound or a bright light is commonly referred to as "salient" by psychologists—this is not how we will use the term. *Salience* is sometimes used to mean something unexpected, representing precipitous change or novelty—this is not how we will use it either. Finally, *salience* may mean something of considerable importance or relevance—this is how we will use the term throughout the book. Because some authors (but not I) may use the term "salience" interchangeably with "novelty," differences in wording do not necessarily imply contradictions in intended meaning.

What compelled Albert Einstein to focus on the relationship between space and time and not on any number of other possible relationships between physical variables? What compelled Lev Tolstoy to write a literary masterpiece about the Napoleonic invasion of Russia as opposed to any number of other possible subjects (incidentally, he refused to refer to it as "a novel," and *War and Peace* probably is a mistranslation; *War and Society* may have been truer to the author's intent, even though in Russian the title is, very likely intentionally so, creatively ambiguous).

At a less exalted level, imagine a group of students taking notes while listening to a lecture. The group behavior will be highly asynchronous. Different students will be taking notes at different points in the course of the lecture because their judgment about the relative importance of various facts or ideas presented by the professor—which ones are more salient and which ones are less—will vary. This is *salience-driven behavior*, guided by the subjective judgment of what's important rather than by an explicit, externally imposed instruction.

In order to understand the brain machinery of salience determination, we need to consider the prefrontal cortex and related structures. The proper function of these structures is necessary to ensure the central prerequisite of a creative process leading to innovation: that it addresses something of societal consequence and not something frivolous, inconsequential, and marginal. Without this ability, an individual may be talented and driven, but his or her labors will be "much ado about nothing" and will thus fail the first litmus test of creativity and will be ignored. In this chapter, we will examine the role of the brain's central players in deciding what is important and what is not: the frontal lobes, the left hemisphere, and dopamine.

Most real-life situations are ambiguous and do not come with externally prescribed "marching orders." It is up to the individual to decide, within certain constraints, what action to take, what problem to focus on, or how to prioritize one's time and resources. Faced with the same set of circumstances, different people are likely to make different choices; one set of choices not necessarily better than another in some "objective," absolute sense. If, upon graduating from college, Jane decided to go to medical school and John to law school, who is to say that one choice is "correct" and the other one is "wrong" in some absolute sense? Salience determination is intrinsically subjective.

Therein lies a paradox and a challenge. Most research paradigms used by scientists to study the functions of the prefrontal cortex in healthy people have been traditionally based on specific tasks with precise instructions to find the "correct" response or the "best" solution, where the definition of "correct" or "best" is built into the task. Even in experiments aimed at understanding the brain machinery of salience, it is common for the subjects to be told ahead of time what the "salient" aspects of the task, which need to be attended to, are: "Press the button only when a red circle appears," "Press the button if the stimulus is the same as before," and so on. The same is true for most neuropsychological tests designed to diagnose frontal-lobe dysfunction in traumatic brain injury, dementia, or other conditions. These paradigms have been quite useful and informative in studying a number of other functions supported by the frontal lobes (planning, mental flexibility, impulse control), but they taught us precious little about the brain mechanisms of real-life salience determination. At the risk of being redundant, let me repeat that in most real-life situations, there is no mental cop to direct our cognitive traffic: it is up to us to decide what is salient and what is superfluous.

Therefore, a real mismatch has existed between a very important aspect of frontal-lobe function and the tools, both research and clinical, available to study it. It was as if we were trying to measure blood pressure with a thermometer. The failure to distinguish between salience as determined by the individual and the "salience" imposed by the experimenter has resulted in a great deal of confusion in neuroscientific literature. This distinction will be very important in our forthcoming discussion; so in order to avoid further confusion, let's refer to salience as determined by the individual as "internal salience" and salience imposed by the experimenter as "external salience." Remember: an even greater potential for confusion is created by a very loose use of the word "salience" in research literature. A stimulus is often called "salient" when it is strong (loud or bright) or unexpected, attributes that may portend "salience" in the sense of "importance" but don't have to. When I walk down the street in midtown Manhattan, I pay attention to new restaurants because I tend to eat out; but I do not pay attention to new bank branches because I have been using the same branch of the same bank for many years and have no reason to be interested in others. This selectivity of attention allocation is driven by internal salience. But if an out-of-town houseguest asks me for directions to the nearest ATM machine, I will pay attention to the bank branches the next time I am on the street. Now the selectivity of my attention allocation will be driven be external salience. Most experiments conducted by cognitive scientists are of the second kind.

Paradoxically, the paradigms commonly used to study animal cognition are closer in some important ways to how human cognition operates than the paradigms used in human research. Unlike in a human study, you cannot "instruct" a monkey or a rat to do whatever it is you want it to do. What you can do, instead, is to set up your experiment in such a way that the animal must discover the variables you want to study as being important from its own perspective, which of course are the variables linked to the reward. You may think that you are studying the rat's spatial memory, but as far as the rat is concerned, it is looking for ways to get the morsel of food. It is up to the animal to determine what is salient in the environment in the context of its needs. So, in reality, what you are studying is not just the rat's spatial memory, but also its ability to select the maze's layout (as opposed to the color of the examiner's dress or the light intensity in the room) as the salient feature whose mastery leads to the reward. The rat may fail the test, not because its spatial memory is impaired (implicating the hippocampi) but because its capacity for salience determination is impaired (implicating the frontal lobes, such as they may be in a rat).

Until relatively recently, the lack of interest in subjective salience determination and its neural mechanisms has led to a great deal of confusion in cognitive neuroscience. This is particularly true when it comes to the trendy but opaque construct of "working memory." As I argued in my earlier book *The New Executive Brain*, and also in Chapter 4 of this book, it may be necessary to consider salience in order to bring clarity to this construct and to the understanding of working-memory breakdown following damage to the frontal lobes. It is only over the last few decades that the studies of the human frontal lobes began to focus on "agent-centered" decision-making driven by subjectively determined salience.[2]

As we already know, the prefrontal cortex and a few structures closely interconnected with it are particularly important for salience determination in ambiguous, not clearly defined situations, when it is up to the individual to decide what choices to make out of many possible ones. It turns out that among the various subdivisions of the prefrontal cortex, the orbitofrontal cortex (sometimes referred to as the ventral) and the closely linked anterior cingulate cortex are particularly important for salience-driven decision making[3]; and the dysfunction of these areas is implicated in several disorders characterized by impaired salience judgment, like schizophrenia and frontotemporal dementia.[4] It also turns out that these two regions are larger in the left than in the right cerebral hemisphere (Figure 5.1).[5]

From this, it may be tempting to surmise that the salience determination is particularly closely linked to the prefrontal cortex in the left hemisphere, and perhaps to the left hemisphere in general. The line of inference is premised on the "bigger is better" assumption, and it may sound too simplistic, almost offensively so, to elucidate the functions of something as exalted as the human brain. But a growing number of morphometric neuroimaging studies have demonstrated that, simplistic as it may sound, the relationship between a neural structure's size and its function often does exist. It makes sense, at least to me, because after all, the brain is a neural net, and computer simulations have shown that the computational power of a neural net is, up to a point, a function of its size.

Salient Default

We learn more about the brain machinery of internal salience-driven cognition by examining the "default mode network" in the brain, already mentioned in

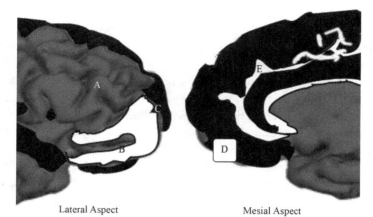

Lateral Aspect   Mesial Aspect

FIGURE 5.1 **Regional asymmetries in the frontal lobes.** Solid black areas are larger in the left hemisphere; white areas are larger in the right hemisphere. (A) Dorsolateral; (B) Ventrolateral; (C) Frontopolar; (D) Ventromedial/orbitofrontal; (E) Anterior cingulate.

Adapted with permission from E. Goldberg et al., "Hemispheric Asymmetries of Cortical Volume in the Human Brain," *Cortex* 49 [2013]: 200–210.

Chapter 4. The interest in the default network is relatively recent, and it is a result of two major paradigm shifts in cognitive neuroscience. The first paradigm shift was the realization that complex mental functions arise, not from isolated brain regions, but from interactions among multiple interconnected distributed *networks* of regions. The second paradigm shift was the realization—to a large degree owing to the work of Marcus Raichle and his colleagues at Washington University in St. Louis—that the activation patterns in a brain at rest are every bit as interesting as the activation patterns in a brain engaged in an externally imposed cognitive task.[6] The findings prompted by these paradigm shifts triggered a profound reconsideration of what we mean by the brain "at rest." A truly idle brain would probably generate a relatively random pattern of activation, but this is not what neuroscientists discovered. It turned out that a distinct pattern of activation emerged, involving the orbital and medial aspects of the frontal lobes, posterior portion of the cingulate cortex, and certain aspects of the parietal and temporal lobes. This network of functionally interconnected brain regions, which we already encountered in Chapter 4, became known as the "default mode network" (Figure 4.3).[7]

The default network is sometimes also referred to as the "task-negative" network, but this is a bit of a misnomer, stemming from the failure to distinguish between external and internal salience. The default network is active when the brain is not challenged with an *externally* imposed task. But far from slumping into idleness or randomness, it is now free to engage in cognitive activities of its own choosing. Its activities are now driven by *internal salience*. Notably, the default network is active during the mental states known as *mind wandering*, when, liberated from the imposition of externally imposed tasks, the brain has the luxury of focusing on the organism's own internally generated priorities: thinking about the future, about the past, about oneself and one's relationship to others. One can argue that it is precisely during these states that the most consequential, even existential dilemmas are confronted and decisions are made by an individual.[8]

For all these reasons, the default network can be justifiably called "internal salience network," even though in the neuroscientific literature the term "salience" is usually reserved for a very different network, namely the Salience Network (SN),[9] which was mentioned briefly in Chapter 4. I would argue that this, too, is a misnomer stemming from an ambiguous use of the word "salience," and that the network commonly referred to as the "salience network" can be more aptly described as the "novelty-detection" or "change-detection" network. That the default network is far from random is also reflected in the fact that it is more pronounced and more distinctly lateralized in the left hemisphere than in the right hemisphere,[10] and that it exhibits more efficient organization in the left than the right frontal lobes.[11] These findings are especially interesting in the context of our discussion, since they again point toward a critical role of the left prefrontal structures in internal-salience driven cognition.

The dynamics between the two "brain states"—one driven by external task demands (the "task-positive" external salience network) and the other by intrinsic states of the organism (the "task-negative" internal salience network)—is particularly interesting. Using a novel "dynamic graph" methodology, John Medaglia and his colleagues at University of Pennsylvania have shown that normal development in humans is characterized by an increasing amount of time the brain spends in these two states and by an increasing flexibility in switching between them. They speculate that these neurodevelopmental changes correspond to the development of executive functions as the developmental process progresses from childhood, to adolescence, to young adulthood.[12]

Salience, Dopamine, and Frontal Arousal—or Lack Thereof
Salience Signaling

There is another, biochemical, player in the brain machinery of salience, and that is dopamine. Dopamine, usually referred to in the scientific literature by the acronym DA, is a neuromodulator. Several biochemical systems operate in the brain and play an essential role in the communication between neurons. Among these biochemical systems, it is common to distinguish between the rapidly acting neurotransmitters and slow-acting neuromodulators (even though both are often referred to as "neurotransmitters"). Dopamine belongs to the second kind. Arguably the only one among the neurotransmitters, dopamine has drawn interest among the general public, almost to the point of tabloid prominence. If there is such a thing as a "trendy" neurotransmitter, dopamine is it. It has been implicated in addiction, in attention deficit hyperactivity disorder (ADHD), and in a host of other conditions. Its exact function (and dysfunction) has been a matter of intense interest, also both scientific and popular. It has been called "the pleasure transmitter" and "the reward transmitter"—colorful designations more likely to breed an illusion of understanding than true understanding.

But dopamine is merely a chemical that by itself does not conduct any neural computations. Its function is in facilitating communication between various brain structures and in facilitating the computations taking place in those structures. In order to understand its function (and dysfunction), it is important to examine the anatomy of dopamine pathways and the relationship between the structures whose communication dopamine facilitates. Patricia Goldman-Rakic, whose work we already discussed in Chapter 4, was among the first to recognize the role of dopaminergic pathways in the proper function of the prefrontal cortex, as well as in its dysfunction when dopamine transmission is disrupted.

An important dopamine hub is the so-called ventral tegmental area, or VTA. The neurons found in this area send dopamine projections to a number of brain structures, including the prefrontal cortex, the hippocampi, the amygdala, and the nucleus accumbens. Damage to this area interferes both with decision making, usually associated with the prefrontal cortex, and with memory. The projections *emanating from* VTA have drawn much research attention, and their role in executive functions and long-term memory was the subject of my own early work.[13] Damage to the VTA and its bidirectional projections to and from the prefrontal cortex results in a clinical condition practically indistinguishable from direct frontal-lobe damage. A distinct possibility exists that subtle damage to these pathways, which may be difficult to visualize with commonly used neuroimaging methods, is responsible for the elusive behavioral and affective consequences of "mild" traumatic brain injury often dismissed as "personality changes." Among other things, an improved ability to detect such damage may help us distinguish between the effects of two conditions often conflated in clinical diagnosis: traumatic brain injury (TBI) where damage to these pathways is likely to be present; and post-traumatic stress disorder (PTSD), where it is not. My colleagues and I described the effects of structural damage to the VTA and its projections many years ago, and we termed this condition the "reticulo-frontal disconnection syndrome."[14] Depletion of dopamine in the frontal lobes mimics the effects of the "reticulo-frontal disconnection syndrome" and also results in the impairment of frontal-lobe functions.[15]

But in order to understand its functions, it is equally important to consider the projections VTA *receives*. Some of the projections *received* by VTA originate in the prefrontal cortex and in the amygdala. We already know that the prefrontal cortex is critical for salience determination, and so is the amygdala. The difference between the two is that the prefrontal cortex determines salience on the basis of cognitive processing, and the amygdala on the basis of emotional resonance.

Let us assume that once a certain stimulus or information is recognized as salient, relevant to the broadly defined organism's success or avoidance of failure, by the prefrontal cortex or by the amygdala, a signal is sent by them to the VTA along the descending pathways, instructing it to put that stimulus or information "ahead of the neural line," so to speak. In response, the VTA sends a signal along the ascending pathways to the neocortex, nucleus accumbens, hippocampi, and other structures, tagging the stimulus or information in question as particularly significant or "salient," drawing attention to it, "urging" the organism to focus on it, and facilitating its commitment to long-term memory storage and reinforcement. So dopamine is a messenger of the message originating in the prefrontal cortex or in the amygdala, rather than the message's author. The surge of dopamine originating in VTA marks certain events or bits of information as "important." It is probably not too far-fetched to assume that the real-time decisions by students listening to a lecture in our earlier example, and selecting on the spot certain information as worthy of being recorded in their notes, are triggered by surges of dopamine. The distribution of major dopamine pathways in the brain is depicted in Figure 5.2.

Different components of the dopamine system play different roles in salience-driven learning. Using positive emission tomography (PET), a team of scientists from McGill University in Montreal have demonstrated that approach behavior driven by positive experiences and avoidance behavior driven by negative experiences are linked to two different dopamine receptors in the cortico-striatal system—D_1 and D_2, respectively. One of the implications of the study is that variability in D_1 and D_2 receptor binding may account for the individual differences in learning from experience styles.[16]

A series of experiments by Karl Deisseroth and his colleagues at Stanford University has provided a particularly elegant demonstration of the importance of specific dopamine receptors in salience-guided decision-making assessment. They found that the ability of the rat to learn from experience in choosing between two levers (one with a steady food supply and the other one with usually

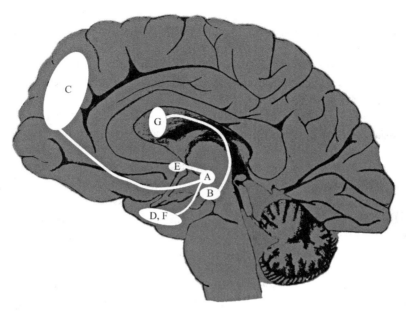

FIGURE 5.2 **Dopaminergic pathways.** (A) Ventral tegmental area (VTA); (B) Substantia nigra; (C) Prefrontal cortex; (D) Amygdala; (E) Nucleus accumbens; (F) Hippocampus and parahippocampal structures; (G) Striatum.

The network of connections between A, C, D, and E is particularly important in salience determination.

small but occasionally very generous supply) was guided by the signal emanating from neurons with D2 receptors in the nucleus accumbens, a brain region on the boundary of the ventral striatum, anterior cingulate, and orbitofrontal cortex, which is known to be the hub of the brain's reward system. Rats with a strong signal generated by these neurons learned from negative experience and adopted a conservative strategy, staying mostly with the lever providing a steady food supply. In contrast, rats with a weak signal generated by the D2 neurons continued to cling to the lever that occasionally released a very generous reward while releasing very little food most of the time. But this stubborn obliviousness to negative experience could be reversed in the risk-taking rats when the D2 neurons in the nucleus accumbens were stimulated optogenetically (a relatively new and highly promising experimental technique, where neurons are genetically modified to become light-sensitive and respond to stimulation with light).[17]

Dopamine signaling serves another important function: it is part of the arousal modulation system in the brain. The "salience" signal conveyed by dopamine modulates the prefrontal cortex, contributing to its optimal arousal state, which we discussed in Chapter 4 and will revisit in Chapter 7. Building on the earlier work by Patricia Goldman-Rakic, Amy Arnsten and her colleagues demonstrated that the arousal modulation provided by dopamine and another neurotransmitter, norepinephrine, plays an essential role in the functions of the prefrontal cortex and that the breakdown of this modulation is responsible for a wide range of cognitive disorders.[18]

I believe that the dual involvement of dopamine and norepinephrine in frontal arousal reflects two complementary types of arousal modulation: one based on perceived stimulus importance (dopamine) and mediating the use of well-established cognitive routines with previously established salience; the other one based on stimulus novelty (norepinephrine) and in tasks requiring mental flexibility and departure from previously established cognitive routines. The rationale behind this assumption can be found in my earlier book *The New Executive Brain*.[19] Complementary effects of noradrenergic and dopaminergic modulation on cognitive functions seem to support this assumption. Pharmacological modulation of the noradrenergic system enhanced the subjects' performance on a range of difficult, novel verbal tasks requiring mental flexibility, such as anagrams and verbal fluency. In contrast, administration of bromocriptine (a dopamine agonist) fails to result in this effect.[20] On the other hand, modulation of the dopaminergic, but not noradrenergic, systems facilitates performance on lexical tasks, which are based on more automatic processing and require the use of well-established semantic relationships.[21]

An important distinction has been made in the neuroscientific literature between intra-dimensional and extra-dimensional processing and set shifting, referring to the degree of mental flexibility required by the task. It appears that the dopaminergic system plays more of a role in the relatively constrained intra-dimensional set shifting involving transition between stimuli of a similar kind, whereas the noradrenergic system plays more of a role in the extra-dimensional set shifting involving more sweeping transitions between stimuli of a different kind.[22]

Later in the book, we will discuss how a dynamic interplay between different states of frontal activation—hyperfrontality and hypofrontality—is essential to the creative process and to the ability to generate new ideas. The brain's capacity for attaining and maintaining a wide range of prefrontal activation and deactivation levels appears to be a highly desirable trait and an important ingredient of complex cognition. To the extent that this range may vary from person to person, such individual differences may reveal themselves as the individual differences in the properties of the ventral brainstem nuclei and their projections emanating from the locus coeruleus, which is involved in the synthesis of norepinephrine, and VTA, which is involved in the synthesis of dopamine. I will argue in Chapter 7 that the wider this range of modulation, the more it benefits the processes of innovation and creativity.

More on Dopamine

The importance of the interaction between the prefrontal cortex and ventral brain stem in ensuring optimal cognitive performance was made clear by the work of Takeuchi and his colleagues at Tohoku University in Japan. Using a common method of measuring the size of different brain structures—MRI voxel morphometry—they demonstrated that individual differences in the performance on a divergent-thinking "creativity" test were related to the size of the right dorsolateral prefrontal cortex and the VTA: better performance was associated with the larger sizes of these structures.[23] "Bigger is better" again!

A relationship has been found between dopamine levels and individual differences in psychological traits, but the opinions regarding the exact nature of this relationship vary. It has been proposed that high dopamine levels are associated with enhanced mental focus and decreased mental flexibility. In contrast, low dopamine levels are associated with increased mental flexibility and novelty seeking.[24] Several human and animal studies lend support to this idea: increase in dopamine levels through pharmacological manipulations results in repetitive stereotypical behaviors.[25] And in the previously described study by Karl Deisseroth and colleagues, individual differences between the rats with a strong or a weak signal emanating from the D2 neurons in the nucleus accumbens translated into the differences between conservative and risk-taking decision-making styles.[26]

Yet the scientific literature is inconsistent, and other studies suggest an association between the dopamine system and novelty seeking.[27] These inconsistencies may reflect different contributions of multiple brain structures influenced by manipulations of dopamine levels. Alternatively, it may reflect the fact that novelty-seeking and salience-driven reward-seeking components of behavior may be so closely interwoven that distinguishing which of the two is more affected by a pharmacological manipulation is very difficult. In an animal experiment, where the animal behavior is by definition driven by reward, the distinction may be particularly difficult to make.

A more nuanced view of the DA role in maintaining an adaptive balance between the stability and flexibility of mental operation distinguishes between tonic and phasic activation within the DA system, the former promoting the stability of mental operations and the latter their plasticity. Different DA receptors may be involved in maintaining the tonic and phasic effects (D1 and D2 receptors, respectively); and possibly also different alleles (variants) of the enzyme

COMT (Catechol-O-methyltransferase), which plays a role in the breakdown of dopamine and norepinephrine, may affect this balance differently.[28]

It turns out that dopamine pathways (see Figure 5.2) are more abundant in the left hemisphere than in the right hemisphere, and this asymmetry has been demonstrated in several mammalian species, including our own.[29] So it appears that several important players in the brain machinery of salience determination are more prominent in the left than in the right hemispheres. These include the orbitofrontal cortex and anterior cingulate cortex (see Figure 5.1), and dopamine pathways, particularly those projecting to the frontal lobes. In combination, these findings suggest that the left prefrontal system and its pathways are particularly closely involved in internal salience-driven cognition.

Salience Diluted

The ability to identify and tag important information, events, and objects is central to the organism's survival and well-being. But this ability may go astray in various ways. Two of them are particularly interesting: *salience diluted* (exceptional memory and inability to forget) and *salience hijacked* (addiction). It is highly uncommon to discuss them in the same breath, but let's consider the possibility—at least as a heuristic proposition—that the neurobiology underlying these two conditions has an important feature in common: dysfunction of the salience machinery.

Unable to Forget: The Curse of Indelible Memory

Human memory is highly selective; our ability to forget being as important as our ability to remember. You remember the events of the day before, but if someone were to ask you what you did on a randomly chosen ordinary day ten years ago, then the odds are that you would be at a loss—unless perhaps you won a multi-million dollar lottery or were awarded the Nobel Prize on that day. The upshot of this observation is both simple and profound: most of the information that is registered in our brain and remembered for a period of time never makes it into our long-term memory (neuroscientists often use the term "long-term store")—only a small subset of such information does. William James was probably the first to point out that selectivity is essential to memory and that remembering everything would be tantamount to remembering nothing.[30] This is selectivity in action—a blessing without which our heads would be veritable information garbage bins, as I argued elsewhere.[31] The way the relatively small subset of information gets admitted into our long-term memories is far from random; it has been "selected" either by dint of the frequency of its use (I call this "*a posteriori salience*") or because it was tagged as important at the time of being encountered (I call this "*a priori salience*," even though this "judgment" by the brain usually reflects some prior experiences). The *a posteriori salience* mechanism works painstakingly slowly, and the odds of getting into the long-term memory via this route are stacked against any particular bit of information.

It is the *a priori salience* mechanism of selectively giving certain information the green light by the brain in ushering it into the long-term memory that is likely to involve dopamine. Evidence exists that dopamine plays a role in the formation of stable long-term memory representations, which involves the proliferation of new synapses[32]; and that such long-term representations tend to particularly depend on the left hemisphere, where dopaminergic pathways abound, for both verbal and non-verbal information.[33] The latter observation is particularly interesting and important, since it challenged the notion that the left hemisphere is narrowly specialized for language processing.

But some people are denied the blessing of forgetting. One such person was described in exacting detail by Alexander Romanovich Luria in his *Mind of the Mnemonist: A Little Book About Big Memory* (I have the book in its original Russian with Luria's inscription in my personal library to this day and occasionally show it to my students).[34] This remarkable "little book" was arguably the first of its kind in the "romantic science" approach to neuropsychology and, according to the late Oliver Sacks, served as an inspiration to him in forging his own unique genre.

The mnemonist in question was Solomon Shereshevsky, to whom Luria referred as "Sh", a man of practically limitless memory. His peculiar gift was first noticed by the editor of a provincial newspaper, where "Sh" worked as a reporter. The editor brought Sh to Luria's attention sometime in the 1920s, and the collaboration between a neuropsychologist and his subject continued for several decades. Sh's ability to memorize long lists of items—words, numbers, drawings—was practically limitless, and having concluded that any attempts to quantify it were basically futile (there seemed to be no ceiling), Luria turned his attention to Sh's ability to forget. Because of the length of their collaboration, Luria was able to test Sh's memory for various stimuli years and even decades after the initial exposure. To Luria's amazement, not only did Sh remember everything, but he also never forgot anything. This inability to forget was at times so oppressive—particularly once Sh embarked on the career of a professional mnemonist-performer—that in desperation he used to write the word lists he wanted to "delete" from his memory on scraps of paper and burned them.

What was the mechanism of this double-edged memory gift-curse? In his book, Luria links Sh's unusual memory to another peculiarity of his subject's mind—propensity toward synesthesias, the ability to link images across different modalities. Letter A was "white and long," and number 2 was "flatter, rectangular, whitish or sometimes a little grey." The voice of the great developmental psychologist Lev Vygotsky (who participated in some of the experiments) was "yellow and flaky," and the voice of Sergey Eisenstein (the famous film director and a close friend of Luria's) was "like flames with capillaries inside moving toward me." This propensity may have enhanced Sh's ability to employ the technique often used by other professional mnemonists of "attaching" stimuli (words, images, or whatever) to the elements of a familiar environment, like buildings on a familiar street or objects in a familiar room.

But in several discussions of the subject, Luria conceded that such a strictly cognitive account probably did not capture the whole essence of the phenomenon. I agreed with him and continued to mentally revisit our discussions occasionally during the years—decades, in fact—that passed since those conversations around the antique table with massive lion-shaped brass legs in Luria's apartment on Frunze Street in Moscow, Russia. Sh's unusual mnemonic abilities had to be rooted in biology, at least in part, since several other members of his family also had exceptional memory, even though perhaps not nearly so remarkable; but Luria's experiments with Sh were conducted decades before neuroscience coalesced as a mature discipline equipped with the concepts and technologies necessary to crack the riddle. We are better prepared to address it today.

Memories and Salience

Today we recognize that "memories" are networks of strongly interconnected neurons—mostly cortical—which tend to be activated together. As such neuronal groupings begin to consolidate, the process must be supported by their ongoing co-activation—a process in which hippocampi and related structures in the mesial temporal-lobe regions play a critical role. Unless facilitated by the recognition of *a priori salience* mechanisms, the process is excruciatingly slow, measured in weeks, months, years, or even decades, during which the connectivity within the network is fragile and subject to decay. The evolutionary "wisdom" (if there is such a thing) of this process is that it ensures forgetting of the superfluous information. But a relatively small number of such networks survive and consolidate in a more robust and stable way through the proliferation of new synapses connecting the neurons within the ensemble, at which point the participation of the hippocampi and related structures is no longer essential, and the network becomes strictly "corticalized." The process occurs either through the painstaking reiteration of "fire together wire together" principle for the frequently used information (*a posteriori salience*) or through the surge of dopamine tagging the information as important at the time of its presentation (*a priori salience*). Since most information is neither important nor frequently used, it goes by the wayside in most people—the blessing of forgetting.

Now imagine an individual in whom most, or perhaps even *all*, incoming information is consolidated—transformed into a stable, synaptically mediated connectivity—orders of magnitude faster than in most people. This super-fast synaptic proliferation leading to abnormally rapid memory consolidation may have various mechanisms behind it.

One possible mechanism is where all incoming information is treated by the brain as if it were salient in an *a priori* way—by the dopamine signal's being released indiscriminately. You will have a Shereshevsky in whom every memory—no matter how ridiculously insignificant—will rapidly become indelible. This is, of course, only a hypothesis, and Mr. Sh is no longer around to be studied with the tools of modern neuroscience, but other individuals with exceptional memory (which they often also find to be a mixed blessing) exist and are being studied.[35]

Another possible mechanism behind Sh's indelible memories may in fact be related to synesthesias. Vilayanur Ramachandran and his colleagues proposed that the propensity toward synesthesias is caused by neural hyperconnectivity.[36] Is it possible that neural hyperconnectivity also drastically facilitates and speeds up the formation of long-term memories, causing it to lose its selectivity in the process? According to this scenario, Sh's synesthesias and indelible memories are the two consequences of the same underlying cause—neural hyperconnectivity.

Either way, the indelible memory and inability to forget is a byproduct of the salience machinery's going astray and losing its selectivity, its ability to distinguish between the important and the superfluous. And Sh's whole life was shot through by this handicap. He was indecisive, and oftentimes befuddled, unsure of what he wanted in life and how to achieve it. Had it not been for his association with Luria, which helped establish him as a professional mnemonist, he would have probably floundered in life miserably.

Salience Hijacked

The salience machinery stripped of its selectivity is bad enough, but this ability may also be subverted, and then the urge to engage in maladaptive, self-injurious, or even self-destructive behaviors may develop. We refer to such urges as *addictions*.

Addiction may take numerous forms and involve different behaviors or objects of desire. Addiction to illicit substances—cocaine, heroin, and others—is the most commonly studied, but alcohol and tobacco can also be addictive, as are certain behaviors like gambling, pornography watching, and even playing video games. Society's attitudes toward addiction have frequently been intertwined and conflated with broad social and legal issues. Certain addictive substances are illegal (cocaine, heroin), while others are perfectly legal (tobacco, alcohol). In certain authoritarian and totalitarian regimes, addiction on a massive scale has been not only tolerated but tacitly encouraged as a distraction and a pressure valve in a deprived society. In the former Soviet Union, vodka prices were deliberately kept low by the state, despite the fact that alcoholism on a massive scale was the bane of the economy. Evidently keeping the masses drunk on their march toward Communism was more vital to the ruling clique's preservation of power than keeping them productive. In today's Iran, opium addiction is so widespread and tolerated, despite otherwise sanctimonious policies, that many believe that the Ayatollahs' government tacitly encourages it.[37]

Until relatively recently, addictions were regarded mostly in righteous moralistic terms, as bad personal choices and lack of self-control or moral fiber; or in socioeconomic terms as an unfortunate consequence of social ills. But the biological underpinnings of addiction are increasingly recognized, and it is increasingly common to understand it as the brain's salience machinery gone astray. At least in the eyes of the general public, legal profession, and society at large, however, it is next to impossible to completely remove the moral, "personal responsibility" taint from any consideration of addiction as long as personal choices can be presumed to be free and available—really, lay common sense dictates that one doesn't *have to* snort cocaine, shoot heroin, or gamble. Having been addicted to cigarettes for many years (and smoking is a form of addiction, never mind its perfectly legal status in society), I recall the sneering stares and righteous admonitions directed at me; and even though I quit more than a quarter of a century ago and now find cigarette smoke unpleasant in the extreme, I still don't have it in me to reproach the occasional smokers in my environment, remembering how offensive it had felt to be the target of such reproaches myself.

But a condition exists where addiction may develop under the circumstances entirely outside the person's control, and the issues of "personal responsibility" or "socioeconomic ills" do not even remotely arise. This in turn highlights the essentially biological nature of addiction and opens an additional window into its mechanisms. The condition in question is a relatively common neurological disorder, and addiction is the last thing evoked in the minds of most people when its name is mentioned. That disorder is Parkinson's disease.

Parkinson's disease (PD) has been traditionally associated with resting tremor (pronounced when the patient's hands are at rest rather than engaged in some activity), difficulty with initiating motor acts ("bradykinesia"), peculiar masklike face devoid of expression, and a host of other symptoms. PD is caused by atrophy of two twin nuclei in the brain stem called (because of their black coloration) *substantia nigra (SN)*, which are a source of dopamine projections into the subcortical collection of nuclei called "the striatum," particularly to its dorsal part consisting of the caudate nucleus and putamen.[38]

The dorsal striatum plays an important role in initiating and maintaining movements as well as in more complex behaviors, and it depends on dopamine for its proper function; so it comes as no surprise that the disruption of dopamine supply results in motor symptoms. More recently it has been discovered that, in PD, atrophy also affects the VTA, which as we already know sends projections into the prefrontal cortex, amygdala, nucleus accumbens, and other structures. Even though PD is usually diagnosed on the basis of motor symptoms, cognitive impairment is also common in this disorder. The pattern of cognitive impairment is somewhat different in different forms of PD, in the so-called left vs. right hemi-Parkinsonian syndromes.[39]

A number of medications exist to treat PD, but their therapeutic effect may come at a cost: the patients sometimes develop addictions. The addiction may take various forms, including pathological gambling, compulsive shopping, and hypersexuality. In a poignant piece written for *The New York Times*, Marc Jaffe describes the transformation of his middle-aged physician wife from a reserved workaholic with modest libidinal interests to one consumed by an insatiable desire for sex when she developed Parkinson's disease and was put on medications.[40]

A team of scientists from London's famous Institute of Neurology in Queen Square provide a dramatic description of what they call "hedonistic homeostatic dysregulation" in fifteen patients with PD.[41] Like in other forms of addiction, these patients kept feeding their addiction by increasing the dosages of dopamine-replacing medications contrary to medical advice and despite the side effects inevitably associated with the excessive doses. As they became hypersexual and embarked on gambling or shopping sprees, they often started hoarding their medications. The patients also developed peculiar motor stereotypies, like repetitive arrangement of objects or manipulation of gadgets: "They ritually dismantle their infusion pumps, or other electrical equipment, even though they realize that this is a senseless and unproductive habit."[42] These stereotypies, called "punding," are particularly interesting because they shed light on the mechanisms of addiction in these patients, and perhaps of addiction in general, since "punding" has also been reported in cocaine and methamphetamine addiction, along with pathological gambling and hypersexuality.[43] Punding is a form of perseveration, a maladaptive clinging to a particular behavior and an inability to let go of it. Even though addiction in Parkinson's disease is usually interpreted as a form of impulsive behavior, "punding" points to the perseverative aspect of this phenomenon, this being suggestive of its more complex nature than often assumed.

Why would medications prescribed to treat a movement disorder cause addiction? Standard treatment of PD involves stimulating the dopamine system in order to increase the dopamine levels in the brain. But the dopamine system is complex, with different dopamine receptors characterized by different concentration levels in different parts of the brain. Addiction as an untoward side effect is especially common for medications such as Pramipexole and Ropinirole, which stimulate a particular class of dopamine receptors—D3 receptors.[44] The D3 receptors are abundant in the nucleus accumbens (part of the so-called ventral striatum), whose role in the reward system we already discussed.[45] The role of nucleus accumbens in reward-driven behavior has been known since the classic work in the 1950s by James Olds and his associates, who discovered that the rats continuously pressed a lever controlling an electrode implanted in this area, presumably because this behavior induced pleasure.[46] More recent studies have shown that nucleus accumbens becomes active when subjects are shown pictures of sexually desirable individuals, when they listen to music, when they expect a monetary gain, and when a mother is in the presence of her offspring.[47]

Nucleus accumbens receives dopamine projections from the VTA. This means that when a certain stimulus or behavior is tagged as adaptive and desirable, the nucleus accumbens is activated by the dopamine-mediated signal sent from the VTA. But whereas in the usual scheme of things this signal reflects a cognitive or affective appraisal coming from the prefrontal cortex or the amygdala, in Parkinson's disease, this appraisal is mimicked by the medication effect. Overstimulation of the projections from VTA to nucleus accumbens and other brain regions (the so-called mesolimbic dopamine pathway) has also been implicated in cocaine addiction and other forms of substance abuse. Presumably, such overstimulation—whether it is a result of cocaine use or Parkinson's medication side effect—results in long-term alterations of this pathway, possibly even through altered gene expression.[48]

This, in turn, predisposes the individual toward addictive behaviors. The pathway that normally serves the admirable function of signaling adaptive salience has now been hijacked and put in the service of self-defeating and self-destructive cravings. And the story may not end there. Because the mesolimbic dopamine pathway is so critical for salience determination in virtually every context, its alteration may result in altered salience judgment in affected individuals above and beyond their susceptibility to addictions, changing their cognitive makeup in profound and far-reaching ways and affecting virtually every aspect of their mental life. These broader implications of the salience machinery hijacked in addiction have yet to receive their full attention by neuroscientists.

As mentioned earlier, addiction in Parkinson's patients (and addiction in general) is often attributed to poor impulse control.[49] The common-sense reason for this assertion is obvious: sound impulse control would have protected an individual from engaging in maladaptive behavior. Indeed, impaired impulse control most likely does play a role in addictive behavior, but the underlying mechanisms are probably more complex. It can even be argued that the emphasis on impulse control in understanding the mechanisms of addiction tacitly reinforces an essentially moralistic interpretation sneaked into the narrative through the back door. It is like saying that sound impulse control would have prevented a patient with Tourette's syndrome from engaging in tics, or would have prevented a stutterer from stuttering.

In reality, understanding addiction merely as a deficit of impulse control probably captures only half of the story. Addiction is also a form of perseveration, extreme loss of mental flexibility, and propensity toward stereotypical behavior, which interacts with poor impulse control. This point is brought home by the fact that addiction in Parkinson's patients often goes hand in hand with punding—a form of perseverative stereotypical behavior described earlier. I believe that any addiction must be understood as a combination of perseveration and poor impulse control.

The link between addiction and perseveration is not limited to Parkinson's disease; "prolonged, purposeless and stereotyped behavior," has also been described in chronic amphetamine users. A similar relationship between addiction and perseveration was demonstrated in a study of cognitive styles in heroin addicts.[50] The propensity toward mental rigidity and perseveration in addicts may take various forms not limited to punding; it seems to be a common motif across different types of addiction in different parts of the world. A former student of mine, Eric Lane, who has had extensive experience with treating recovering alcoholics in the United States, shared an interesting observation: his clients tended to always order the same food in a restaurant and were reluctant to try anything new—a form of perseveration, albeit a benign one. And colleagues from the Philippines shared an observation that pathologically repetitive perseverative behaviors are common among amphetamine abusers in their country. Furthermore, such behaviors are present in other forms of addiction as well. This is how Luz Casimiro-Querubin, professor of psychiatry and former president of the Philippine Psychiatric Association, described them in a personal communication to me:

The phenomenon of perseveration is something I personally observed in gambling addiction and alcohol addiction. The behavior is almost ritualistic, bordering on superstitious in some. Perseveration is also evident in the process of recovery, when patients tend to repeat irrational behavior patterns with an underlying belief that doing so helps them "avoid" the substance that they are addicted to.

It is the combination of impulsivity and perseveration driving the maladaptive behavior of an addict that makes it so difficult to overcome. This is not that different from the behavior of a patient with bilateral frontal-lobe damage in whom perseveration and field-dependent behavior are intertwined in odd collages. Perseveration is usually a product of left frontal damage, and field-dependent behavior a product of right frontal damage.[51] Likewise, the cognitive style of patients with the right hemi-Parkinsonian syndrome (left nigro-striatal dysfunction) gravitates toward perseveration, and the cognitive style of patients with the left hemi-Parkinsonian syndrome (right nigro-striatal dysfunction) gravitates toward field-dependency (more about it in Chapter 6).[52] From this it would follow that the PD patients with significant nigro-striatal dysfunction on both sides, and thus with the propensity toward both field-dependency and perseveration, are particularly prone to developing addictions once the salience circuit has been hijacked.

On a broader note, frontal-lobe and striatal dysfunction is commonly implicated in so many forms of addiction that it appears to be a cardinal feature of the disorder; and so is the combination of perseveration and impulsive field-dependent behavior. Based on the foregoing discussion, a common link most likely exists between the neuroanatomical and cognitive features across multiple forms of addiction and not just in PD: perseveration is caused by the left fronto-striatal dysfunction and field-dependent behavior along with impulsivity by the right fronto-striatal dysfunction. Indeed, the neuroimaging studies of addiction show that the prefrontal dysfunction is often bilateral.[53] This further suggests that both perseveration and poor impulse control play a role, which is precisely what the work by Antonio Verdejo-Garcia and his colleagues has shown.[54] Before impulse control comes (or fails to come) into play, an urge must develop in need of being controlled and contained. Understanding the irresistible urge at the center of any addictive behavior as a form of perseveration, and introducing perseveration into the narrative about the mechanisms of addiction, is more than a semantic flourish. It expands our understanding of the mechanisms of addiction and has important implications, both for elucidating the critical neural circuits involved and for developing effective treatment approaches. And the recognition of the lateralized mechanisms of fronto-striatal dysfunction leading to perseveration and field-dependent behavior may help us better understand the neurobiology of different forms of addiction, as well as their natural history—the changes that accompany addiction over time.

6

The Innovating Brain

The Novelty Challenge

A great city stands firm despite a draining siege, its walls impenetrable, and its defenders unbowed. Meanwhile, the attacking army is in disarray. Achilles is dead, Agamemnon is despised by his own troops; the Greeks, dispirited and mutinous, are ready to give up. A cunning ruse is then devised, a huge hollow horse built and placed conspicuously in front of the city gate while the besieging Greeks pretend to have lifted the siege and departed. The city inhabitants, thinking the horse to be a worthy trophy, carry it inside. Then, in the dark of night, the few élite Greek soldiers hidden inside the horse creep out and open the city gate. The besieging army pours in, and a savage orgy of destruction begins. The unsuspecting city is sacked and burned, its inhabitants put to the sword. . . . I think I hear Homer and Virgil turning in their graves . . . I had better stop. . . .

After ten years of siege, Troy was brought down, not by Agamemnon's military leadership, nor by Achilles' marshal prowess, but by Odysseus' ingenious invention, even though we cannot be sure whether the innovation in question was a military one by a real-life crafty king of Mycenaean-period Ithaca, or a literary one by a Greek poet spinning his epic centuries later. When we talk about innovation and creativity, we usually invoke great scientists and artists of modernity or of relatively recent history, but this is a very narrow perspective. Innovation has propelled human civilization since its very dawn in its every manifestation and continues to do so to this day.

Creativity continues to fascinate both scientists and the general public, and the notion that the right hemisphere is "the seat of creativity" has been around for some time. Yet, on closer examination, it turns out to be a product of popular lore more than of rigorous research. In its origin, this notion is probably an offshoot of an equally loose (and factually incorrect) popular notion that the right hemisphere is the "emotional" hemisphere, as opposed to the "coldly rational" left hemisphere (in fact, both hemispheres are involved in emotional control). As we already concluded earlier, creativity is a very complex process ultimately involving the whole brain, as well as its interaction with culture, and linking it to any single brain structure is an oversimplification that flies in the face of serious science. This, by the way, is true for any complex mental process, so whenever we link a complex cognitive process to a particular brain structure—a hemisphere, a lobe, or a nucleus—we really mean that that brain structure plays a *particularly important* role in the cognitive process in question, which is not the same as to say that it is the *only* structure involved in that process. This is an important caveat for the reader of this book—or of any book about the brain—to keep in mind. Whenever a statement is made that "cognitive process X depends on brain structure Y," it is important to realize that this is merely shorthand for a more nuanced statement. It is for this reason that I tend to take claims made in scientific literature linking very specific functions to very specific brain regions with a grain of salt and tend not to make such statements in my own work. Because of its complexity, creativity is best approached by identifying its more tractable components and trying to understand them first.

Understanding how the brain deals with novelty will take us a long way toward understanding the brain mechanisms of creativity. Clearly, creativity cannot be reduced to novelty-seeking alone, but no creative process can exist without it. The ability to deal with novel challenges is an essential component of a creative mind, and it refers to a more fundamental and more universal cognitive asset. This makes it an attractive and tractable target of scientific investigation and a promising stepping stone toward understanding creativity. Novelty is something we encounter in things small and big, including the tale of two empires.

In 334 BC, an audacious youth by the name of Alexander, aged 22, crossed the straits known then as the Hellespont and today as the Dardanelles, and invaded the Persian Empire, in those days the preeminent power of the Mediterranean world. In the Battle of Gaugamela, Alexander and his troops found themselves facing Indian war elephants. This had to be an utterly novel experience for the Macedonian troops; nothing in their prior experience in Greece prepared them for this kind of adversary. Yet Alexander was not stymied by a novel challenge, found a way of mastering it, and the decisive battle was won. King Darius fled, only to be murdered by his own satraps; and a few years later the conquest of the Persian Empire was completed. Alexander created the largest and most diverse empire of his time and an unprecedented cultural fusion of East and West followed, which left an indelible mark on the subsequent course of history both in Europe and in Asia. In the process, he did not hesitate to scandalize his parochially minded Macedonian followers time and again with his embrace of new and different cultures and with his vision of cultural fusion. All this was geopolitical innovation on the grandest of scales, which is why Alexander of Macedon is also known as Alexander the Great. He is remembered as one of the most innovative military commanders in history, whose battles are studied in military academies throughout the world to this day; and also as one of the most visionary state builders of all times.

In contrast, the Aztecs did not fare well when confronted with a military novelty from the animal kingdom. Horses, unknown at the time in Mesoamerica, played a decisive role in the conquest of Mexico by Hernan Cortes. Throughout numerous battles, the vastly outnumbered Spaniards were able to prevail largely because of their cavalry; faced with this novel challenge, the Aztec warriors panicked and were unable to forge an effective strategy to oppose it. As a result, the Aztec Empire, up to that point the dominant power in Mesoamerica, crumbled; its emperor, Montezuma, was captured by the Spaniards; and its capital, Tenochtitlan, was renamed Mexico City, which it remains to this day.

The tale of the life and death of two empires shows clearly that the ability to cope with novelty matters. It may lead to a glorious victory when it is effective and to a crushing defeat when it is not. So it is time to find out how novelty is handled in the brain.

Hemispheres Misunderstood

A very direct link exists between the ability to tackle novel situations and the right hemisphere, and it is precisely through its affinity for novelty that the right hemisphere contributes to the creative process. This is not to say, however, that creativity resides in the right hemisphere, tempting as it may be to disregard nuance for the sake of a catchy soundbite.

The ideas about the division of labor between cerebral hemispheres evolved over time. Early observations linking damage of the left hemisphere to language impairment date back to antiquity, but the first such well-documented observations were made in the nineteenth century. These observations by the French neurologist Broca and German neurologist Wernicke are often regarded as the beginning of modern neuropsychology, and they helped confirm the link between the left hemisphere and language.

In contrast, the right hemisphere has been linked to the visual and spatial ("visuo-spatial") processes. Because of the paramount role of language in human cognition, the left hemisphere has often been referred to as the "dominant hemisphere," and the right hemisphere maligned as the "subdominant" hemisphere, often with the implications that it was more dispensable. As we will find out in this chapter, the right hemisphere is far from dispensable and is in charge of particularly heavy neural lifting.

The distinction between the "language" left hemisphere and the "visuo-spatial" right hemisphere remains the prevailing view of the division of labor between the two hemispheres to this day, despite numerous reasons to believe that, while not incorrect, this distinction is certainly incomplete. First, there are plenty of exceptions to this rule. Certain aspects of language are equally represented in the two hemispheres, and some, like prosody (inflections used to emphasize meaning), are even better represented in the right than the left hemisphere. Likewise, certain visual and spatial processes (like the ability to recognize visual images of meaningful objects) are better represented in the left hemisphere. We discussed some of these findings in Chapter 3.

Even more to the point, there appears to be a deep conceptual flaw in the prevailing understanding of hemispheric specialization. If the link of language to the left hemisphere is the cardinal feature of hemispheric specialization, then hemispheric specialization has to be unique to humans, since only humans have language, at least in its rigorous definition. This point of view may flatter the collective narcissism of our self-indulgent species, but it flies in the face of basic biology; and in fact it may reflect the insularity of psychology from natural sciences, which was pervasive until relatively recently.

Remember: the division of the brain into two hemispheres is not unique to humans; is a ubiquitous feature of all mammalian and even non-mammalian species inhabiting the earth. This alone suggests that there should be certain functional differences between the hemispheres that are universal across species. One might counter this concern by assuming that only human cerebral hemispheres are biologically asymmetrical, whereas the hemispheres of other species are mirror images of each other; but this was proved to be an incorrect assumption. A number of morphological, cellular, and biochemical differences between the two hemispheres have been discovered, some of them exhibiting strong similarities across several mammalian species, including our own.[1] We already came upon one of them, the asymmetry of dopamine pathways which we share with several mammalian species, and we will encounter others later in the book.

But if cerebral hemispheres are structurally and biochemically asymmetrical in many species, and furthermore, if the nature of these asymmetries is similar across those species, including the humans, then it is only logical to assume that the functional differences between the two hemispheres also exist in many species and that the nature of these differences is similar across species. This in turn means that the nature of such differences cannot be fully captured by a distinction between language and nonverbal functions, because the rats and monkeys in question do not have language!

These questions began to bug me many years ago, when I was still a student at Moscow State University in the early 1970s, and I felt that an entirely new approach to hemispheric specialization was needed, one premised on the assumption of evolutionary continuity, which would be meaningful across species. I came up with the idea that the fundamental difference between the functions of the two hemispheres is based on the distinction between cognitive novelty and cognitive familiarity. The left hemisphere excels in processing information by applying well-formed cognitive patterns and strategies. In contrast, the right hemisphere steps in when the organism encounters a truly novel situation to which none of the previously formed patterns, strategies, or ready solutions can be successfully applied.

The Novel and the Routine

Over the years, I began to refer to this idea as the "novelty-routinization" theory of hemispheric specialization. Unlike the more traditional approaches, the novelty-routinization theory is meaningful across all the species capable of learning and provides a framework for studying hemispheric differences across species. Without negating the left hemisphere's dominance for language in humans, one can view it as a special case of a more fundamental relationship between the left hemisphere and cognitive routines. And unlike the concept of "creativity," the concept of "novelty" can be operationalized in a relatively straightforward and unambiguous manner.

Creativity in humans is studied by asking subjects to solve puzzles requiring "out of the box" solutions. But what is or is not "out of the box" is a matter of opinion and of subjective judgment. In contrast, novelty can be more easily defined empirically for any given individual by surveying his or her prior experience. The use of the ability to deal with novelty as a proxy measure of creativity also provides the basis for animal models, which adds a broad evolutionary perspective to creativity research. One may be hard pressed to figure out what "creativity" is in a rat or a monkey, but it is much easier to design a novel task for these creatures based on our knowledge of their ecological environment and typical experience. In fact, a growing body of research exists studying the ways various animals deal with novelty, and this research informs us about the evolutionary roots of creativity. We will review it later in the book, in Chapter 8.

How much evidence is there to support (or refute) the "novelty-routinization" theory? This question was posed to me by Louis Costa a few years later when I settled in New York. Lou was an important influence in my life when I came to the United States as a Soviet émigré at the age of 27, and we became close friends. Lou was older, already an established neuropsychologist, a departmental chair and later dean at a major university, and by temperament more cautious and methodical than I. When I first shared my novelty-routinization idea with him, he was skeptical; it was too radical a departure from the prevailing understanding of hemispheric specialization. But instead of dismissing it out of hand, Lou helped me outline the kind of evidence that was needed to test the hypothesis and perhaps design the appropriate experiments. As is common in science, we, with the help of my then–research assistant Bob ("Chip") Bilder, now a professor at UCLA, conducted extensive literature reviews before embarking on our own experiments, and it turned out that much of the data we were looking for was already out there in bits and pieces awaiting someone to integrate them into a coherent point of view.

Together Lou and I wrote a paper, which was probably the first scientific publication articulating the novelty-routinization idea, with a cumbersome title "Hemisphere Differences in the Acquisition and Use of Descriptive Systems."[2] Whenever I come across this very old paper, I hear my Russian accent come through in an occasional awkward turn of phrase. But "old" does not always mean "wrong" or "outdated" (think of the multiplication table!) and much of my subsequent research, including more recent work, has been based on this idea—developing it further with modern neuroimaging methods and applying it to our understanding of several neurological disorders.

The novelty-routinization idea leads to several predictions, which is precisely what makes it testable through rigorous research. Let's make these predictions:

- A complex, specialized skill that takes a long time to acquire will rely mostly on the right hemisphere in a novice and on the left hemisphere in a professional.
- A highly practiced skill will rely mostly on the left hemisphere, while a comparable but less practiced skill will rely mostly on the right hemisphere in the same people.
- A cognitive task will be controlled mostly by the right hemisphere while it is new and unpracticed, but it will fall under the predominant control by the left hemisphere with increased familiarity and practice in the same individual.

Indeed, this is what happens. In a study that has since become classic, Bever and Chiarello at Columbia University presented musical recordings to the left or right ears of their subjects in order to find out which hemisphere was better at processing music (this was possible because of the sensory, in this case auditory, pathway-crossing in the brain: information from the left ear travels mostly to the right hemisphere, and vice versa). It had been assumed for years that music is processed in the right hemisphere in all right-handed individuals. The findings by Bever and Chiarello were more nuanced, however: indeed, the right hemisphere excelled in processing music in most people, but the opposite was true for trained musicians. In trained musicians, the left hemisphere excelled.[3]

Bever and Chiarello compared performance on the same task in competent (trained musicians) and naïve (the rest of humanity) subjects. Marzi and Berlucci made the same point by comparing performance in the same subjects on comparable tasks, but in this case, one novel and the other one familiar. To this end, they projected two sets of facial images to the left or the right hemispheres (this, too, was possible due to crossing of the visual pathways in the brain). The first set consisted of unfamiliar faces (like a random assemblage of strangers you meet on the street). The second set consisted of the faces of famous individuals who have been staring at you from magazine covers and newspaper pages for years. A striking dissociation emerged: the novel faces were processed more accurately by the right hemisphere, and the famous faces by the left hemisphere. This finding, too, challenged the entrenched old-school notion, that faces are better recognized by the right than the left hemisphere. Like the music experiment by Bever and Chiarello, it suggested that, contrary to the old-school notions linking certain cognitive functions in inviolate ways to one or the other hemisphere, what matters is the degree of familiarity and task mastery. When a task is novel, it is supported mostly by the right hemisphere, but the left hemisphere takes over as the task is being mastered and becomes increasingly familiar.[4]

These experiments suggest the changing hemispheric roles in the acquisition of a cognitive skill gradually extended over a long time: the right hemisphere plays the leading role at early stages, and the left hemisphere at late stages. Indeed, it takes years for a person to become a musician, and it usually takes years for an individual to acquire a celebrity status, for his or her face to become "famous." But the advances in functional neuroimaging allow us to make and test yet a different type of prediction:

• It is possible to see a right-to-left shift in the pattern of cortical activation in real time within a matter of hours or even minutes, by imaging the subject's brain while he or she is performing a novel cognitive task that becomes familiar in the course of the experiment.

Functional neuroimaging has changed the face of cognitive neuroscience over the last few decades, and with the constant improvement of neuroimaging methods and techniques, this change is ongoing. Several such techniques exist, giving us a window into the human brain in action. Among these methods, functional magnetic resonance imaging (fMRI) has become particularly popular, but other techniques exist, such as positron emission tomography (PET) and optical neuroimaging. Using different physical principles and measuring different biological variables (oxygenated blood levels in fMRI, glucose metabolism levels in PET, and near-infrared light in optical neuroimaging) these techniques make it possible to examine the patterns of brain activation in a subject performing a cognitive task while in the scanner. The approach is called "cognitive activation" functional neuroimaging (as opposed to "resting state" functional neuroimaging, more about which later in the book).

Suppose now that the cognitive task starts out as novel and the subject is basically clueless, but in the course of the experiment, the task becomes increasingly familiar and the subject gradually masters the task. The whole experiment may take 20–30 minutes. In fact, many such experiments have been conducted using fMRI and PET. The cognitive tasks employed in these experiments are all different—both verbal and nonverbal, both perceptual and motor—but most of them reveal a similar pattern of change: as the task novelty decreases and subjects learn the task, the activity in the right hemisphere decreases and the activity in the left hemisphere increases, at least in a relative sense.

This was demonstrated with great elegance in a study by Alex Martin and colleagues at the National Institute of Mental Health (NIMH) using PET. Subjects (all neurologically healthy individuals) were asked to attend to the pictures of real objects, pictures of nonsense objects; to silently read real words, nonsense words; and to stare at meaningless visual "noise" (similar to static on a TV screen). Quite reasonably, the authors assumed that whatever the subjects' prior experiences may have been, performing cognitive tasks lying supine in a scanner was not one of them. This meant that the task was novel in the beginning of each of the five experiments but became at least somewhat familiar in the course of the experiment. What was the effect of such familiarization on the brain? To answer this question, for each of the five conditions, PET scans were performed twice, in the beginning and the end of the experiment. And guess what—regardless of the nature of the stimuli, the activation was greater in the right temporoparietal cortex and the mesial temporal lobe in the first scan (when the task was novel) compared to the second scan (when the task was more familiar).[5]

An experiment by my former student Vasilisa Skvortsova made the point with the subjects performing the Wisconsin Card Sorting Task (WCST) while in the MRI scanner (Figure 6.1). WCST is one of the most popular neuropsychological tests used in cognitive neuroscience research to study the healthy brain, and in clinical neuropsychological practice to help diagnose various brain disorders. The subject is shown a number of cards with geometrical designs and must figure out the hidden classification principle. The experiment starts as a guessing game: the subject receives a "right" or "wrong" response to every guess and is supposed to infer the hidden principle based on these responses. But the task contains a trick: the classification principle changes in midstream, and this change happens five times in the course of the experiment, thus requiring the "discovery" of six classification principles. The subject is not forewarned about the changes and

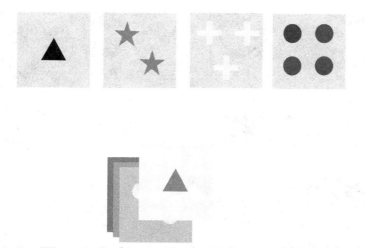

FIGURE 6.1 Wisconsin Card Sorting Test (WCST). Every new card is placed under one of the four cards on top, based on the similarity by color, shape, or number of items.

must switch from the old to the new classification principle as rapidly as possible once the change has taken place. The ease with which the subject is able to catch on is supposed to reflect the degree of his or her mental flexibility.[6] In order to do well on WCST, the subject must accomplish two things: (1) arrive at a general realization that the classification principle changes in the course of the experiment, and (2) discover each of the six specific classification principles.

Vasilisa's experiment was designed to discern the brain mechanisms of dealing with cognitive novelty; therefore, she compared the activation levels in different parts of the brain at different stages of learning the task. To that end, she conducted two kinds of comparisons. To capture the change in the neural activation pattern accompanying the discovery of the general principle, she compared the average activation levels for the first three and the last three segments of the task. And to capture the change in the neural activity accompanying the discovery of specific categories, she compared the average activation patterns for the first and second halves of each of the six segments of the task.

The results of this analysis confirmed that the right hemisphere is particularly active at the early stages of discovering both general and specific rules of the WCST, as predicted by the novelty-routinization hypothesis. More specifically, the right prefrontal regions are active at the early stages of both types of "discovery," bringing the frontal lobes into our story again (Figure 6.2).

The findings are consonant with those reported in a number of published fMRI studies. According to Corbetta and Schulman, the right ventrolateral prefrontal cortex is critical for switching and redirecting attention toward a novel

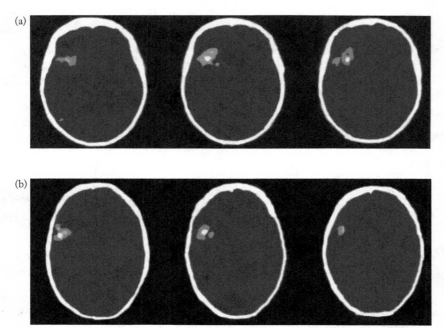

FIGURE 6.2 Functional magnetic resonance imaging (fMRI) of Wisconsin Card Sorting Test (WCST) performance. (a) Area more active during the first three categories than during the last three categories. (b) Area more active during the first than the second half of each category.

target. In contrast, the left ventrolateral prefrontal cortex is critical for retrieval of previously consolidated information from long-term memory, in keeping with the idea developed in Chapter 3, linking the left hemisphere to the conservation of previously acquired information.[7] Consistent with these findings, the "attention networks," which are presumably directed toward the external world, are better articulated and more specialized in the right hemisphere.[8]

Sridharan Devarajan and coauthors conducted a complex analysis of co-activation patterns of multiple brain regions as the subjects listened to classical music. Any "movement transition" (transition between distinct sections of a symphony or a concerto) was associated with right fronto-insular activation followed by right posterior parietal activation.[9] Trevor Chong and colleagues found particularly strong activation in the right inferoparietal cortical regions when the subjects observed a novel action, but an attenuated activity in response to previously observed actions.[10]

Nancy Kanwisher and colleagues studied the activation patterns in the visual cortex as the subjects learned to discriminate between the exemplars of novel object categories. Indeed, learning was accompanied by the changes in the activation patterns, which varied significantly across different regions of the right versus left hemispheres.[11] In a similar vein, training on complex arithmetic multiplication problems results in the shift of the activation patterns toward the left hemisphere, particularly the left parietal regions.[12]

As we already discussed in Chapter 4, the thrust of functional neuroimaging research, particularly one employing fMRI, has shifted from isolated brain regions to networks and their interactions. Several such studies have shown that an abrupt, precipitous change in the midst of a cognitive task triggers activation in a network of regions in the frontal and parietal cortex, and this activation is lateralized to the right hemisphere. The specific nature of change does not seem to matter, as long as a precipitous change of any kind takes place. In one such experiment, change took the form of "musical movement" transition (transition from one distinct segment of a complex composition to another). In another experiment, the "oddball" paradigm was employed, when a sequence of visual stimuli is punctuated by a distinct "oddball" stimulus infrequently and unpredictably. It appears that any abrupt change in the environment activates a network of regions in the right hemisphere.[13]

The take-home message from these studies is both simple and profound: the neural mechanisms of cognitive processes are not static, they cannot be understood simply as fixed networks of regions. Instead, the networks are constantly modified by experience, and the relative roles of the two hemispheres change in the course of learning.

Unfortunately, it is not particularly common in functional neuroimaging research to do what Vasilisa did in her experiment: to examine performance characteristics at different stages of a cognitive activation task separately and to compare them. It is much more common to average across the whole sequence, combining the data points acquired in the beginning, middle, and end of the experimental sequence. This would be a reasonable approach if one could safely assume that the neural machinery underlying task performance remained unchanged throughout the process of task mastery. But as we saw earlier, this assumption is often flawed, since as the subject learns the task, the underlying brain machinery changes.

Scientists are often eager to combine as many data points from an experiment as possible in order to enhance the power of their analysis, but this can only be done if all the data points come from the same "population" of data points. If they don't, then the results of the analysis are meaningless, even if they look plausible on the surface. Suppose Johnny weighed 50 pounds when he was a little boy. Because he was so fond of his beer and hamburgers, his weight shot up to 300 pounds by the age of 40. But now that he is an old man, Johnny has shriveled down to 100 pounds. So you add up 50, 300, and 100, divide it by three, and conclude that Johnny's weight is 150 pounds. Plausible on the surface, but utterly meaningless and misleading! In contrast, documenting *changes* of brain activation patterns over time in the course of learning a new cognitive task may tell us a lot about normal and abnormal cognition, including the individual differences in novelty seeking and perhaps even in creativity. You learn much more about Johnny by examining the trends in his weight changes over time than by averaging Johnny's weights across different points in his life.

Failure to consider novelty as a critical variable in cognition has been a persistent source of confusion and data misinterpretation. When performance on typical neuropsychological "verbal" and "visuo-spatial" tasks is compared, the fact is usually ignored that the "visuo-spatial" tasks are likely to be inherently more novel than the "verbal" ones, because the latter are composed of familiar elements, words. And any task involving "salient" stimulus detection is also a task of novelty detection if the stimulus is infrequent (as in the commonly used "oddball" paradigm). We will learn more about the neural machinery of learning in healthy people and the ways it may become impaired in various brain disorders by examining how patterns of brain activation change over time across multiple cognitive tasks as they cease being novel and become familiar.

How about evidence from other branches of neuroscience? Convergent evidence—evidence derived from multiple diverse sources—is particularly important in testing a scientific hypothesis. Does such evidence exist for the novelty-routinization hypothesis in addition to the cognitive studies described here? It does, and it comes in two varieties: biochemical and computational.

Earlier we discussed the neurotransmitter dopamine. It is time to introduce another neurotransmitter, norepinephrine (or NE). If dopamine is involved in the machinery of salience, then norepinephrine appears to be involved in novelty seeking. It has been shown that by stimulating the NE system in animal models, you enhance the animal's exploratory behavior.[14] Consistent with this, novelty seeking is associated with noradrenergic transmission in humans as well.[15] And guess what—norepinephrine pathways are more abundant in the right than in the left hemisphere.[16] This converges with the activation neuroimaging evidence linking the right hemisphere to cognitive novelty. In contrast, you will recall that dopamine pathways are more abundant in the left hemisphere, and by stimulating them you enhance the animal's stereotypical, highly practiced behavior.

Another source of convergent evidence comes from computational neuroscience—a rapidly developing field using mathematical models and computer simulations to understand the brain. One of the daunting challenges encountered in such brain models is how to reconcile two essential properties of the brain without which no cognition is possible: the ability to acquire new information, and the ability to preserve previously acquired "old" information.

When these two kinds of processes inhabit the same neural real estate, they seem to compete and trip over each other. As a result, the acquisition of new information is often associated with the erosion of previously formed representations. One way of combining these seemingly irreconcilable processes in the same brain model without having them clash is by separating them in the model, a solution proposed by several computational neuroscientists.[17] It may be that the evolution has solved this design conundrum by doing precisely that: by differentially investing the right hemisphere with a particular propensity toward processing novel information and the left hemisphere toward preserving "old" information.

A growing body of evidence exists that hemispheric specialization allocating cognitive routines to the left hemisphere and cognitive novelty to the right hemisphere is not unique to humans. Quite the contrary, it has been documented in a wide range of species and seems to be a universal principle of brain organization across evolution. These and related findings are so intriguing—and so deflating to the notion of the human species' exclusivity—that a whole chapter (Chapter 8) is devoted to them later in the book.

Wired for Novelty

What is it in the structure of the right hemisphere that makes it especially adept at processing novel information? Certain parts of the neocortex (the youngest in evolutionary terms and the most advanced type of cortex) are critical for particularly complex cognitive processes. They are the lateral prefrontal cortex (which is often divided into dorsolateral and ventrolateral) and inferoparietal heteromodal association cortex (Figure 6.3).

These two areas work in intimate concert, and together they serve as the brain machinery tackling the most complex problems arising from the outside world. They are connected through direct pathways enabling continuous rapid communication between them. The lateral prefrontal and inferoparietal regions are known to be activated together, and they form the so-called central executive network. Remember, we talked about it briefly in Chapter 4, and it is depicted in Figure 4.3.

The two hemispheres contain the same types of cortex, but subtle differences exist in their relative sizes. Several studies, including our own, have shown that both the lateral prefrontal regions and the inferoparietal regions are significantly larger in the right than in the left hemisphere (Figure 6.4). In addition to being larger, these regions are also more robustly interconnected, and thus are better able to work in concert in the right than in the left hemisphere. The connectivity between the frontal lobes and the cortical regions located toward the back of the head ("posterior cortex") relies to a large extent on von Economo cells, also

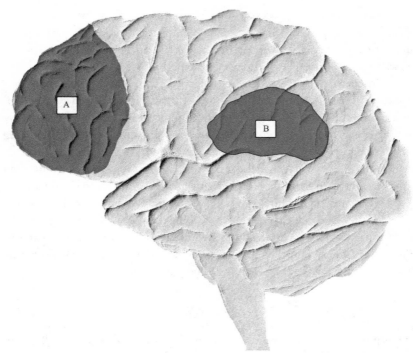

FIGURE 6.3 Lateral prefrontal and inferoparietal heteromodal association cortex. Lateral prefrontal (A) and inferoparietal (B) regions.

known as "spindle cells." These cells originate in various parts of the prefrontal cortex, both orbital and lateral; in the anterior cingulate; and in the frontoinsular regions, and they send very long projections to the posterior cortex. Spindle cells arose late in evolution and are found only in a few species known for their high intelligence, large brains, and highly developed social behaviors: in the great apes, in certain dolphin species, and in elephants. But of all the species, they are particularly abundant in humans. It is commonly assumed that spindle cells play an especially important role in complex cognition, including social cognition. It has been shown that spindle cells are more abundant in the right than in the left hemisphere.[18] Since the spindle cells are uniquely equipped to provide very rapid communication between distant cortical regions, their relative abundance in the right hemisphere makes it particularly well equipped to deal with the unforeseen, unexpectedly arising challenges.[19]

So it appears that both the cortical regions and the cortical pathways implicated in particularly complex cognition are more abundant in the right hemisphere. Far from being "subdominant," the right hemisphere is especially well equipped for dealing with daunting cognitive challenges, which novel situations

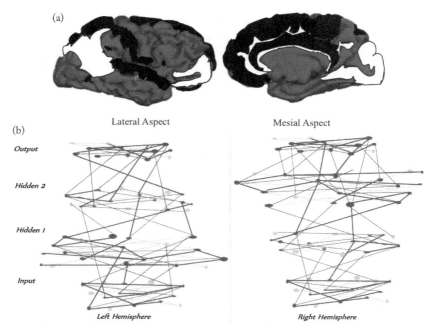

FIGURE 6.4 **Regional hemispheric differences.** (a) Regions larger in the left hemisphere in black. Regions larger in the right hemisphere in white. Lateral prefrontal and inferoparietal heteromodal association cortex is larger in the right hemisphere.

Adapted with permission from E. Goldberg et al., "Hemispheric Asymmetries of Cortical Volume in the Human Brain," *Cortex* 49 [2013]: 200–210.

(b) Schematic representation of the cortical space allocation in the two hemispheres. Heteromodal cortex is schematically represented as Hidden Layer 2.

Reprinted with permission from E. Goldberg, *The New Executive Brain*, Oxford University Press, 2009.

by definition are. The right hemisphere is uniquely adept at dealing with novel situations, which are unlike any prior situations encountered by the organism, and for which no ready-to-use solutions are available in the organism's cognitive repertoire.

Certain clinical disorders exist, characterized by cognitive rigidity and aversion to novelty. Nonverbal learning disability is one such condition. The late Byron Rourke, one of the most influential developmental neuropsychologists in North America, proposed that right-hemispheric dysfunction is particularly common in this condition. Some of Byron's work on nonverbal learning disabilities was influenced by our novelty-routinization theory, a fact that he generously acknowledged in his now-classic book *Nonverbal Learning Disabilities: The Syndrome and the Model.* The dedication in the book goes as follows:

In the late 1940's and early 1950's Ralph M. Reitan launched a research program that revolutionized the manner in which the scientific and clinical aspects of human neuropsychology were to transpire for the next 40 years. In 1975, Helmer R. Myklebust published a chapter, entitled "Nonverbal Learning Disabilities," that has had a profound effect on the direction of our research program. In 1981, Elkhonon Goldberg and Louis Costa published a landmark theoretical paper that has formed the basis of my theoretical and model-building activities since that time. Without the seminal works of these scientists, the present work would not have seen the light of day. For these and other reasons too numerous to mention, this book is, with affection, dedicated to the four of them—whether they like it or not.[20]

Extreme mental rigidity, obsession with routines, and intolerance of novelty are also hallmarks of Asperger's syndrome, a diagnostic category that strongly overlaps, and some researchers believe is virtually identical, with nonverbal learning disabilities.

When my then–postdoctoral fellow Allan Kluger and I compared cognitive impairment caused by diffuse brain damage equally affecting the two hemispheres with the cognitive impairment caused by lateralized brain damage affecting either the left or the right hemisphere alone, striking similarities were noted between the effects of diffuse and right-hemispheric damage.[21] Why would diffuse brain damage, where from a structural standpoint both hemispheres are equally affected, disrupt the function of the right hemisphere more than the dysfunction of the left hemisphere? Most likely, it is because of the right hemisphere's link to cognitive novelty. As each of us undoubtedly discovers through everyday experience, any source of general disruption—be it illness, inebriation, or lack of sleep—will affect novel tasks more than the overlearned tasks.

Changes in the brain occurring throughout the lifespan are also revealing. The right hemisphere matures faster, and is more active, than the left hemisphere at early developmental stages in children. In an elegant study using SPECT (single photon emission computerized tomography), a group of French scientists led by Catherine Chiron demonstrated a greater activity in the right than left hemispheres in children ages one to three years old, but this asymmetry was found to be reversed after the age of three.[22] This may very well be related to the fact that the ability to process novel information is particularly important in childhood when the world has yet to be discovered. But the right hemisphere succumbs earlier than the left hemisphere to the effects of age-related atrophy as we grow old.[23] This may well be a reflection of the fact that, barring some drastic discontinuities, life falls into increasingly familiar routines as we age, and exposure to novel challenges decreases, thus depriving the right hemisphere of the neuroprotective effects of activity-driven neuroplasticity. At least, this is how it has been so far. Whether it will remain to be the case in the brave new world of ever more rapid informational and technological societal changes, and what implications such changes may have for brain aging, is an intriguing question, which will be addressed in some detail in Chapter 11.

To summarize, all the observations reviewed in this chapter point in the same direction. They highlight a particular role of the right hemisphere in dealing with novel cognitive challenges.

Driven by Novelty

According to some sources, Alexander the Great was left-handed. This, of course, has to remain a matter of conjecture, and it has been challenged; but if indeed it was true, then he was one of the more fortunate ones. Left-handedness, a condition characterized by right-hemispheric dominance at least in a motor sense (albeit not usually in the sense of language dominance), and shared by about 10% of the population, was regarded as somehow inferior and even evil in most traditional societies. This prejudice is codified in many languages. *Right* means both spatial orientation and value judgment (*correct* or *true*) in English. The same relationship between *rechts* and *richtig* exists in German; and between *pravij* and *pravda* in my native Russian, the implication being that *left* is somehow *incorrect* or *false* (this implication is made explicit in the Russian street slang, where *left* means *shady* or *underhanded*). In Latin this assumption is made explicit: *sinister* (*sinistra* in Italian) means *left*. This is the case also in French, where *gauche* means both *left* and *vulgar* (the latter is true in English as well). In many traditional cultures, left-handedness was "exorcised" and left-handed children were forced to switch handedness. This is exactly what happened to me when I was growing up in the old Soviet Union. And in my clinical practice, I encountered several cases over the years, when the mere question about handedness addressed to an older immigrant from a traditional culture was met with extreme umbrage as a personal insult: "How dare you even think that I could be left-handed!"

Left-handedness has existed in every human society, including the Neanderthal one, and historically it has been repressed in most societies. It often runs in families, which suggests a genetic basis, but its prevalence varies from society to society and in the same society over time, which suggests strong cultural factors as well.[24] The attitude toward left-handedness began to relax only recently and only in societies that became less rigidly driven by tradition and more open to change. In fact, striking differences have been reported between the prevalence of left-handedness in the societies of East and Southeast Asia (very low) and in the Americans of Asian descent in the United States (much higher).[25]

Why were the left-handers stigmatized through most of human history? Was it merely because they were a minority, or was there a less obvious, but perhaps deeper, more profound reason? Of course, in left-handed individuals, the right hemisphere is more "dominant" than the left hemisphere, at least in some sense. In the "practicing" left-handers, for instance, the right hemisphere exists in a relatively more activated state because it is involved in most motor activities (a thought fraught with the deflating possibility that my Russian kindergarten handlers stripped me of any hope for creative potential by "converting" me to right-handedness). And we know by now that the right hemisphere is part of the novelty-seeking machinery of the brain. Anecdotal accounts of an association between left-handedness and creativity, and of a disproportionately high number of left-handers among exceptionally accomplished individuals across various walks of life—science, literature, the arts,—have abounded for years. Nonetheless, rigorous statistics remains elusive, not the least because in most cases it is impossible to calculate the total group memberships, and thus impossible to calculate the ratios of unusually gifted individuals to the total number of individuals both in the right- and left-handed population subsets. Presidents of the United States are a notable exception, since we know exactly what the total membership of this exclusive club is. Indeed, depending on the source, eight or nine out of 44 American presidents (there have been 45 presidencies but 44 presidents, since Grover Cleveland served two non-consecutive terms) were left-handed—twice the proportion of left-handers in the general population. If we accept the common assumption that the rate of left-handedness in the general population is about 10%, then the probabilities of this happening by chance are 0.068 (for eight or more out of 44) or 0.028 (for nine or more out of 44). Among the post–World War II presidents, where more reliable handedness data are available and the likelihood of forced handedness conversion is lower, the ratio is even more intriguing: six out of 13 are left-handed. They are Harry Truman, Gerald Ford, Ronald Reagan, George H. W. Bush, Bill Clinton, and Barack Obama.[26] The probability of six or more individuals out of 13 being left-handed by chance is a miniscule 0.00092, which strongly suggest that factors other than chance played a role. Whatever one's attitude toward party politics is, it would be silly to deny that American presidency is an exceptional feat of personal accomplishment.

To the extent that income is another, and more ubiquitous measure of accomplishment, while in the general population, left-handers earn 10–12% less than the right-handers, among the college-educated people (who are presumably more likely to make a living by their brain than by their brawn) the ratio is reversed, the left-handers earning 10–15% more than their right-handed counterparts.[27] The latter findings are particularly impressive because some of the left-handers in the sample were likely to have been so-called "pathological" (an unkind term not of my creation) rather than "natural" left-handers, in whom hand preference shifted early in life as compensation for the effects of early damage to the naturally "dominant" hemisphere as opposed to having been born left-handed. In "pathological left-handers," some degree of cognitive impairment is likely, diluting the positive relationship between "natural left-handedness" and accomplishment.

Could it be that left-handedness is often associated with a restless dissatisfaction with the status quo, a quest for change, and rebellious novelty-seeking, and that these personality traits were perceived as threatening in stagnant traditional societies? I wonder if, by examining artistic representations of humans in ancient statues, frescos, and ceramic paintings, it may be possible to gauge the prevalence of left-handedness during different historic epochs, and if this prevalence was elevated during the cultural "bursts" described earlier in the book and was lower during the periods of cultural stasis. (For instance, which hand did Alexander use to cut the proverbial Gordian knot; or to hold the javelin with which, in a haze of drunken rage, he killed Cleitus, a valiant officer in his army who had saved his life earlier?) This could be an interesting project on the interface of biology, history, and cultural anthropology, but perhaps difficult to realize.

Meanwhile, my former student Ken Podell and I undertook a much humbler project asking right- and left-handed individuals to make choices in an intentionally ambiguous situation. The options were to either choose an item more similar to the target, unrelated to the target, or more different from the target. All the right-handers chose more similar or unrelated items, but a number of left-handers chose more different items. Contrarian on a modest scale but contrarian nonetheless![28]

Numerous attempts have been made by neuropsychologists to relate left-handedness to certain cognitive traits, but as long as these attempts revolved around the old hackneyed distinction between verbal and nonverbal cognition, they failed. The majority of left-handers are still left-hemisphere-dominant for language. In contrast, the association between left-handedness and novelty seeking is intriguing and it may be real. Am I saying that left-handedness is always associated with novelty seeking? This may be too extreme a claim. But I am proposing something more nuanced: that novelty seeking may be more common and more pronounced among left-handers than in the general population. Later in the book, in Chapter 10, we will encounter the neuroimaging finding that may provide at least a partial explanation for the mechanisms that may underlie these differences.

Is there an evolutionary advantage to having both right-handedness and left-handedness represented in the population, and in a particular ratio at that? Perhaps there is. In order for a society to be stable, a certain continuity and conservatism must be maintained, since too numerous or too frequent perturbations will bring about instability and chaos. On the other hand, progress requires change and disruption of established paradigms and order. Whatever the neural peculiarities associated with handedness are, the approximately 9:1 ratio of right-handers to left-handers in the population may have evolved as maintaining an optimal balance between stabilizing conservation and disruptive innovation in society. And the degree of acceptance of left-handedness may reflect the variation around this average favoring a bias toward change or toward stasis in a particular society at a particular time in history.

Novelty Overdrive

Like most good things, attraction to novelty is good up to a point. But a clinical condition exists when it may go overboard and result in excessive, extreme, uncontrolled exploratory behaviors. Is this condition ADHD? No, but it is often mistaken for ADHD. I believe that an unrecognized form of Tourette's syndrome (often referred to as "Tourette syndrome") exists, which is dominated not by tics but by irresistible attraction to novelty and excessive exploratory behaviors. To recognize it, one must cut across the traditional boundaries dividing clinical neuroscience.

The field of clinical neuroscience has grown by leaps and bounds over the last few decades, and the flip side of this expansion has been its increasing fragmentation, or to borrow a geopolitical term, "balkanization." Different diseases are studied by different clinical "tribes" who attend different conferences, publish in different journals, and draw their salaries from different medical school departments. Cross-talk is limited and often nonexistent. This is very unfortunate for reasons too obvious to belabor here, but it is a fact of life in many clinical environments. This is particularly unfortunate in the neurosciences, because what often determines the nature of a disorder's clinical manifestations is its neuroanatomy more than its etiology. In plain language, this means that, even if the pathophysiological mechanisms of two brain disorders are different, the symptoms may be similar, as long as they affect the same neuroanatomical structures. This also means that a lot can be learned by crossing the boundaries between traditional areas of clinical neuroscience, and a lot can be missed by perpetuating the existing balkanization of the field.

An example of such balkanization in neurosciences is close at hand. If evidence for consistent hemispheric specialization across species abounds, challenging the notion that the distinction between language and nonverbal functions is fundamental to laterality, why has it not made much of a dent in the prevailing *Zeitgeist* about hemispheric specialization among neuropsychologists, neurologists, psychiatrists, and other tribes dealing with the human brain and its disorders? It could be the same accursed balkanization, perhaps inevitable given the sheer volume of scientific information accumulated today, but lamentable nonetheless.

Maybe because I was born left-handed, and despite the efforts of my Soviet kindergarten handlers to exorcise the contrarian tendencies that go with it, I have always been inclined to disregard the established taxonomic boundaries between clinical disciplines and moved across them my whole professional life in neuropsychology, for better or worse. In that spirit of "anti-balkanization," let's consider a multi-layered neural hierarchy. It consists of three types of brain structures: (1) the prefrontal cortex, (2) the subcortical structure called the *dorsal striatum,* consisting of a number of nuclei, and (3) the substantia nigra and ventral tegmental area nuclei in the brain stem, which send projections rich in the neurotransmitter dopamine to the cortex and the striatum. All these structures come in twin pairs, one in each hemisphere. As a result, we have a three-level twin hierarchy, depicted in Figure 6.5. We will refer to it as a "triple decker." The hierarchy may be broken at different levels, resulting in different disorders; and each of these disorders is shoehorned into a different diagnostic pigeonhole. But we are about to cross the boundaries of our infuriatingly balkanized clinical world.

The breakdown at the juncture between the brain stem and the dorsal striatum results in Parkinson's disease, where atrophy of the dopaminergic nuclei

The Triple Decker

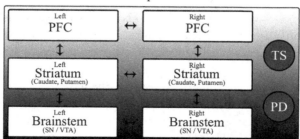

FIGURE 6.5 **The triple decker.** Three levels of the hierarchy: prefrontal cortex (PFC), striatum, and ventral brainstem. Caudate and putamen nuclei are found in the dorsal striatum. Two major dopaminergic nuclei, substantia nigra (SN) and ventral tegmental area (VTA), are found in the ventral brainstem. Parkinson's disease (PD) involves dysregulation at the brainstem–striatum junction. Tourette's syndrome (TS) involves dysregulation at the fronto–striatal junction.

substantia nigra and ventral tegmental area results in the depletion of dopamine supply to the caudate and putamen nuclei of the striatum. In contrast, the breakdown at the juncture between the striatum and the prefrontal cortex results in Tourette's syndrome. The two disorders are related not only neuroanatomically, but also, it would seem at least in some cases, genetically, since both disorders sometimes show up in the same individuals and in the same families.[29] And since perfect symmetry exists only in mathematical abstractions and in the arts, in any individual case of Parkinson's disease or Tourette's syndrome, the interface is likely to be somewhat more affected on one side of the triple decker than on the other. We know this to be the case in Parkinson's, so why would it be any different in Tourette's syndrome? Do such slightly asymmetrical variants of these disorders result in different cognitive symptoms? And can our insights into the disorders at one level of the triple decker inform our understanding of the others?

My interest in Parkinson's disease and Tourette's syndrome was triggered by precisely these questions. Based on the earlier research with my then–graduate student Ken Podell, I knew that damage to the left and right prefrontal cortex results in very different symptoms, at least in males. Damage to the left prefrontal cortex results in perseveration, a pathological propensity toward repetitive behaviors, toward routines. In contrast, damage to the right prefrontal cortex results in field-dependent, excessive exploratory behavior, a pathological attraction to every incidental novel object in one's environment. In many clinical conditions (like severe traumatic brain injury), these symptoms co-occur because the frontal lobes are affected on both sides, but they can be very clearly dissociated when the damage is limited to one side, like in stroke. The difference between the consequences of left and right frontal damage may be very dramatic in males. A very different picture emerged in females, however, where both left and right frontal lesions resulted in exploratory behaviors.[30]

Those familiar with Parkinson's disease know that its signature characteristic, resting tremor, is usually lateralized, more severe on one side than on the other, this resulting in the so-called hemi-Parkinsonian syndromes. Either side can be affected, but the dominant hand more likely so. Based on the clips from the old documentaries, in Adolph Hitler, arguably the most infamous Parkinson's patient (or perhaps even any kind of patient) in history, the tremor was mostly on the left side. In contrast, anyone watching CNN on a regular basis may recall a clip of the anchorwoman Hala Gorani interviewing an elderly man with a resting tremor on the right side.

Even though Parkinson's disease is traditionally classified as a movement disorder, known mostly for its resting tremor and difficulty initiating movements, cognitive impairment, sometimes quite severe, is frequently present as well. So, in the spirit of cutting across taxonomic boundaries, a team of colleagues at

New York University School of Medicine and I conducted a study to find out if the knowledge of the effects of left and right frontal lesions (breakdown at the top layer of the triple-decker) can provide a window into the understanding of cognitive impairment in the right and left hemi-Parkinsonian syndromes (breakdown at the juncture between the bottom two layers of the triple-decker).

And indeed, just as we expected, the cognitive peculiarities of the left and right hemi-Parkinsonian syndromes paralleled in important respects the cognitive profiles of the right and left prefrontal lesions. The right hemi-Parkinsonian syndrome (where the left substantia nigra is more severely affected) was characterized by more perseverative behavior than the left hemi-Parkinsonian syndrome (where the right substantia nigra is more affected). And like in the prefrontal lesions, sex differences emerged when males and females with Parkinson's disease were compared.[31] These findings may have multiple implications, not the least related to the risk of addiction in Parkinson's disease, which was discussed in the previous chapter.

The success in predicting the cognitive profiles of hemi-Parkinsonian syndromes provided an encouraging "proof of concept" for the triple decker's heuristic value. The next step was putting the triple decker to use in understanding Tourette syndrome. Tourette's is an intriguing condition accompanied by a whole range of colorful manifestations. The most commonly mentioned among them are motor and vocal tics, which take the form of forced, jerky movements and odd vocalizations, like throat-clearing or grunting. The symptoms usually start in early childhood, peak around the age of 10–12 years old, and often (but not always) abate after that. The majority of people with Tourette's—anywhere between 50% and 90% depending on the source, and approximately 60% according to the Centers for Disease Control—have also been diagnosed with ADHD. This gave rise to the notion of a high Tourette's/ADHD "comorbidity"—a notion that I have had a hard time embracing for quite some time.[32]

The root of my longstanding skepticism had to do with the very definition and diagnostic criteria of Tourette's. These criteria are based exclusively on the presence of motor and vocal tics and leave out another type of symptom common in people with Tourette's: unusual and excessive exploratory behaviors. The duality of Tourette's symptomatology was eloquently described in the paper by Oliver Sacks titled "Tourette's syndrome and creativity," which appeared in *The British Medical Journal* in 1992.[33] Sacks distinguished between the "stereotypic" form of Tourette's dominated by tics, and the "phantasmagoric" form of Tourette's dominated by excessive exploratory behaviors. But if Sacks was right, then, since the "phantasmagoric" symptoms never made it into the "official," commonly used definition of Tourette's, this definition captured only half of the cases of the disorder and left out the other half! Because the definition was too narrow, it failed to account for the complete range of the manifestations that the disorder could take, in effect splitting it in the middle and ignoring one half.

When considered as part of the triple decker, the duality of Tourette's symptoms made perfect sense. Just as Parkinson's disease is almost never perfectly symmetrical, neither would be Tourette's. In any particular case, the fronto-striatal dysfunction is likely to be more severe on the left, which would result in the preponderance of tics, a form of perseveration; or (perhaps less commonly) on the right, which would result in the preponderance of excessive exploratory behaviors. Because of the overly narrow diagnostic criteria, only the former will be correctly diagnosed as Tourette's, whereas the latter will be misdiagnosed as some other condition.

This leads to an intriguing possibility that just as there are left and right hemi-Parkinsonian syndromes, there are left and right "hemi-Tourette's" syndromes, and because of the unduly narrow diagnostic criteria, only one of them is recognized as Tourette's, whereas the other one is routinely misdiagnosed as something else, particularly often as ADHD, not least because of the casual thoughtlessness, frequently bordering on the unethical, with which this diagnosis has come to be given in our clinical culture.[34]

To make matters even more confusing, "excessive exploratory behavior" is not recognized as a distinct diagnostic category in any of the commonly used diagnostic systems. As a result, because clinicians so often feel obligated to squeeze every clinical presentation into a "recognized" diagnostic category, a neglected symptom like excessive exploratory behavior will be forced into one of the "officially sanctioned" pigeonholes whether it belongs there or not. Regrettably, "sanctioned" does not always mean "accurate," and people with an exploratory behavior–dominated form of Tourette's may be routinely misdiagnosed as suffering from ADHD or from some other condition.[34]

In reality, excessive exploratory behaviors and hyperactivity are very different. Exploratory behavior is driven by incidental, often random external stimuli in the environment. In contrast, hyperactivity is an excessive amount of motor activity not necessarily directed at anything in particular. While the distinction between excessive exploratory behavior and hyperactivity is conceptually important, it is all too often ignored. This confusion is also a product of balkanization. Excessive exploratory behavior is well known among neuropsychologists and behavioral neurologists under the names of "field-dependent behavior" and "utilization behavior."[35] But it is not nearly so well known in the clinical circles concerned with either Tourette's or with ADHD. Numerous diagnostic scales exist for hyperactivity and for tics, but none exists for excessive exploratory behaviors.[36]

Once the conceptual difference between the hyperactivity and excessive exploratory behavior is clarified and explained, it becomes easily recognizable to a practiced clinical eye, resonates with one's clinical experience, and is in hindsight self-evident—a sure sign that the distinction is real, consequential, and captures important aspects of clinical reality. While less well described than tics, exploratory behaviors can be quite extreme and oppressive. People with Tourette's syndrome sometimes experience an irresistible urge to touch random objects in their environment, even at the expense of hurting themselves, like when grabbing a hot light bulb; to touch total strangers, even when this violates social norms and is fraught with unpleasant consequences, including being arrested by police; to sniff, lick, or even swallow inedible objects just to experience their taste and find out what they feel like on the palate, and so on. They may also experience an irresistible urge to mimic other people's movements (e.g., imitating the peculiarities of someone's gait or a posture), this resulting in echopraxia; or vocalizations (e.g., imitating someone's accent or a tone of voice), this resulting in echolalia. Even though these two forms of propensity toward imitation are often classified as tics or hyperactivity, in reality they are neither; they are exploratory behaviors. The patients also report a peculiar dynamics involving exploratory behaviors and tics: what begins as imitative echopraxia or echolalia gradually becomes a repetitive motor or vocal tic. This is strikingly similar to the dynamics between field-dependent behavior and perseveration which is often observed in patients with bilateral prefrontal damage (an example of such dynamics in a patient with bilateral damage of the frontal lobes can be found in Chapter 7).[37]

A whole category of patients may even exist in whom excessive exploratory behaviors dominate the clinical picture unaccompanied by tics, due to a strongly lateralized right fronto-striatal dysfunction. These patients will not be recognized as having Tourette's syndrome at all. Instead, they are likely to be misdiagnosed as cases of ADHD, despite the fact that the underlying mechanism is one of Tourette's, albeit with a right- rather than left-lateralized neuroanatomical expression.

All this appeared to make perfect sense, but there was a major problem with my "hemi-Tourette's syndromes" idea: how to actually recognize them in patients? In Parkinson's disease, you don't need any sophisticated equipment to note that the tremors are more pronounced in the left or in the right hand. No such cut-and-dry lateralized symptom exists in Tourette's syndrome.

When I mentioned my "hemi-Tourette's" idea in a lecture in Oslo a few years ago, my Norwegian hosts suggested that together we take a look at a body of data acquired by them on a sample of children and adolescents with Tourette's. One way of designing a proxy index of "hemi-Tourette's" syndromes was by comparing motor speed in the two hands. In right-handed individuals, the right hand is usually somewhat, but not hugely, faster than the left hand. Disparity in the opposite direction (left hand faster than right) suggests left-hemispheric dysfunction, and a huge disparity in favor of the right hand suggests right-hemispheric dysfunction. This is precisely the analysis that two Norwegian neuropsychologists, Kjell Tore Hovik and Merete Øie, and I conducted on a sample of boys with Tourette's syndrome who were studied at University of Oslo. As a result, three groups emerged: right hemi-Tourette's (in whom the left hand was faster than the right hand, presumably due to the mostly left fronto-striatal dysfunction); left hemi-Tourette's (in whom the right hand was abnormally faster than the left hand, presumably due to the mostly right fronto-striatal dysfunction); and a symmetrical pattern (presumably reflecting a roughly equal severity of left and right fronto-striatal dysfunction). When we looked at the diagnoses the boys had received in earlier evaluations, the data spoke for themselves: most "right hemi-Tourette's" cases had the diagnosis of Tourette's syndrome pure and simple; all "left hemi-Tourette's" had the diagnosis of Tourette's syndrome "comorbid" with something else—mostly with ADHD; and the "symmetrical" cases were evenly split between these two kinds of diagnoses.[38]

Failure to recognize excessive exploratory behavior as a distinct symptom, and overly narrow diagnostic criteria for Tourette's, may also help explain a vastly uneven prevalence of Tourette's syndrome in boys and girls. According to the Centers for Disease Control, this diagnosis is made three to five times more often in boys than in girls.[39] Why is this so? One possible answer is provided by the studies of sex differences in the effects of lateralized frontal lesions. Whereas in males, left and right prefrontal lesions result in distinctly different symptoms (perseveration in the former and field-dependency in the latter), in females, field-dependent behavior, but not perseveration, is caused by lateralized prefrontal lesions regardless of the side.[40] So, in the spirit of the triple decker, is it possible that while in boys left and right fronto-striatal dysregulation results, respectively, in tics and exploratory behaviors, in girls both lead to excessive exploratory behaviors? If that is the case, the underdiagnosis of Tourette's would be much more common in girls than in boys.

The implications of the foregoing discussion are quite provocative: they suggest that many cases (mis)diagnosed with hyperactivity are in fact cases of excessive exploratory behavior, of abnormal attraction to novelty no longer serving any constructive purpose and utterly counter-productive. This, in turn, implies that many cases diagnosed as ADHD are in fact misdiagnoses, that they are really cases of Tourette's syndrome. It is not uncommon for a child who is put on stimulant medications as a result of ADHD diagnosis to develop tics. According to some sources, this happens in up to 25% of children and adolescents receiving the diagnosis, even though the causal nature of this association has been challenged.[41]

These may be the cases of Tourette's misdiagnosed as ADHD, and they may be merely the tip of an iceberg. The issue takes on particular importance because of the oft-misguided casual ease with which the ADHD diagnosis has come to be made and stimulant medications prescribed in our society. Excessive exploratory behavior, a condition where attraction to novelty becomes uncontrolled and self-defeating, is an under-recognized disorder in need of further investigation, hopefully leading to improved diagnosis and treatment.

7

Directed Wandering and the Ineffable Creative Spark

No Monkey Business

How do multiple brain structures conspire to propel human innovation and creativity? We have already concluded that any attempt to pin this process on a single part of the brain is an exercise in futility. Nor does it seem likely that it can be reduced to a single mental operation. Exploration of the nature of creativity has a much longer history than the systematic research into its cognitive attributes and brain mechanisms. Long before creativity became a trendy subject of formal investigation by psychologists and neuroscientists, the elusive mechanisms of the creative process had intrigued some of its most consequential practitioners. Wolfgang Amadeus Mozart, Albert Einstein, Henry Poincaré, Jacques Hadamar, and a few others attempted to capture its effervescent dynamics through introspection and to communicate their observations in essays and private correspondence. Some of their writings, compiled in a volume edited by Brewster Ghiselin, will be referred to later in this chapter.[1]

It became clear a long time ago that, at a minimum, it is important to distinguish between the generation of novel ideas and the subsequent selection among those generated; and it seemed logical that the former task must precede the latter. Both parts of the process were shrouded in mystery, generation probably more so than selection. While the selectivity of cognitive processes has been the subject of systematic research for years, the question of how novel content is generated was not nearly so actively pursued, nor was this inquiry anchored in any established cognitive psychological tradition. So it comes as no surprise that a paradigm was imported to the rescue from a different discipline—evolutionary biology. First introduced into creativity research by Donald Campbell (1916–1996), the paradigm is sometimes referred to as *blind variation and selective retention*, or BVSR.[2]

According to BVSR, novel content is generated essentially randomly, this being followed by a selection process whereby wheat is separated from chaff: a small fraction of randomly generated content is judged as good and retained, and the bulk of the randomly generated content is discarded.

The notion that a creative process begins with random, unconstrained idea-generation was appealing mostly because it relieved the cognitive scientists from the daunting challenge of figuring out what is really taking place; a conceptual copout of sorts, embraced out of exasperation. On closer examination, however, the BVSR idea runs into several problems.

The first problem is combinatorial. Given the practically infinite number of "blindly" generated ideas, it may take too long to generate anything useful for this mechanism to be realistic. In the beginning of the twentieth century, the French mathematician Emile Borel came up with the "infinite monkey theorem," based on the idea of a monkey (or a collection of monkeys) in front of a typewriter hitting the keys randomly. Given an infinite amount of time, the monkey would sooner or later (later rather than sooner) come up with William Shakespeare's whole *oeuvre*, among numerous other, far less exalted outputs. But the real monkey's life is finite, as is the life of a creative human scientist, author, or artist, so good luck! It is almost certain that a mortal monkey will go to monkey heaven well before a single sonnet is typed, and a similar fate is likely to await a mortal human random-idea generator.

The notion of "mental wandering" at the heart of the creative process has been around for some time. But while powerful computers are good at rapidly going through all the possible options and selecting those that meet certain criteria, human beings are not. As the work by Allen Newell and Herbert Simon with chess players has shown, in order to be effective, human decision making has to be constrained from the outset, and even trial and error processes have to be somewhat selective.[3] On strictly informational grounds, then, it would appear that in order to be manageable by human beings, the mental wandering at the heart of the creative process needs to be somewhat constrained from the beginning. Decision making is no monkey business!

The other problem is one of the reality of the creative process. It is not as if great ideas in any field were arrived at by some quixotic naïfs without any prior interest in, or knowledge of, the field, idly generating mental chaff in order to arrive at a few grains of wheat, with any luck. No, in real life the creative breakthrough is usually the culmination of a sustained intellectual or artistic effort extended over a long period of time. The creative breakthrough usually comes to an individual who has toiled in the field of his chosen pursuits for years or even decades, and who is its accomplished master. The ability to generate the new is usually rooted in an excellent grasp of the old, even if in the end it leads to the rejection of the old. This by definition implies that some constraints are operating on the creative process.

In this chapter, we will introduce the novel (pun intended!) idea of a creative process and its brain machinery, where the constrained and under-constrained components are interwoven, the former preceding the latter instead of following it. We will refer to this process as *"directed wandering."*

The Extreme Frontal Lobes
Bistability

In order to understand how the brain approaches novelty and arrives at a creative solution, consider the concept of *bistability,* a concept that has been borrowed by neuroscientists from mathematics and that continues to be extremely influential in shaping the way we think about the brain. The concept of bistability is invoked here as heuristic metaphor only, and it is useful in that sense.

Bistability (usually spelled in the scientific literature without a hyphen) is a fundamental phenomenon both in the natural world and in manmade devices; and the concept is widely used in physics, chemistry and biology. A system is called *bistable* if its behavior is characterized by transitions between two states. An electronic system storing information in binary form is based on bistability. A spring that controls the position of the retractable ballpoint in your pen is bistable. In biology, cell differentiation is also a bistable process (Figure 7.1).

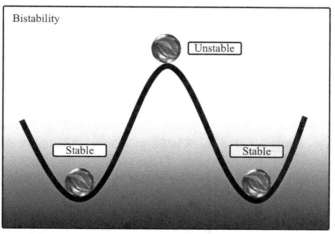

FIGURE 7.1 Schematic representation of a bistable system. The system gravitates toward one of the two stable states.

Certain essential interactions between the prefrontal cortex and the rest of the brain are also characterized by a relationship that, while probably not a strong bistability in a literal sense, functionally approaches bistability. Introducing this concept into the narrative is more than a semantic flourish; it ushers in a level of conceptual clarity and may be particularly productive in guiding the designs of computational models of the frontal interaction with the rest of the brain.

Hyperfrontality and Hypofrontality

During wakefulness, and particularly during active mental states, the prefrontal cortex is more physiologically active than the rest of the cortex much of the time in normal people. This phenomenon is called *hyperfrontality,* and it has been demonstrated with a number of neuroimaging techniques, such as PET scans measuring levels of glucose metabolism, and electroencephalography (EEG) measuring electric activity in different parts of the brain. We already encountered hyperfrontality when we discussed the central executive network and the "task-positive" brain state in Chapter 4. But in certain states, the level of frontal activation is diminished, and the relationship between the levels of physiological activity in the prefrontal cortex and the rest of the cortex may even sometimes be reversed, in a condition known as *hypofrontality.* In healthy people, the brain is in a state of hypofrontality during much of sleep, under hypnosis, and in trancelike states. Certain psychiatric disorders, like schizophrenia and severe depression, are also characterized by hypofrontality. And the brain is often hypofrontal if the prefrontal cortex has been affected by traumatic injury or by atrophy due to dementia. We will discuss a number of such conditions later in this chapter.

Even in healthy individuals, both hyper- and hypofrontality may take extreme forms. Problem-solving under conditions of high stakes and time constraints is associated with extreme hyperfrontality. In contrast, meditative states are associated with hypofrontality.[4]

In the next sections, we will consider an example of each of these two states. Even though no actual recording of brain states was conducted in either case, I am convinced that both episodes were associated with extreme (but opposite) levels of frontal-lobe activity. And the advantage is that both episodes were not artificial, staged, laboratory experiments, but events from real life—my own. In one of them (hypofrontality), I was a bewildered but passive observer; and in the other one (hyperfrontality), I was the hapless actor who, thankfully, has survived the encounter to tell the story.

Hypofrontality: Deep Trance in Indonesia

In my capacity as a clinician, I encounter the effects of hypofrontality in patients all the time, but my most striking encounter with hypofrontality was as a traveler many years ago. As addictions go, this one of mine was relatively benign: I was (and still am) addicted to Southeast Asia, particularly to Indonesia. I crisscrossed this inexhaustible archipelago on foot, by car, by boat, and by plane. I have seen elaborate Hindu temple processions on the island of Bali, and sacrificial Tana Toraja ceremonies on the island of Sulawesi. I have spent a night in the company of a dragon loitering between the stilts supporting the ranger guest house in which I slept on the island of Komodo. And in Eastern Java, I encountered a mysterious dance.

I had just had a meeting at the Gadjah Mada University in the old royal city of Yokgyakarta and now decided to spend the rest of the day as an unabashed sightseer. While passing through a rather nondescript village, I stopped my jeep to check out a crowd gathered on the side of the road for what I thought would be five or ten minutes. Instead, I ended up spending the remainder of the day there, mesmerized by what I saw.

In a circle made by the local villagers, a group of young men were mounting what looked like flat wooden horses (I later found out that they were made of woven rattan), of the sort that children ride. Once mounted, they began to "ride" them in an increasingly mechanical, robot-like fashion under the rhythmic and increasingly intense sounds of *gamelans* (traditional percussion instruments of Indonesia) emanating from the crowd. A few older men emerged from the crowd and began to flash bright objects in front of the horsemen's eyes in a pendulum-like fashion. As the gamelan and the pendulum rhythms were getting faster, so was the pace of the young men riding their rattan horses. Their eyes were getting glassy and their postures rigid and mechanical. They were immersing into a state of trance.

As their trance deepened, the young men's actions were getting increasingly, for the lack of better word, wild. They were jumping off their horses, dashing up the smooth trunks of the surrounding palm trees in ways that defied the laws of gravity, ripping the coconuts open with their teeth, and descending with the same physical law–defying agility. They were grabbing slabs of glass that somehow appeared in their midst and chewing the glass without suffering any discernible injury. And they were eating fire. Then they were mounting their horses again, and the wild ride continued. I had read about similar feats by the *fakirs* of India but had always thought this to be a product of poetic license or staged-for-the-tourists gimmicks—until I saw it with my own eyes. What was particularly remarkable was that the protagonists were clearly not "professional" performers, nor was the whole event a staged tourist show. The performers were village youths casually and unexotically dressed in T-shirts and jeans, and I was the only outsider in the crowd.

Meanwhile, the young horsemen were getting visibly exhausted yet unable to break the ride. The intensity with which a few older men in the crowd were watching them suggested that their condition was approaching a dangerous state (I was not sure what the nature of this anticipated danger was, but suspected that the trancelike state with its hypersynchronized electrical brain activity combined with the rhythmic movements of shiny pendula and rhythmic gamelan beat could set off seizures in the young horsemen). All of a sudden, as if reacting to some abrupt change in the young men's demeanor, the older men stepped into the circle and pulled one, then another of the horsemen off his horse, while the young man continued to jerk rhythmically and with catatonic-like rigidity even when off the horse, unable to break out of the trance. Then two older men lifted the horseman, rigid as a wooden board, by his feet and shoulders, and a third one jumped on the middle of his torso, breaking the rigidity and literally folding him. Unsteady on his feet, with his eyes glassy, the young man staggered in the direction of the village, disappeared from sight, and returned half an hour later, still unsteady, to join the crowd of spectators. Meanwhile, different youths stepped out of the crowd, entered the circle, mounted the vacated horses, and the dance continued. And I went back to my hotel in Yogyakarta trying to digest what I had just seen.

The mysterious event I witnessed is called the *Jathilan* (or Horse Dance). A traditional Eastern Javanese dance, it is full of symbolism and implications of mystical powers. It involves immersion into a deep trance, of the sort that is generally associated with temporary ("transient") hypofrontality. More recently, I watched a similar dance on the island of Bali, where it is known under the name of *Sanghyang Jaran*. Here a single performer, immersed in a state of trance under the rhythmic chanting of a chorus of sorts, trampled a bonfire barefoot, his movements mechanical, his posture rigid, and his facial expression remote and contorted. He, too, must have been in a state of transient hypofrontality (Figure 7.2).[5]

Hyperfrontality: Near-Drowning in Italy

In the presumed hyperfrontal episode, I was the hapless protagonist, aged 27. Having just emigrated from the Soviet Union, I was spending a few months in Rome on my way to the United States. It was the middle of July, the city was getting scalding hot, and a swim in the Mediterranean sounded like an excellent idea. I took the suburban train to the seaside town of Ostia, headed for the

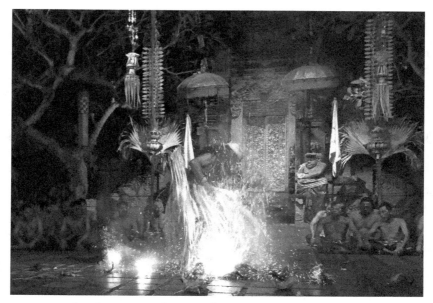

FIGURE 7.2 **Sanghyang Jaran dance performance in Bali.** Photo by the author.

beach, and went straight into the water. The next thing I knew, I was being pulled out by a powerful rip current. Having grown up on the Baltic Sea, I was a reasonably good swimmer, but this current was unlike anything I had encountered before, and my efforts to resist only resulted in more helpless thrashing. As I was being pulled out, and as it felt, under, a distinct thought went through my mind, virtually articulated in words, cold and detached: "What is happening to me is drowning, and I have only a few seconds to sort this out." I did not experience any emotion. There was a sense of detachment bordering on depersonalization, but also a sense of intense focus. A thought came to mind as if by itself, something I must have read somewhere a long time before, that in such situations you don't try to get above water but do the opposite, go as deep under the water as you can and swim toward the shore. This is what I did, and a few moments later I was thrown out by the surf onto the pebbly beach. Once safely on land, I looked around. The beach was packed with sunbathers, but no one in the water; the locals must have known that the spot was treacherous. I have no idea how I knew about the maneuver that very likely saved my life; not even sure that I had read about it, it may have been an act of sheer improvisation, but here I am to tell the story. And in retrospect, I can hardly think of any other event in my life characterized by such an intense mental focus condensed in a heartbeat of time, yet so depersonalized and devoid of any feeling. I am convinced that had my brain been imaged at the time, a state of extreme hyperfrontality would have been recorded.

These two examples of transient states of presumed extreme hyper- and hypo-frontality were triggered by unusual circumstances in generally ordinary and healthy people. In contrast, persistent hyper- or hypofrontality is indicative of brain disorder. Pathological hyperfrontality is seen in certain forms of schiz-ophrenia when the patient is challenged by a cognitive task.[6] It has also been reported in retired National Football League (NFL) players with a history of multiple head injuries, when performing tasks designed to challenge the frontal lobes.[7] In these cases, it probably reflects a greater-than-normal burden placed on the frontal lobes by tasks that healthy people do not find particularly chal-lenging or stressful. It has also been observed in people while taking certain hal-lucinogenic substances, although hypofrontality is a more common finding in addictions.[8]

Pathological hypofrontality is much more common than pathological hyper-frontality. As mentioned earlier, it has been documented in numerous neuropsy-chiatric and neurological disorders and may take a variety of forms.[9] Later in the chapter, we will discuss the case of a young man who suffered severe brain trauma. The cognitive deficit evident in his performance on a memory task is a result of the loss of much of the prefrontal cortex—an extreme case of hypofrontality.

Dorsolateral Bistability: Inspiration and Perspiration

So far, we have discussed hyper- and hypofrontality as if they were global phe-nomena. But it is unlikely that either of them affects the whole frontal lobe equally. We already know that the frontal lobes consist of different parts that are distinct both anatomically and functionally, and both hyper- and hypofrontality may take more specific, and less extreme, forms in different parts of the frontal lobes. The area of the frontal lobe of interest to us here is the lateral aspect of the prefrontal cortex. As mentioned earlier, it consists of the dorsolateral and ventrolateral components, but for the purposes of this discussion, we will con-sider them together under the name "dorsolateral prefrontal cortex," or DLPFC for short. DLPFC may also function in such a way that distinct hyperfrontality is intertwined with distinct hypofrontality in a fashion approaching bistability, and this will be of particular interest to us here.

This brings us to the perennial conundrum of "inspiration" versus "perspira-tion." What are their respective roles in the creative process? The issue has been inconclusively debated for years, both seriously and in jest, both in scientific liter-ature and particularly in the popular media. Opinions differ and often gravitate toward the extremes. Is it the proverbial "95% perspiration and 5% inspiration" and "practice, practice, practice" that will get you to Carnegie Hall? Or is crea-tivity a godsend, a blessing unfairly showered on the fortunate few without any effort on their part? And what is the neurobiological meaning of "inspiration" and "perspiration" anyway?

I will argue that both perspiration and inspiration are required to ignite the creative spark through a sequence of events in the brain, culminating in what we will call "directed wandering." We will examine a possible scenario of how this "directed wandering" happens. It turns out that this process is driven by an intricate dance between hyper- and hypofrontality. The role of hyperfrontality in any vigorous thought process is almost self-evident, and the sustained, goal-directed effort that we casually refer to as "perspiration" probably requires the brain to be in a hyperfrontal state. To put it more succinctly, perspiration implies hyperfrontality. The role of hypofrontality, however, is far less apparent, and the very suggestion that it plays a constructive role in cognition may come across as counterintuitive. Nonetheless, it has been proposed that temporary ("transient") hypofrontality plays an important role in the creative process,[10] and that more broadly, so does the temporary general lowering of arousal mediated by reduced levels of the neurotransmitter norepinephrine.[11]

By themselves, hypofrontal states or generally under-aroused brain are not likely to result in anything useful. Their role becomes productive only as part of that neural dance involving also transient hyperfrontality and a host of other neural events. This means that a wide range of modulation of frontal arousal by the dopaminergic and noradrenergic systems of the ventral brain stem (ventral tegmental area and locus coeruleus) is essential for the creative process. Enhanced capacity for such modulation may be an important ingredient of a creative mind, and the individual differences in the range of such modulation are likely to be related to the capacity for creative innovation, with wider ranges benefiting this capacity. Indeed, according to a cogent review by Allison Kaufman and colleagues, EEG studies suggest that both higher-than-average cortical basal arousal level *and* low arousal level (increased alpha-frequency activity) are present during solving divergent thinking tasks, which, according to many scientists, require creativity, and which are often used in creativity research.[12]

Lego® Master at Work: Creative Perspiration

During *hyperfrontal* states, the dorsolateral prefrontal cortex is hard at work. It manipulates mental representations stored in the brain like Lego pieces, assembling them into new configurations through a deliberate goal-driven process, some aspects of which were sketched in Chapter 4 and will not be repeated here.

The deliberate process of the dorsolateral prefrontal cortex in accessing and manipulating information stored in other parts of the brain is reflected in the central executive network (as we discussed in chapters 4 and 6), which becomes active in our brain when we strain, consciously and deliberately, to solve a particular, well-articulated cognitive task at hand; this is why this network is sometimes referred to as "task-positive." When scientists examined the temporal sequence in which different components of the network became active, it became clear that the activation within this network is driven by the prefrontal cortex.[13] Hyperfrontality at work!

The goal-oriented systematic machinery of the prefrontal cortex often goes a long way toward driving the creative process to fruition, even though it does not always succeed. But even when insufficient in and of itself, the goal-directed search for solutions guided by the prefrontal cortex is necessary in most cases to prepare the grounds for that proverbial "creative spark."

Lego® Master at Rest: Creative Inspiration? Not Yet

What happens when the dorsolateral prefrontal cortex is in a state of hypofrontality, and what is the dynamic between the networks we discussed in the previous chapters? What happens then to the posterior cortical circuits, which were controlled by the frontal lobes while the central executive network was on? They do not disappear, and they do not go to sleep. Quite the contrary: according to the scenario we are exploring here, what happens in those parts of the brain during dorsolateral hypofrontality may hold the key to the mystery of the creative process.

When the central executive network is no longer active, the default mode network may become active instead (the two networks are "anticorrelated": when one is on, the other one is off), but these two networks think different thoughts and engage different circuits in the posterior cortex. The posterior—temporal, parietal, and occipital—circuits, which were activated while the central executive network was on, are now on their own, no longer directed and supervised by the prefrontal cortex—like orchestra musicians without the conductor, or a company's employees without the chief executive officer. The activation spread within these regions is now guided strictly by their internal connectivity within the posterior cortex, and not by a superimposed goal or plan of action laid down by the prefrontal cortex. We can think of these processes as *undirected mental wandering*. This is what a healthy individual probably experiences in sleep or in any dreamlike state, whether in trance or under hypnosis. The processes unfolding in the posterior cortex unsupervised by the frontal lobes are best understood by examining the clinical cases of frontal-lobe pathology. Let us examine the case of a young patient of mine from many years ago who, because of an accident resulting in head injury, had to undergo neurosurgery removing much of his prefrontal cortex around the frontal poles bilaterally (Figure 7.3).

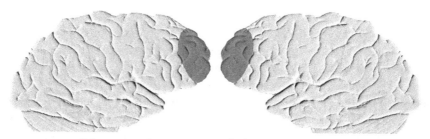

FIGURE 7.3 Schematic representation of the patient's bilateral frontal pole resection.

I asked the patient to listen to a story and immediately recall it from memory, while I sat facing him and taping his recall on a portable tape-recorder. The story, a version of a timeless fable titled "A Hen and Golden Eggs" went as follows:

> A man owned a hen that was laying golden eggs. The man was greedy and wanted more gold at once. He killed the hen and cut it open hoping to find a lot of gold inside, but there was none.

Here is the patient's recall:

> A man was living with a hen . . . or rather the hen was the hen's owner. She was producing gold . . . the man . . . the owner wanted more gold at once . . . so he cut the hen into pieces but there was no gold. . . . No gold at all . . . he cuts the hen more . . . no gold . . . the hen remains empty. . . . So he searches again and again. . . . No gold . . . he searches all around . . . in all places. The search is going on with a tape recorder . . . they are looking here and there, nothing new around. . . . They leave the tape recorder turned on, something is twisting there . . . some digits 0, 2, 3, 0 . . . so they are recording all these digits . . . not very many of them . . . that's why all the other digits were recorded . . . turned out to be not very many of them. . . so, everything was recorded. . . . I'll tell you what . . . there were only 5–6 digits there. . . . (*I ask: Have you finished?*). . . Not yet, I will finish soon . . . so, there were only 5–6 digits there. . . . When they took bus #5, so you get there and transfer to bus #5 and get to Bauman Square, you go further on, further on, here you take off. . . . And again you take bus #5 . . . (*The monologue continues*).[14]

The recall is not particularly bad in the beginning, which suggests that the patient's memory itself is not terribly impaired. But instead of terminating the recall once the gist of the story has been conveyed, the mental wandering continues, the patient is unable to stop it, and superfluous content is creeping in. A close look at the superfluous content suggests that it comes in two kinds. First, there is incessant repetition of the same content, words and phrases over and over again. The patient is "stuck" in the same content, unable to move on. This phenomenon is called *perseveration*, a common symptom of frontal-lobe pathology. Second, the patient's recall diverts toward the description of incidental external objects or events and internal associations completely unrelated to the story, as they keep creeping into the narrative—like the description of my tape recorder and bus #5. This phenomenon is called "field-dependent behavior," another common symptom of frontal-lobe pathology. They resemble "loose associations" observed in many patients suffering from schizophrenia. Schizophrenia, of course, is a disorder very different from traumatic brain injury suffered by my patient, but the frontal lobes are affected in schizophrenia as well, which is what accounts for the field-dependent behavior.

My patient suffered bilateral frontal damage, and the two types of symptoms—perseveration and field-dependent behavior—were intertwined and intermingled in the same performance. How about unilateral frontal damage? Remember the triple-decker in Chapter 6? According to our earlier research, when damage to the frontal lobes affects only one hemisphere, the two symptoms become dissociated, at least in males: damage to the left prefrontal cortex results in perseveration, and damage to the right prefrontal cortex results in field-dependent behavior.[15] And our subsequent research, briefly described in Chapter 6, has shown a similar dissociation in subcortical disorders indirectly affecting the left or right frontal lobes: in Parkinson's disease and Tourette's syndrome.[16]

It looks like when they are deprived of the "adult" supervision by the DLPFC and abandoned to their own devices, the two posterior cortices—left and right parietal, temporal and occipital lobes—slip up in very different ways. What does this tell us about the differences in their organization?

The left hemisphere, left to its own devices, ends up being stuck in a particular process and unable to switch to other processes, even when such a switch is required by the cognitive task at hand. The right hemisphere, left to its own devices, exhibits a very different behavior: it flits from one thing to the other, unable to "stay in place" even when staying in place is required by the cognitive task at hand. The left hemisphere gets stuck in place; the right hemisphere wanders. The left hemisphere is ponderous, the right hemisphere is flighty. Neither one is able to carry the task well by itself, but they fail in different, in a sense, opposite ways.

The Brain's Small World

What are the differences in the neural makeups of the two hemispheres that make them behave in such different, even opposite ways? To understand this, we need to introduce the concept of a *small-world network*. Like the concept of bistability, the concept of the small-world network was imported by neuroscientists from mathematics. A network (or a graph) possesses small-world properties if its structure combines two seemingly irreconcilable properties: it has a high degree of local node clustering ("cliquishness"), and at the same time even the nodes that are not close neighbors can be connected by a relatively small number of steps. In a typical small-world network, certain nodes are hubs on which particularly numerous connections converge (Figure 7.4).[17]

The small-world network concept has been developed within an abstract mathematical discipline called the *graph theory*, and it provides a powerful tool for describing a wide range of diverse systems: a traffic network with subway stations as nodes, a social network with people as nodes (think of "six degrees of separation"), or a neural network modeling the brain. In the latter case, neuronal groupings or even individual neurons are the nodes and synaptic contacts between them are the steps. One of the advantages conferred by small-world properties is an optimal balance between local processing and global integration within the network,[18] and it has been proposed that these properties arise when the networks evolve to process highly complex information, as has been the case for mammalian brain evolution.[19]

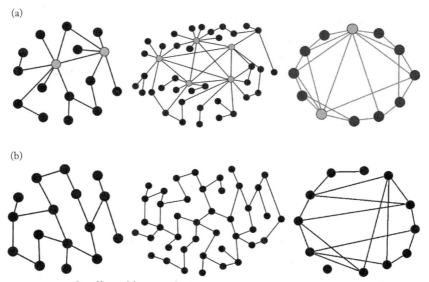

(a)

(b)

FIGURE 7.4 Small-world networks vs. random networks. (a) Small-world networks. (b) Random networks. In a small-world network, even distant nodes are connected with a minimal number of steps. Light gray nodes are hubs. Networks designed by Anton Shapovalov.

It was the development of neuroimaging and of complex computational methods that brought the graph theory into neuroscience. As the realization was growing that, in order to understand how the brain functions, it is necessary to understand how different parts of the brain are connected, several cutting-edge neuroimaging methods have been developed to study connectivity in the brain with a degree of precision and detail that was formerly unthinkable. As a result, huge and complex data sets were generated, characterizing the intricate connectivity patterns in the brain, and graph theory provided a mathematical method for uncovering the principles and regularities hidden in these data.

It turned out that many connectivity patterns within the cortex are indeed small-world networks. Furthermore, it turned out that the connectivity within the right hemisphere follows the small-world rules to a greater degree than connectivity in the left hemisphere. In contrast, the left hemisphere consists to a greater degree of tight local neighborhoods with dense connections within the neighborhoods but sparser connections between them. This difference between the connectivity patterns in the two hemispheres seems to be quite robust. Moreover, it is not unique to humans; it was found also in nonhuman primates, this being consistent with the broad observation of the similarities in the nature of hemispheric asymmetries across species which we made in Chapter 6 and will examine further in Chapter 8.[20]

In keeping with much of the argument developed in this book, the subtle differences between the connectivity patterns in the two hemispheres appear to reflect a computational adaptation present throughout evolution, rather than one uniquely linked to human cognition. The gray:white matter ratio is also higher in the left than in the right hemisphere, which suggests a greater reliance on far-flung long connections in the right than in the left hemisphere.[21] This explains why, abandoned to their own devices, the activation patterns in the left hemisphere are more likely to get stuck within a particular neural neighborhood, resulting in perseveration, and activation patterns in the right hemisphere are more likely to wander within a much wider cortical territory.

Directed Mental Wandering: The Creative Spark

Is mental wandering a useful process or merely a neurological aberration? As with many things in life, the answer is "yes and no." There are good reasons to believe that mental wandering saves the day when a conscious, systematic effort to solve the problem comes up short. *But in order for this to happen, it must be preceded by a period of a "hyperfrontal" deliberate go at the problem.*

"Coming up short" does not mean an outright failure. Deliberate effort plays an important role in the creative process in synergy with mental wandering. It is precisely the combination of the two processes, one deliberate and guided by the "hyperfrontal" frontal lobes, the other one spontaneous and "liberated" from frontal-lobe control in hypofrontal states, and going back and forth between these processes, that makes the creative process productive and ultimately successful. Abandoned entirely to its own devices, mental wandering is devoid of any direction and is unproductive; we see it in certain forms of schizophrenia and following massive damage to the frontal lobes, as was the case in my patient. The conscious, effortful part of the creative process guided by the frontal lobes provides the anchoring points for the mental wandering that follows, by constraining it and giving it direction.

Here is a rough, hypothetical sketch of what all this means neurobiologically. A creative process usually begins with a conscious idea of what needs to be accomplished, however vague and imprecise. As we already established, an innovative idea usually does not occur to someone who has never pondered the subject matter before; even when the subjective experience is one of the idea "appearing out of nowhere," it occurs to a prepared mind. The birth of a creative idea begins through the frontal lobe–driven process by activating certain regions within the vast cortical network distributed to a large extent throughout the posterior (parietal, temporal, and occipital) association cortex. The brain is in a state of task-specific ("task-positive") hyperfrontality. The activated regions are likely to be quite disparate within the cortex; they are not integrated into a single strongly interconnected network, and their disparate nature is the source of the subjective feeling that while you have some vague sense of what you want to accomplish, you don't have a clear idea how to get there. But these disparate regions activated during the hyperfrontal state will constrain the "mental wandering" that will come later. We will call the disparate locations activated within the network during the "hyperfrontal" state *neural anchoring points.*

When the hypofrontal mental wandering steps in, it almost literally "fills the gaps." It finds pathways between the initially disjointed neural anchoring points, which had been formed earlier during the "hyperfrontal" states. Clearly, this can be more readily accomplished in a network endowed with small-world properties. The cortical regions along these paths become integrated with the anchoring points, which were tagged earlier during the hyperfrontal state into a single interconnected network, which, with any luck, embodies the desired solution for a scientific puzzle or an artistic yearning. The mental wandering is a product of spontaneous activity within the vast cortical regions, particularly in the posterior (parietal and temporal) association cortex. Meanwhile, the frontal lobes are either globally inactive (as in sleep, under hypnosis, or in some dissociated state), or they are inactive with respect to the task at hand because they switched to doing something else. The experience of waking up with a sense of a breakthrough insight, which had eluded the creative individual before, has been often mentioned by creative individuals and is probably not coincidental. But in order for the mental wandering to be successful in finding the solution, it has to have been directed, and for that to happen, the problem had to be tackled first in a deliberate "hyperfrontal" state. It is the combination of the two processes that results in *directed mental wandering.*

Because mental wandering is not a product of a conscious, deliberate effort, the creative individual has little awareness of it unfolding. As the single interconnected network is emerging and the activation within it is still weak and fleeting, there is a feeling of being on "the verge" of the solution without consciously knowing yet what it will be. And when the network finally coalesces and the activation within it reaches a certain level of intensity and duration, the solution reveals itself at a conscious level. The "ineffable creative spark" is somewhere in between being "on the verge" and consciously knowing the solution. The process is likely to be iterative, with multiple candidate solutions produced by "frontalless" mental wandering critically reviewed, and accepted or rejected through a more deliberate and conscious process driven by the frontal lobes.

The character of mental wandering in the two hemispheres is constrained by the differences in their organization. In the left hemisphere, consisting of tightly knit local neighborhoods with less interaction between them, mental wandering is likely to get stuck within a few such neighborhoods and is less likely to result in connecting the anchoring points if they are far-flung within the neocortex. In the right hemisphere, because of its better articulated small-world properties, mental wandering is likely to spread over a vaster territory with a much greater likelihood of success in connecting the far-flung anchoring points of the network. The crucial importance to the creative process of the ability to connect "elements drawn from domains which are far apart," to quote Henri Poincaré, has been commented on by several individuals whose opinions are noteworthy, not because they were "creativity researchers," but by virtue of being top-tier creative minds in their chosen fields, as Poincaré was in mathematics and physics.[22]

The right hemisphere is better equipped for efficient mental wandering and for connecting the distant dots, which makes it a probabilistically more likely site of producing that "ineffable creative spark," hidden from introspection and resulting in the magical subjective feeling of sudden revelation. But it is the left hemisphere that by dint of its more tightly organized local circuitry is more efficient at storing well-developed representations once they have been developed. The subjectively vague combinatorial nature of this process preceding the emergence of an explicit "logical construction" has been captured in an introspective account of the creative process given by Albert Einstein to Jacques Hadamard, a French mathematician and an exceptionally creative individual in his own right.[23]

While the brain is seemingly (and deceptively) at rest, in the default mode state, which as we already know is more (but not exclusively) pronounced in the *left* hemisphere and is driven by the previously formed ideas and concerns, the mental wandering unfolding mostly (but also not exclusively) in the posterior cortex of the *right* hemisphere connects the anchoring points, the "neural dots" activated during the hyperfrontal state that came before. This does not necessarily mean that the default mode network plays no role in the process. The nature of the interplay between the central executive network (CEN) and the default mode network (DMN) in directed mental wondering is not well understood, but it is safe to assume that CEN drives the effortful part of the process, which is dominated by lateral prefrontal hyperfrontality and results in tagging the neural anchoring points. In contrast, during the seemingly effortless mental wandering, the lateral prefrontal cortex is in a hypofrontal state while DMN takes over. You will recall that in DMN, different parts of the frontal lobes are active instead, the orbitofrontal and ventromedial areas. They also project into the posterior association cortex but activate different networks, which reflect different thoughts and preoccupations. As a result, the neural anchoring points activated while CEN was at work find themselves embedded in very different neural networks when DMN becomes active, permitting all kinds of not previously possible connections to be made. So it may be that the spontaneous processes occurring in the posterior cortex, "liberated" from the control exerted by the lateral prefrontal cortex when CEN is no longer at work, and the gentle prodding by the now-active DMN combine, this increasing the probability of the ineffable creative spark and a creative breakthrough taking place.

Now comes the time for another caveat. Any discussion of hemispheric specialization runs the risk of leaving the reader with the impression that the two halves of the brain are organized in a radically different fashion. They are not. The differences discussed here are subtle, and each hemisphere has both the local and small-world properties discussed earlier. But the emphases are subtly different: the local properties are more strongly expressed in the wiring of the left hemisphere, and the small-world properties in the wiring of the right hemisphere. The emphasis on local properties favors the emergence of a "deeply indented" network with a multitude of distinct neighborhoods, and the emphasis on small-world properties favors the emergence of a "shallower" network with less articulated neighborhoods and greater connectivity throughout (see Figure 7.5). Computational models of the human brain using the *semantic neural networks* have demonstrated that a network endowed with small-world properties is capable of generating a richer and less predictable array of novel activation

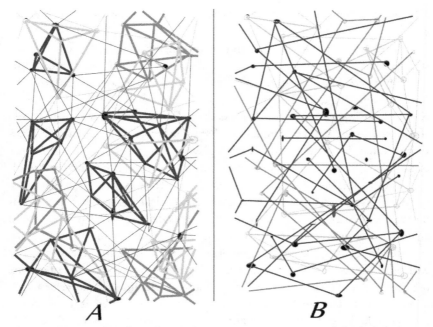

FIGURE 7.5 Deeply indented vs. shallow network connectivity. (A) Deeply indented connectivity is more articulated in the cortex of the left hemisphere. (B) Shallow connectivity is more articulated in the cortex of the right hemisphere.

Reproduced with permission from *The New Executive Brain*, Oxford University Press, 2009.

patterns—a neural basis for new-idea generation.[24] Endowing the two hemispheres with these subtle differences in their wiring properties may have been evolution's solution of reconciling and enhancing the two fundamental cornerstones of successful cognition—the ability to generate new solutions, and the ability to preserve previously accrued knowledge.

The intricate relationship between the deliberate hyperfrontal and wandering hypofrontal states in the creative process is implicitly recounted in the famous anecdotes about the moments of creative epiphany with which the history of science abounds: Archimedes discovering buoyancy while taking a bath, or Newton discovering gravity by watching a falling apple. None of these moments would have happened had these great minds not been ruminating about these subjects all along. Albert Einstein is closer to us in time, and explicit accounts exist about his spending long hours thinking through his problems systematically before the moments of epiphany appeared as if out of nowhere. At the turn of the twentieth century, Jacques Hadamard approached a number of leading physicists of the time, Einstein among them, with a questionnaire aiming to capture the nature of their creative process. Below are the excerpts from Einstein's response.

My dear Colleague,

In the following, I am trying to answer in brief your questions as well as I am able. I am not satisfied myself with these answers and I am willing to answer more questions if you believe this could be of any advantage for the very interesting and difficult work you have undertaken

(A) The words or the language, as they are written or spoken, do not seem to play any role in my mechanism of thought. The psychical entities which seem to serve as elements in thought are certain signs and more or less clear images which can be "voluntarily" reproduced and combined. There is, of course, a certain connection between those elements and relevant logical concepts. It is also clear that the desire to arrive finally at logically connected concepts is the emotional basis of this rather vague play with the above-mentioned elements. But taken from a psychological viewpoint, this combinatory play seems to be the essential feature in productive thought—before there is any connection with logical construction in words or other kinds of signs which can be communicated to others.

(B) The above mentioned elements are, in my case, of visual and some of muscular type. Conventional words or other signs have to be sought for laboriously only in a secondary stage when the mentioned associative play is sufficiently established and can be reproduced at will.

(C) According to what has been said, the play with the mentioned elements is aimed to be analogous to certain logical connections one is searching for.

(D) Visual and motor. In a stage when words intervene at all, they are in my case purely auditive, but they interfere only in a secondary stage as already mentioned.

(E) It seems to me what you call full consciousness is a limit case which can never be fully accomplished. This seems to me connected with the fact called the narrowness of consciousness (*Enge des Bewusstseins*).

Remark: Professor Max Wertheimer has tried to investigate the distinction between mere associating or combining of reproducible elements and between understanding (*organisches Begreifen*); I cannot judge how far his psychological analysis catches the essential point.

With kind regards,
Albert Einstein[25]

The relationship between the deliberate and the "wandering" states in the creative process is iterative: the deliberate state precedes the "wandering" one and also follows it. Einstein's sense that his account fails to capture the essence of the process is revealing, as is his sense that "words of language . . . do not seem to play any role in my mechanisms of thought" and that "conventional words or other signs have to be sought for laboriously only in a secondary stage when the mentioned associative play is sufficiently established and can be reproduced at will." This is suggestive both of "afrontal" and of the predominantly right-hemispheric nature of the "creative spark," followed by a more conscious and deliberate formulation in symbolic terms—essentially a left-hemisphere mediated enterprise. In my own humble way, I can relate to this owing to my early studies at University of Moscow where I had a dual psychology-mathematics major. I recall noting as a student (and marveling at this) that the mental process of *formulating* a mathematical statement, a theorem, often had very little to do with the process of *proving* it once it had been formulated.

Many creative individuals report almost dreamlike states with solutions to daunting problems or artistic images appearing effortlessly, as if by themselves. But they also report hard, focused mental effort preceding these magical moments. The revelation of the benzene structure as a vision of a snake devouring its tail that came to August Kekulé in a dreamlike state is an oft-cited experience of mental wandering, seemingly effortless and "afrontal." But what is less often mentioned is that the revelation came to Kekulé after years of grinding work on the subject—very much a frontal-lobe-driven activity. You also hear accounts of a creative individual spending a day of mentally exhausting struggling with an intractable problem, going to bed and waking up with a solution the next morning. These are all manifestations of the synergistic interaction of the two sides of a creative process: one conscious, driven by the frontal lobes, and the other one unconscious, or at least less conscious—directed mental wandering. In the creative process characterized by an essential duality, the frontal-lobe driven conscious part intertwined with the "afrontal" mental wandering, trying to figure out which component is more important than the other is an idle exercise. The epiphany, that incomparable triumph of birthing something new and important, arises from the synergistic interplay between the two.

Einstein's mention of Max Wertheimer's work is interesting and in a way prescient. Wertheimer was one of the three founding fathers of Gestalt psychology (Kurt Koffka and Wolfgang Köhler were the other two). In an uncanny way, the process of arriving at a creative solution through the combination of the "frontal" and "afrontal" processes outlined earlier in this chapter resembles experiments of Gestalt psychologists in the beginning of the twentieth century. They discovered that human perception tends to "connect the dots": presented with a set of dots arranged along the imagined contour of a familiar shape—a triangle or a circle—an observer tends to mentally connect the disjointed dots and perceive them as a continuous image (Figure 7.6).

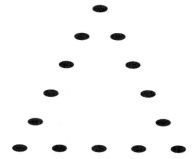

FIGURE 7.6 An example of Gestalt phenomenon. The dots are mentally "connected": they are perceived as a triangle.

And it has been said that the right hemisphere perceives environment in "gestalts." It appears that the old intuition about the psychological properties of the right hemisphere, which for decades was merely a heuristic metaphor, may have presciently captured some important properties of the creative process that could only be grasped with the benefit of neuroscientific discoveries made many years later: the frontal lobes help identify the dots by activating disparate regions within vast and far-flung neural nets, and the afrontal mental wandering connects them into a coherent network. An allusion to the Gestalt-closing nature of the creative moment, evocative of the coalescence of a cohesive neural net, is found in a letter written by the great Wolfgang Amadeus Mozart where he attempts to capture the process of creating a musical composition. At a certain point, Mozart does not hear in his imagination "the parts successively, but . . . as it were, all at once (*gleich alles zusammen*)."[26]

Gestalt-psychologists' prescience is remarkable but not unique. It is not uncommon for a modern scientific concept or theory to have an early, vague prefiguration decades and even centuries earlier. Remember, we all stand on the shoulders of giants, and the discontinuity in the intellectual history of society is closely intertwined with continuity. Early antecedents of the atomic theory of matter had existed already in ancient India and Greece, more than two millennia before modern chemistry came into being; an early antecedent of calculus was practiced already by Archimedes almost two millennia before it coalesced into a developed branch of mathematics; and if Freud's ideas were prescient and resonate in many ways with modern neuroscience, then why not Gestalt psychologists? This invokes the concept introduced by another giant on whose shoulders we all stand, the philosopher Georg Wilhelm Friedrich Hegel (1770–1831)—the dialectical spiral of progress.

Iteration and Selection

We end this chapter where we started—with blind variation and selective retention, or BVSR. In the beginning of the chapter, we argued that a totally random blind variation is not an informationally realistic scenario for how novel ideas are generated, and most of the chapter was devoted to outlining an alternative scenario that we called "directed wandering." In contrast, selective retention is a necessary, even obligatory part of the process. A creative individual must be extraordinarily lucky to hit upon the winning solution right away. This means that the product of a "creative spark" must be refined and evaluated for its effectiveness and relevance in meeting the goal. This part of the process is more likely to be conscious, to involve language or other symbolic systems as noted by Albert Einstein in his introspective account, and to be guided by the frontal lobes. Selection among alternatives has been more extensively studied, and is less mysterious and better understood than the way in which the alternatives are generated. The role of the prefrontal cortex in the selection and critical appraisal of choices, once the choices have been generated, has been long established.[27] This means that the creative process is an iterative cycle: *hyperfrontality* > *hypofrontality* > *hyperfrontality*, and on and on, often extended over days, months, or years, until the good-enough solution is found and the restless mind is satisfied.

8

Is the Baboon Creative?

Novelty in Evolution

For those who, like myself, don't subscribe to an extreme belief in our species' uniqueness, any exploration of human traits would benefit from being considered in an evolutionary context; and creativity, as well as the ability to deal with novelty, is no exception. In this chapter, we will explore the evolutionary roots of these traits, which opens the door for all kinds of questions, including the following one: "Is the baboon creative?" This could be a difficult question to answer, and the answer depends on how we define creativity. Radical anthropomorphic exceptionalism would imply that creativity is by definition a uniquely human attribute, but one can argue that such reasoning is both circular and outdated. If primatologists like Frans de Waal are right in arguing that cognitive differences—as well as cognitive similarities—between humans and other species are best understood as gradual and incremental, rather than binary and precipitous, then we must assume that some cognitive ingredients of creativity can be traced throughout evolution.[1]

It was precisely my embrace of the premise of evolutionary continuities, rather than abrupt discontinuities, that has prompted the hypothesis of hemispheric specialization based on the distinction between cognitive novelty and cognitive routines, which we discussed in Chapter 6. And no matter where one stands on the issue of "animal creativity," one can be reasonably assured that the baboon is capable of processing novel information in the changing environment of the African savanna, or else it would have become extinct long time ago. Research has shown that the baboon can even learn to discriminate orthographically correct English words from orthographically implausible quasi-words—a hell of a feat of novelty-mastering considering what baboons normally do.[2]

So it is reasonable to ask the question, "Where in the baboon's brain is novelty processed?" It turns out that, like in their human fellow primates, a baboon's right hemisphere is more efficient at processing novel information than its left hemisphere is. And, like in humans, the left hemisphere takes over when the task becomes familiar. This was demonstrated in an experiment requiring the animals to match complex geometric shapes varying in their degree of novelty or familiarity. The shapes were presented to the left or right half of the visual field, projecting respectively in the right or left hemisphere. To participate in the experiment, the baboons (three males and three females) had to learn how to fixate their gaze on a centrally located fixation point and to manipulate a joystick. The experiment is a close replica of the typical experiments designed to study hemispheric specialization in humans, some of which were described in earlier chapters; and the fact that the baboons were able to learn "the rules of the game" and to follow them is in itself a remarkable demonstration of their intelligence. The findings were also remarkably human-like. In the beginning of the experiment, when the task was novel, the baboons' performance was faster when the stimuli were presented to the left half of the visual field and consequently projected to the right hemisphere, but by the end of the experiment, this effect disappeared. The authors concluded that "hemispheric lateralization changes with practice and that the right hemisphere of the baboon plays a critical role in the processing of novelty"—very much like the conclusion we reached in Chapter 6 with respect to the human brain.[3] And this remarkable similarity of hemispheric specialization in humans and baboons is no longer a joke; it suggests an evolutionary continuity in the way novelty is handled in the brain.

Creativity Across Species

What is the baboon doing in a book about human innovation and creativity? Since Darwin's times, scientists have recognized that we are better able to understand our own species by placing it in the evolutionary context, and the fact that novelty-processing in the baboon also relies on the right hemisphere helps accomplish precisely that. The search for evolutionary precursors of human creativity is an attractive research target, but defining creativity in other species is a dicey proposition, particularly since we are often at a loss how to define it in our own. Novel behaviors are easier to recognize, define, and measure. When it comes to the ability to generate novel behaviors, the baboon is not alone. In a 2009 paper in *Scientific American,* Peter MacNeilage, Lesley Rogers, and Giorgio Vallortigara proposed that the division of labor linking novelty to the right hemisphere and established routines to the left hemisphere has been the defining feature of brain organization for the 500 million years of vertebrate evolution.[4] Indeed, already in rodents, the right and left hippocampi serve different functions at different stages of memory formation.[5]

The club of brain-lateralized species capable of generating novel behaviors is not limited to terrestrial creatures; it includes also *cetaceans*—an order of marine mammals consisting of whales, dolphins, and porpoises. Dolphins are particularly interesting in several respects. Apart from humans, great apes, and elephants, they are the only creatures whose brains contain von Economo (or "spindle") cells, the neurons with very long axons capable of providing rapid communication between distant brain regions and presumed to be associated with high intelligence and problem-solving capacity and with social behavior. Highly intelligent animals, they are capable of complex problem-solving and perhaps even of creativity of sorts.

To support the latter claim that cetaceans may be in some sense creative, a study conducted in 1965 at the Makapuu Oceanic Center in Hawaii is often cited.[6] Two female rough-toothed porpoises, Malia and Hou, were "encouraged" to generate novel behaviors. On any given day, the only behaviors that were reinforced were those that had not been exhibited the day before. Within a few days, the animals began to exhibit behaviors (various kinds of aerial flips, gliding with the tail above water, "skidding" on the tank floor) that were quite complex, and many of which were unlike anything seen in any rough-toothed porpoise by the marine park staff before. The porpoises appeared to have grasped the idea that to get reinforcement (fish), they had to generate novel behaviors, and they met the challenge in a "creative" way. Since the porpoises were coming up with behaviors different from those exhibited in previous sessions on a number of successive days, it has been argued that, however you define creativity, the porpoises were capable of forming a general concept of "novel" behavior. As in humans, individual differences in "creativity" were also evident: Malia's novel behaviors were "more spectacular and 'imaginative'" than Hou's.[7] Moreover, in order to continue coming up with new behaviors, the two porpoises had to keep in memory which behaviors they had already exhibited in the previous sessions—an impressive feat of working memory as well. In Chapter 4, we discussed how this particular frontal-lobe–dependent form of memory manifests itself in the monkey and in humans, and now we encounter it also in the porpoises, this further attesting to their advanced cognition.

Lateralization Across Species

How are the brains of these creatures wired to enable such prodigious cognitive feats? Tasks involving visual discrimination are particularly instructive, since in cetaceans, visual pathways are completely crossed (unlike in the human brain, where only the nasal pathways are crossed). This makes it easier to make assumptions about the hemispheric specialization on the basis of their behavior: left-eye preference or advantage in performing certain tasks implicates the right hemisphere and right-eye preference implicates the left hemisphere. A number of studies have been conducted, leading to the conclusion that the cetacean brain is functionally lateralized, and that the distinctions between novelty and familiarity, and between unique items and general rules, capture some important features of this lateralization.

Porpoises are not the only cetaceans endowed with considerable intelligence. Their distant cousins, bottlenose dolphins, are capable of forming rudimentary numerosity concepts, and this ability seems to be linked to the left hemisphere.[8] On the other hand, "inquisitive" behavior engages the left eye (right hemisphere) more frequently than the right eye (left hemisphere).[9] Somewhat inconsistently with these findings, the left eye (right hemisphere) was mostly used to examine familiar objects and the right eye (left hemisphere) to examine unfamiliar objects in other dolphin species.[10]

And then there are birds: Contrary to the dismissive scorn implicit in the expression "birdbrained," many avian species are capable of complex learning and problem-solving. Any doubter should read the book by the science writer Jennifer Ackerman *The Genius of Birds*.[11] Various parrot species, like Goffin cockatoos of Indonesia, for instance, exhibit complex cognitive skills, like inference by exclusion, tool making, and solving technical puzzles.[12]

But birds accomplish their cognitive feats by relying on a neural architecture very different from the mammalian one. In mammals, most complex cognition is supported by the cortex arranged in several (usually six) layers—laminae. In contrast, in birds, cognitive complexity—often rivaling the mammalian one—is carried out by a complex collection of nuclei. According to the modern view of the vertebrate evolution, it diverged into the branches eventually resulting in the mammals and birds sometime during Permian period, more than 200 million years ago.[13]

This means that any similarities between the mammalian and avian brains may reflect some evolutionarily very early and very fundamental principles of neural organization. Alternatively, it may reflect "convergent evolution"—an independent development of similar adaptations in vastly different species, which would also attest to the fundamental utility of this principle. So is the avian brain lateralized, and in which way? It turns out that it is, and a more lateralized avian brain solves problems more efficiently than a less lateralized brain in several species, which include the Australian parrot, domestic chick, and others.[14]

Not only is the avian brain lateralized, but the functional differences between its left and right sides strongly parallel those observed in the mammalian brains, including the human. The more a visual pattern is rewarded, the more strongly it activates the bird's left hemisphere.[15] The same is true for learning the importance

("salience" discussed in Chapter 5) of auditory stimuli, when one song was associated with food and the other one was not. Once the salience rule was learned
and neuronal activity was recorded from the two sides of the zebra finch brain,
it turned out that the fast-learning birds had more activity in the left hemisphere
than the slow-learning birds. Both stimulus familiarity and its salience were
encoded predominantly in the left hemisphere![16]

Remember, we have already encountered an association between salience and
the left hemisphere—in the *human* brain. The link between salience and the
bird's left hemisphere revealed itself in an especially dramatic way when mating
behaviors were examined. In choosing a female mate, the male zebra finch relies
on its right eye (and therefore on the left hemisphere) to such an exclusive degree
that when its right eye is occluded, the bird is simply unable to make the choice.[17]

Experiments with bird-song learning are particularly intriguing. They reveal
the contrasting roles of the bird brain's hemispheres in representing familiar as
opposed to novel stimuli, which uncannily resemble those we encountered earlier in the human brain. Youngster zebra finches learn their songs by imitating
an adult "tutor" bird's song. It turns out that the previously learned tutor song
activates the bird's left hemisphere in particular; in contrast an unfamiliar song
does not.[18] And as the song is being learned and memorized, significantly more
neurons become activated in the left than in the right hemisphere.[19]

The baboon, the porpoise, and the finch are far apart on the vertebrate evolutionary tree, yet they exhibit similar patterns of hemispheric specialization: novelty and uniqueness are processed mostly by the right hemisphere, and familiar
patterns and categories by the left hemisphere. This is indeed a general principle
of brain organization that either emerged early in evolution and has been conserved across far-flung branches of the vertebrate evolutionary tree, or (probably
less likely) represented an amazingly consistent point of convergence in the independent evolution of diverse species (Figure 8.1).

How universal is brain lateralization and the distinction between novelty
and familiarity embodied in this lateralization? Can it be observed also in the
invertebrate nervous system? The answer to this intriguing question hinges on
the honeybee's antennae, the two protrusions used by the insect to sample odors.
Despite its unassuming position on the evolutionary tree, the tiny creature is
capable of memorizing and distinguishing odors, and its basic dynamics of learning are uncannily human-like. Once an olfactory memory had been formed using
both antennae, "short-term" recall (one to two hours after training) required the
integrity of the right antenna, but "long-term" recall (23–24 hours after training)
required the integrity of the left antenna (note that the pathways are uncrossed in
the honey bee, which means that the right antenna projects into the right half of
the brain and the left antenna into the left half).[20]

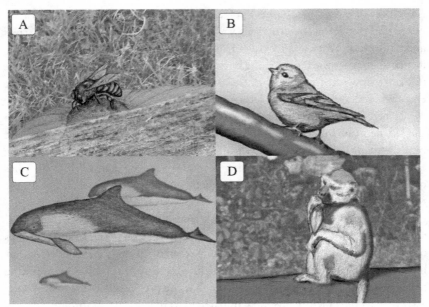

FIGURE 8.1 **Honeybee, finch, porpoise, baboon.** These very different animals have similar brain organizations: entrenched routines are linked to the left half of the brain, and processing novel information, to the right half.

That the nervous systems of such disparate living organisms should exhibit so impressively similar patterns of functional lateralization is nothing short of astounding. Whether this similarity is a result of successive evolution of a common ancestor with a remarkable conservation of certain principles of brain organization across species, or is a product of "convergent" evolution coming up with similar neural architectures independently in different species, is a matter of intense and still-unresolved debate in biology. Nor is the uniformity of lateralization clearly understood. Many scientists believe that this uniformity is peculiar to species engaged in social behavior, and less common in solitary species.[21]

Whichever way these controversies are eventually resolved, the distinction between cognitive novelty and cognitive routines is fundamental, and separating their processing in the brain appears to confer a universal computational advantage. As we already discussed, the distinction between information processing that is or is not driven by previously formed routines is far more fundamental than the distinction between verbal and nonverbal processing, the latter being merely a narrow special case of the former. The results of the functional neuroimaging experiments with human subjects described in earlier chapters find resonance in virtually every niche of the evolutionary tree. The theme of the right hemisphere specialization for tackling novelty and the left hemisphere for guiding routine behaviors pervades much of the vertebrate and even invertebrate evolution. Having examined the brain mechanisms of confronting novelty in other species, we are finding striking parallels with our own.

Human Development and Animal Creativity
Proximal Development

Whatever the brain mechanisms of aptitude for novelty processing are, how do you measure this aptitude in other species to begin with? The idea for a novel approach to measuring novelty aptitude (another pun intended) discussed here is based on "the zone of proximal development"—a concept introduced by Lev Vygotsky, a Jewish Russian psychologist who worked in the Soviet Union in the beginning of the twentieth century. Vygotsky was arguably one of the two most seminal students of cognitive development in children, the other one being Jean Piaget, the Swiss psychologist, whose work is much better known in the West. Through an uncanny coincidence, they were born in the same year, 1896—but their life trajectories were very different. Piaget lived a long and productive life in the stable and protected world of a European academic and educational policy-maker. Vygotsky died young of tuberculosis in the volatile and turbulent environment of post-revolutionary Russia on the verge of the impending Stalin's purges which makes the significance of his intellectual legacy even more remarkable.

Both Vygotsky and Piaget were interested in the stages of cognitive development and their progression, but their approaches were very different, in a way reflecting the disparities in their personal intellectual histories. Piaget's early interests were in zoology, and his first publications were about mollusks. In contrast, Vygotsky's early interests were in the humanities, and his first publications were essays about the psychology of literature and the arts. These essays were posthumously compiled in a book, which, for political reasons, could only be published more than 30 years after his death, titled *The Psychology of Art*,[22] whose copy, inscribed by Vygotsky's widow, was among the few books in my sparse luggage when I came to the United States in 1974 (Figure 8.2).

The different routes that brought them to developmental psychology were reflected in their theories. Piaget thought of the stages of cognitive development as a preordained unfolding driven by hard-wired intrinsic biological rules. In contrast, Vygotsky thought of cognitive development as being prodded by the cultural milieu through explicit instruction, which allows the child to attain the cognitive skills above and beyond those attainable by the child on her or his own. If you think of cognitive development as an expanding space, then "the zone of proximal development" is the area reflecting the difference between the expansion attainable to the child learning on her or his own and the additional

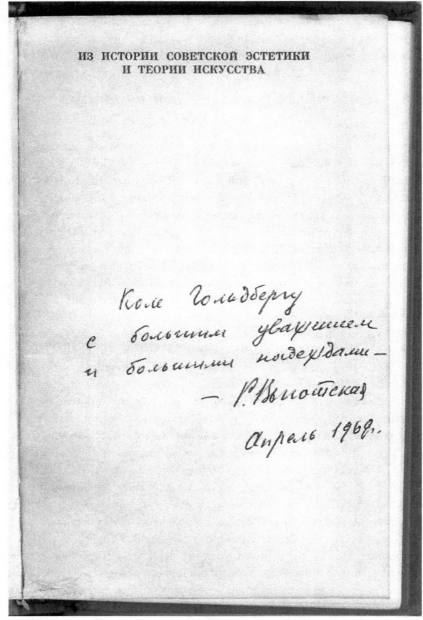

FIGURE 8.2 Lev Vygotsky's *Psikhologiya Iskusstva,* with his widow's inscription. A page from *Psikhologiya Iskusstva* [*The Psychology of Art*] by Lev Vygotsky (2nd edition, published in 1968 in the Soviet Union) with the inscription and signature by the author's widow, Roza Noyevna Vygotskaia. The inscription reads: "To Kolya [*my Russian nickname*] Goldberg with great respect and great expectations. R. Vygotskaia, April 1969."

From Elkhonon Goldberg's personal library.

expansion made possible through instruction. Vygotsky argued that two children (and presumably adults) may perform similarly on tests reflecting their current knowledge and cognitive skills, yet be characterized by very different-sized "zones of proximal development."[23]

Vygotsky believed that the size of the "proximal development zone" varies from person to person, and that this variable captures a crucial attribute of the human mind, as well as the individual differences between human minds. Why so? Because this is how humans learn. Without explicit instruction and introduction to the cognitive tools implicitly crystallized in culture, it is doubtful that any of us would have learned how to read, write, and compute on our own—it would be just too much for any individual, no matter how talented and creative, to reinvent from scratch. At a more exalted level, even the most solitary and daring discovery or conceptual breakthrough by the most talented scientist or artist has been "instructed" by the culture in which it takes place, and it gets ahead of the host culture only so far—the zone of proximal development again. Although Archimedes already used infinitesimals and the method of exhaustion in his work, he did not parlay this into a coherent discipline. Calculus as a well-articulated branch of mathematics had to await its birth almost two millennia longer, until it was finally introduced by Isaac Newton and Gottfried Wilhelm Leibnitz in the second half of the seventeenth century. Here is a prime example of the broad cultural and scientific milieu both propelling and delimiting the mental powers of an individual genius. The concept introduced by Lev Vygotsky to characterize the cognitive development in children can also serve as a useful heuristic device to capture the relationship between the process of individual creativity and capacity for innovation, and the host culture. Vygotsky was one of the first psychologists to explicitly attempt an integration of the biological and cultural perspectives on cognition, which makes his intellectual legacy directly relevant to the studies of creativity.

Vygotsky's Legacy He Did Not Plan

So what is Lev Vygotsky, a student of cognitive development in human children, doing in the chapter on animal intelligence? He is here because, even though Vygotsky's own research was on human cognitive development, the utility of the "zone of proximal development" as an index of the capacity for mastering novelty is not limited to our species (Figure 8.3). It is applicable to any species capable of learning, and in fact we often use it to gauge the cognitive potential of these species without calling it so. When placed in the company of humans, animals often display dazzling feats of novelty-mastering that they would not have accomplished on their own and that are completely outside of their ecologically natural

Zone of Proximal Development

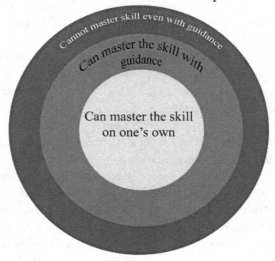

FIGURE 8.3 The zone of proximal development according to Lev Vygotsky.

behaviors or cognitive demands. Ironically, Vygotsky himself believed that the "zone of proximal development" was a uniquely human attribute not found in non-human primates, but the research conducted on a variety of species since his death in 1934 proves him wrong. Paradoxically, by so doing, it only amplifies the importance of Vygotsky's ideas.

The oft-quoted examples of what can be construed as the primate "zone of proximal development" in action include Koko the lowland gorilla, who (yes, she is an individual and not an object!) acquired a large vocabulary of words in American Sign Language and was even able to combine them into novel statements expressing her wishes and even emotional states. Chantek the orangutan, raised by the primatologist Lyn White Miles as her "foster son," also acquired a large vocabulary of signed words and was even able to conjure up composite new ones, like "tomato-toothpaste" for "ketchup," and "cheese-meat-bread" for "cheeseburger."[24] Kanzi the bonobo is also famous for his mastery of cognitive novelty. He (another individual!) learned a vocabulary of 384 or more lexigrams (visual symbols representing things or ideas) and was able to use this knowledge to communicate by pointing at the lexigrams arranged on a keyboard. Kanzi accomplished this feat even without the benefit of explicit instruction but merely by watching his mother, Matata (in fact his adoptive "mother" who stole Kanzi from his natural parents) being taught. Subsequently, Kanzi's sister, Panbanisha, and her sons Nyota and Nathan also learned the lexigraphic language. But Kanzi remains unsurpassed by being the first, and very likely the only so far, bilingual ape, having also learned some American Sign Language by watching videos of Koko the gorilla using it.[25] Not to be upstaged by other great apes, chimpanzees have the cognitive ability to cook, given the appropriate tools and instruction by their human companions, as a recent study has shown.[26] And don't forget the baboon mastering the orthographic rules of the English language.

At a less exalted but closer-to-home level, consider a dog, a family pet, learning a range of verbal or hand commands. This is usually accomplished through explicit training, but not always. My late bullmastiff, Brit (to me he was definitely an individual of great importance whom I miss to this day) learned a number of verbal commands just by my using them in context rather than through an explicit drill, and my new English mastiff puppy, Brutus, is showing a lot of promise in this direction at the tender age of 11 months old. At the same time, I never attempted to teach either Brit or Brutus algebra. Brit did display a rudimentary sense of numerosity in the form of the anticipated number of cookies he was used to getting as a "nightcap" every evening (and objected whenever I came short), but this was probably as far as his "zone of proximal development" could stretch, and I did not attempt to push the envelope.

The capacity for acquiring cognitive skills far outstripping those evident in their natural behavior, through direct interaction with a human "instructor," is not limited to mammals. The long-standing "collaboration" between the Grey parrot Alex and the cognitive psychologist Irene Pepperberg is a remarkable case in point. Under Pepperberg's tutelage, Alex learned how to "name" more than 50 objects, seven colors, five shapes, and quantities up to six (later extended to seven and eight). He even learned how to construct simple phrases expressing his wishes and had some understanding of the relationship between numbers.[27]

The "zone of proximal development" as a measure of novelty-mastering is rich in implications and possibilities. There are two general ways of studying it in other species: by measuring their ability to learn from humans, and by measuring their ability to learn from members of their own species. Indeed, the "instructor" pushing the boundaries of an animal's "zone of proximal development" does not have to be human; it may be a member of its own kind. As a result of such social rather than biological transmission of information from one member of the species to another, and from one generation to the other, certain behaviors and skills may be present and conserved in one animal pack but absent in another pack of the same species. This phenomenon has become known as "animal culture." While the connotations implicit in this term remain controversial, the observations leading to coining it speak for themselves.

Soon after the end of World War II, the Japanese primatologist Kinji Imanishi and his colleagues set out to study Japanese macaques. To their surprise, they noticed that different macaque troops, all members of the same species but living in different parts of Japan, exhibited very different behaviors, ranging from different ways of rearing their babies, to their eating habits. Among the unique behaviors observed in one macaque troop but not in others, was the habit of washing sweet potatoes in a stream before eating them.[28] In a similar vein, 39 different behavior patterns affecting tool use, nest making, grooming, and courtship were documented in several chimpanzee troops, presumably as a result of cross-generational learning within communities, rather than of genetic transmission.[29] Similar "culturally transmitted" behaviors acquired through imitation or even through direct instruction of a baby by an adult animal, have been observed in other primates and even in rodents.[30] Not to be outdone, the Amazon parrots of Costa-Rica also exhibit "culturally transmitted" behaviors: different populations of these birds communicate in different and distinctive "dialects," which their young learn much more easily than the older birds do.[31]

The zone of proximal development has been invoked in primate research, but not often.[32] And despite my best efforts, I was unable to find anything in the scientific literature about extending this concept into the comparative neuroscience of individual differences in various species. But if the concept of a zone of proximal development is equally applicable to human and to animal cognition, then why not do what the neuroscientists have been doing for decades: use animal models as a window into the brain mechanisms of human creativity and capacity for innovation and the individual differences thereof? Research into the neurobiology of creativity is gathering speed in a number of laboratories at leading universities worldwide, but any such project runs into the problem of how to define, and even more thornily, how to measure this elusive construct. These challenges may be more surmountable in an animal study where different members of the same species are compared on the "size of their zone of proximal development," defined as the relative ease with which they master novel cognitive skills through an interaction with either a human or a non-human instructor. Having identified individual species members with relatively large and those with relatively small "zones of proximal development," it may be possible to compare their brains with a degree of detail not easily attainable in human research. And since the basic underlying neurobiology is likely to be fundamentally the same, what can be learned from such animal studies is at the very least likely to offer useful heuristic insights into the nature of the human capacity for innovation and even creativity.

Indeed, available evidence suggests that individual differences in the size of the proximal development zone exist in animal species: Malia the porpoise was more "creative" than Hou the porpoise; Kanzi the bonobo was more receptive to novelty than Matata the bonobo; certain finches learned faster than others;

and Alex the parrot seemed to far outstrip other Grey parrots in his capacity for learning "human" skills. These animals exhibited vast differences in their individual "zones of proximal development." So what are the differences in the brains of animals characterized by large vs. small "zones of proximal development"? Identifying and characterizing these differences in other species morphologically, biochemically, and genetically will open a new window on understanding them in our own. By homing in on the neurobiology underlying the individual differences among the members of these diverse species, we may gain revealing insights into the nature of such differences in humans.

On a more general note, there is a growing realization that humans are not the only species whose members are characterized by a wide range of individual differences in cognition (as a "serial" dog owner, I have known it all along). Take "personality," for instance. The whole proposition of "personality," let alone individual differences in personality traits, in species other than our own would have been met with derision even a few decades ago, but it is gaining traction among serious scientists. In a review published in *Science*, one of the most authoritative scientific journals in the world, Elizabeth Pennisi describes stable individual differences among birds, lizards, and spiders along dimensions such as sociability, reclusiveness, aggression, and propensity toward exploratory behavior.[33] If all these traits are subject to individual differences among the members of a particular species, then why not the capacity for innovation, both on one's own and through instruction? By letting go of the theologically inspired but biologically naïve notion of humans' standing totally apart from the animal kingdom, we usher in the possibility of learning about the neurobiology of such differences in humans by studying them in our close and distant cousins from the animal kingdom.

Why is the zone of proximal development's "size" a good proxy measure of the capacity for innovation and creativity? Because it models the fundamental nature of innovation, described earlier in the book, in a way that the more commonly used methods to measure creativity fail to do. An act of innovation, a creative act is inherently dual. The feat is individual, but it does not take place in isolation. It is embedded in culture: the actor "stands on the shoulders of giants." To a creative primate, his human handler is that giant, and the contact with human culture may not only alter its behavior, but impact the animal's very sense of self in profound ways that we still fail to fully grasp. This was poignantly expressed by Chantek the orangutan, who called himself "orangutan person."[34]

9

The Creative Mind

A Few Worthy Feats

Flush from his early victories over the Persians, Alexander arrived in the Phrygian capital of Gordium in today's Turkey. There he was shown an oxcart tied to a post with an intricate knot. According to an ancient prophecy, the man able to untie the "Gordian knot" would become the "King of Asia." Since this is precisely what the famously superstitious Alexander had in mind, and since his troops were watching anxiously for an omen, the knot had to be untied one way or the other. According to historians, Alexander fumbled with it for a few minutes without success. As to what happened next, the ancient sources diverge. According to the popular lore, Alexander hacked the knot with his sword and sliced it in half. But according to Plutarch and Arrian,[1] Alexander did something more subtle: he pulled out the pin that connected the knot to the pole of the chariot, allowing him to untie the knot. Either way, the Gordian knot was untied, and Alexander went on to conquer the sprawling Persian Empire and become the "King of Asia." In an odd way, the knot episode may have indeed helped him along, since in those superstitious times, an inability to untie the knot would have been perceived by Alexander's troops as a "bad omen" and would have undermined their morale, with self-fulfilling consequences.

Two thousand years later, the great mathematician Johann Friedrich Carl Gauss (1777–1855) cut his own Gordian knot while still in elementary school, when he was ordered by his irate teacher to calculate the sum of all the integers (numbers without fractions) between 1 and 100 as a punishment for unruly behavior. Where most people would have started dutifully adding the numbers one by one (in the age when there were no calculators around), the young Gauss had an instant insight that the sums of any two numbers equidistant from the middle of the sequence were the same: $1 + 100 = 2 + 99 = 3 + 98 \ldots = 50 + 51 = 101$. Since there were 50 such pairs, the solution to the problem posed by the nasty teacher (which in all likelihood the teacher himself was not aware of) was $101 \times 50 = 5050$, and it was reached by the young Gauss within seconds.[2]

One of the things that distinguishes a truly creative process from an intelligent but uninspired one is the parsimony and elegance of its solution. A number of scientists of acknowledged creative mettle have reported that the "Aha" feeling, the sense that the solution of a thorny problem is nearly at hand, is triggered by the sense of parsimony, of a particular elegance of the candidate solution. The ability to find such an unexpected solution leapfrogging over the grinding, laboriously linear line of attack on the problem is a measure of individual creativity. This is why the legend of Gordian knot has enjoyed its iconic status for over two thousand years.

A truly innovative, creative solution is often unexpected, surprising, and even counter-intuitive, at least to an ordinary observer, and so is the creative mind responsible for the solution. A potpourri of personal qualities may play a role, not always consistent or intuitively apparent, and at times even mutually contradictory. A few such qualities of the creative mind will be discussed in this chapter. The ability to come up with creative solutions implies that, aside from the conventionally defined cognitive powers, a creative individual may benefit from certain "personality" traits that are likely to be maladaptive or even outright self-defeating in everyday circumstances, such as a contrarian frame of mind. Since the individual differences in our "personalities" are also to a large extent a reflection of the individual differences in our brains, the following discussion may lead to unexpected speculations about the neural attributes of a creative brain.

Conform or Not Conform?
The Double Edge of Conformism

Kevin Joseph Sutherland lost his life on July 4, 2015, of all days. A graduate of American University, the 24-year-old Sutherland was riding the Red Line Metro in Washington, D.C., on his way to join a group of friends. The 18-year-old Jasper Spires, crazed and probably on synthetic drugs, boarded the same car with very different intentions. He grabbed Sutherland's cell phone, and when the latter resisted, punched him multiple times, knocking him to the floor, then proceeded to stomp and stab him 30 or 40 times with a knife, killing him. Spires then proceeded to rob other people in the car, exited the train on the next station unimpeded, jumped the turnstile and was gone. But while clearing the turnstile, he dropped a bag containing his ID's, and was apprehended and arrested.[3]

The killing of Kevin Sutherland was witnessed by a dozen or so horrified fellow passengers, none of whom interfered or tried to save his life. How was this so? Was it a manifestation of self-preservation bordering on cowardice, perhaps understandable in the presence of a crazed hoodlum brandishing a bloody knife? Not necessarily, opined the TV talking heads. Rather, this could have been "diffusion of responsibility" due to the "bystander effect," according to which members of a group tend to behave in a similar fashion. According to the psychiatrist Gail Saltz, a frequent CNN commentator, an individual witnessing an outrage like this when alone would be likely to intervene 85% of the time, but only about 30% of the time as a member of a larger group of bystanders. This is conformism at its worst.

Indeed, an episode like this makes "conformism" a dirty word. It makes one think of the "banality of evil" in Nazi Germany, children reporting on their parents in Stalin's Russia, and the lemminglike submissiveness of the Jonestown cult members. "Social engineers" in totalitarian regimes and petty cult demagogues like Jim Jones knew very well how to exploit the human propensity toward conformism. Nonetheless, despite its not-uncommon aberrant exploitations, the phenomenon itself is the basic glue of group behavior, with profound prosocial effects. It is the prerequisite of social cohesion both in its benign and in its malignant manifestations. Without a certain degree of coordination and consistency across individual behaviors, a social group simply cannot exist. Counter-intuitive as this may sound, conformism is, for better or worse, the glue of both totalitarian regimes and democracies alike.

Conformism appears to be a universal phenomenon pervading human decision-making in matters big and small, for good or for evil. In a famous experiment conducted by psychologist Solomon Asch, subjects were asked to match a line to one of three other lines according to their relative lengths. Even though the correct choice was obvious, most subjects were swayed at least to some degree by the blatantly incorrect response feigned by fake experiment participants to represent the "majority opinion."[4] On a more malevolent level, totalitarian ideologues have always been adept at practicing the art of "the big lie," bombarding the populace with the same message from every direction. And a cross-cultural study involving 23 countries by Simon Gächter and Jonathan Schultz has shown that the more corrupt the society is as a whole, the more fragile is the individual honesty of its citizens.[5]

Conformism appears to have strong evolutionary roots and is present even in highly hierarchically organized animal species. Ariana Strandburg-Peshkin and colleagues tracked a troop of baboons with the Global Positioning System (GPS) to find out how the decisions about the direction of troop movement are made. It turned out that the troop moves in the direction chosen by the majority of its members and not by the alpha leader—a proto-democracy in action.[6]

Conformism and the Brain

What is a discussion of conformism doing in a chapter about the creative mind? We often gain insight into the nature of things by examining their opposites. That any consequentially creative act is an exercise in nonconformity is a self-evident truth in no need of elaboration. Propensity toward nonconformity is certainly not a sufficient prerequisite of creativity, but it is arguably a necessary one. No matter how original a thinker an individual is, if any disparity between his beliefs and those prevalent in the society at large is likely to spook and stymie him, the creative process will almost certainly be aborted and brought to a screeching halt. Whatever other traits a creative individual must possess, the ability to resist the pressures implicit in such dissonance, to withstand the burden of being an iconoclast, is among them. In some societies, the cost of nonconformity to a creative individual can be shockingly high. Think of the great Galileo Galilei (1564–1642) prosecuted for his heliocentric view of cosmology by the Inquisition and forced to spend the last two decades of his life under house arrest; or of Nikolai Vavilov (1887–1943), the Soviet scientist thrown by the Stalin regime into the Gulag for his research in genetics, where he died of starvation. Think also of the modernist artists prosecuted in Nazi Germany as part of the campaign against "degenerate art" ("*Entartete Kunst*," an endearing turn of phrase coined by Joseph Goebbels); and of a similar, albeit not nearly so harsh a campaign, against Modernism in the Soviet Union under Nikita Khrushchev in the 1960s.

Enter the anterior cingulate cortex (ACC): It has been known for a while that the ACC becomes active when the organism encounters a disparity between its expectations and reality; in other words, when error detection takes place. The ACC also seems to activate preemptively, in situations when an error is *likely* to occur due to increased competition between possible responses.[7] It sounds like the ACC is a weary structure, the worrier in the brain guarding the organism against "stepping in it."

But stepping into what? We know that the emergence of cingulate cortex in evolution was linked to the emergence of social behavior, such as parenting. Mammalians with intact cingulate cortex are good parents, but damage to the cingulate cortex results in the loss of parenting skills or perhaps even of parental inclinations.[8] Damage to the cingulate cortex in the macaque monkey reduces the amount of time it spends in social interactions and increases the amount of time spent in manipulating inanimate objects.[9] Biochemical evidence points in the same direction: vasopressin, a neuropeptide closely involved in social behaviors and the regulation of emotions in mammals, is particularly active in the cingulate cortex.[10] Is it perchance the case that the error detection or error anticipation by the ACC can be best understood in the social context? Is the ACC the conformist in the brain, in charge of bringing the individual behavior into line with that of the group?

In an experiment conducted by Vasily Klucharev and his colleagues at the Donders Institute of Brain, Cognition and Behavior in The Netherlands, subjects were shown an array of female face photographs and asked to judge their beauty on a scale. Having rated a face, the subject was shown a rating presumably reflecting the majority opinion of the subject pool, significantly different from the subject's own. This dissonance between the individual opinion and that of the group resulted in a burst of activation in the ACC, which was recorded both with functional magnetic imaging (fMRI) and with magneto-encephalography (MEG); and the stronger the activation, the more eager the "dissenting" subject was to revise her own rating to bring it into line with that of the group.[11] However, the urge to conform to the majority opinion disappeared when the ACC was temporarily inhibited using a technique called repetitive Transcranial Magnetic Stimulation (rTMS).[12] The dual effect—the propensity toward conformism associated with a strong ACC activation and reversal of the effect with ACC inhibition—directly points to the role of this structure in conformist behavior.

What are the implications of these findings for understanding the differences between the conformist and nonconformist brains? Just as these experiments tell us about the brain mechanisms of conformism, they lead to intriguing hypotheses about the brain mechanisms, or at least prerequisites, of nonconformity. By this light, people with less active, or perhaps even morphologically smaller, ACCs may be less averse to disagreeing with the majority, more tolerant to the pressures of "going it alone," and thus may be better equipped for exhibiting the courage of intellectual, artistic, or possibly even moral dissent that is so important in any creative process leading to consequential innovation. Curiously, but perhaps not coincidentally, cingulate cortex is smaller in the right than in the left hemisphere, this paralleling the relative roles of the two hemispheres in dealing with cognitive novelty (right) vs. cognitive routines (left).[13] And at the risk of sounding two simplistic, I am inclined to entertain the possibility that the ACC is somewhat reduced in size or is less physiologically active in the natural left-handers, a proposition very easily falsifiable in a morphometric study (to the best of my knowledge, still waiting to be conducted).

To further examine the role of the ACC in social conformism, consider the following. In a typical functional neuroimaging experiment, the "error message," the conclusion that a mismatch has occurred between the subject's response and the correct response, which in turn triggers a surge of activation in the ACC, is not established by the subject directly. Rather, it is communicated to him by a "virtual authority figure," usually a computer screen on which one of two appraisals flash: "correct" or "wrong." The presence of the virtual authority figure "judging" the subject's behavior injects a distinct social component into the experiment, which is usually not controlled for. What would constitute an appropriate control? Perhaps a situation when a subject is asked to judge a quantity, say the length of a line, and then gets to measure the line directly and thus reach his own conclusion about the accuracy of his judgment, may serve as a control experiment. Here the dissonance between the subject's response and the correct response will be devoid of the social connotations of nonconformity. Will the degree of ACC activation in response to error detection be the same with and without the social component, or will it be different?

Or in Klucharev's experiment with judging beauty, a control experiment could involve judging age. Here, instead of matching the subject's opinion against a make-believe majority opinion, the subject's estimate would be matched against equally make-believe "actual" ages. Both tasks would involve a prediction–outcome comparison, but in the first case, this comparison will have the social connotations of conforming or not conforming with a "majority opinion," and in the second case it will not, since the individual judgment will be compared with an impersonal "fact" rather than with a group "opinion." It wouldn't be surprising if, in such an error-detection situation, devoid of social-approbation undertones, the ACC activation following a mismatch is reduced or at least different in some respect.

Note that the ACC (as well as the lateral and orbital prefrontal and fronto-insular cortex) is the seat of von Economo neurons (VEN).[14] These neurons (also known as the spindle cells) are remarkable for having very long axons projecting to the posterior cortex. As already mentioned earlier, von Economo cells provide rapid communication between the far-flung brain regions and are found in the mammalian species with very large brains and highly developed cognition and social behavior—in humans, great apes, elephants, and whales. They are more abundant in the right than in the left hemisphere and are presumed to be important in regulating social cognition and social behavior.[15]

Damage to von Economo cells is common in fronto-temporal dementia, and it results in a loss of social judgment, empathy, and self-restraint in interaction with other people.[16] This makes my assertion that reduced size of the ACC (possibly but not necessarily associated with a reduced number of von Economo cells) may be an adaptive, creativity-enhancing trait a bit disconcerting, since one would think that rapid communication between the prefrontal cortex and other parts of the brain is also an important prerequisite of a creative process—and it probably is. But this seeming contradiction may in fact be a reflection of a profound feature of the evolution of the brain and evolution in general. The evolutionary process cannot be expected to have the perfect organization of an orchestral composition. Quite the contrary, as argued the late Stephen Jay Gould, the process is full of contradictions, inconsistencies, and ad hoc adaptations. As we already know, multiple paths to creativity exist, relying on different constellations of neural structures in different creative individuals. The role of the ACC in the creative process has been posited by many authors. It is possible that both a hyperactive/large and a hypoactive/small ACC may benefit the creative process but in very different ways: by facilitating the fronto-posterior interaction via von Economo cells ("bigger is better"); or by liberating the creative person from the clutches of conformity ("less is more").

The Theory of Mind's Mixed Blessing

A true conformist will not only align his views with the declared views of other people, he will also try to anticipate views not yet declared. Such anticipatory conformity is closely intertwined with the capacity for insight into other people's minds, the "theory of mind." Of course, we know that the "theory of mind" is a good thing. We have all learned that it is among the most advanced manifestations of frontal-lobe function, that it is the glue of complex social interactions, and that individuals deficient in the "theory of mind" department are at a huge social disadvantage. It is quite obvious that it is indispensable in many fields of creative endeavor.

A performing artist must have a connection with the audience on a visceral if not intellectual level, and so does a talented "natural" politician. The ability to "read" the audience is essential to the success of either. This is probably true in any pursuit where a creative individual must resonate with the general public. An entrepreneur must not only have a good sense of the consumers' current collective frame of mind, but must be able to anticipate the direction of its change. Steve Jobs, the founder of Apple, has been celebrated not only for his technical acumen but even more so for his ability to anticipate, and even "create" the public's perceived needs. On the other hand, when George Boole (1815–1864) first introduced what is known today as Boolean algebra or Boolean logic in the middle of the nineteenth century in a book with the lofty title *An Investigation of the Laws of Thought*, how much was he guided by the prescience that, a century later, his mathematical invention would become the foundation of the brave new world of computers and other digital technologies? Probably not so much.[17] "Nothing is more practical than a good theory," is an oft-quoted maxim attributed to the psychologist Kurt Lewin (1890–1947), and it is generally true. But this does not always mean that the creative mind behind a "good theory" was necessarily driven by the anticipation of its practical applications; more likely than not, it was driven by the internal logic of the discipline and a personal sense of intrinsic intellectual importance.

So, is it perchance possible that a ground-breaking mathematician or theoretical physicist may find obliviousness to the majority opinion of his peers—both declared and particularly anticipated—liberating? After all, too keen an awareness of such opinions may be intimidating and invite conformism. A keenly developed capacity for the "theory of mind" may be an indispensable asset in certain creative pursuits and a stymying liability in others.

How do we measure the capacity for insight into other people's minds, the "theory of mind" ability? A number of paradigms to study it exist, and they usually focus on "duets," on the insight of one individual into the mind of another. But it is equally or more interesting, particularly in the context of our discussion, to measure the ability of an individual to form insight into a "collective" frame of mind, a weighted average of sorts, capturing the group opinion, attitude, or thought processes. How does one measure an individual insight into a group's collective mind?

Consider a game "2/3 of the average." A player is asked to choose a whole number (an integer) between 0 and 100 which is 2/3 of the average number picked by other people playing this game. In effect, the game is about the theory of mind, but of a group rather than an individual mind. Someone completely devoid of this ability may simply pick 67. This is the highest number one can pick without breaking the rules, but to pick it, one must be completely oblivious to other players. The game participants are unlikely to make this choice, since individuals that obtuse are not likely to be interested in a cerebral game of this sort to begin with; they are more likely to be having a beer in the neighborhood bar. Someone who considers other people's mental states would assume that other players' number has to be no greater than 2/3 of 67, or 45. Someone who credits other players with a deeper "theory of mind" will consider yet another step (resulting in 30), or even more such steps. A collection of totally "rational" players will continue this iteration to its logical end, each reaching the solution of 0, an outcome known in game theory as an example of the "Nash equilibrium."[18]

But as behavioral economics has taught us, real flesh-and-blood human beings are almost never "infinitely rational," and "rationality" comes in vastly different doses in different individuals. It may have taken academic economists decades to discover that the models built on the assumption of "perfect rationality" rarely capture the behavior of real people, but practical decision-makers have known it all along. One of them, arguably an exceptional individual in his own right, named Napoleon Bonaparte was reported to have famously commented that winning a battle had less to do with having a "perfect" battle plan and more with accurately anticipating the opponent's imperfect moves. Accordingly, a thoughtful player of the "2/3 of the average" game will make the choice based on his assumptions about other players' assumptions.

In that spirit, when I first played the game online, I made a set of arbitrary assumptions that in a typical sample of players, 10% would pick 45; 20% would pick 30; 40% would pick 20; 20% would pick 13; and the remaining 10% would pick 9. This resulted in an estimate of 22 as the average number picked by a typical sample of players, and 14 or 15 as my choice for the puzzle solution. How accurate were my assumptions about the mental processes of my fellow players? To find out, I visited the game's website, where the results for the most recent hundred players were displayed daily.[18] On five consecutive days, they were on the average 10, 9, 10, 10, and 12. It looked like the other players had a slightly more flattering view of me than I of them. I underestimated the group "theory of mind" of my fellow players, but not by a lot.

But this is me, a rather ordinary clinical neuropsychologist. How would individuals with a recognized record of consequential innovation and creativity perform on a test like this? Would the results be uniform, or "domain-specific," perhaps even vastly different for different brands of creativity? Would different performance profiles on such "theory of mind" tasks be reflected in distinct differences in the players' brains revealed in neuroimaging findings? Would an exceptional capacity for innovation and creativity be reflected in a distinct "theory of mind" profile at all? Or would there be no relationship between the two, and performance on games like "2/3 of the average" be the same in brilliant individuals and in ordinary Joe Blows? To the extent that there is a difference, will there be a positive correlation between creativity and the "theory of mind" insight, or will it take the counter-intuitive form of more creativity associated with less "theory of mind" insight? These are interesting questions that have yet to be systematically asked, and the games like "2/3 of the average," while they have been used in behavioral economics research, have yet to be imported into the research arsenal of broader cognitive neuroscience.

My sampling of the average "2/3" response by 100 players over several days produced extremely stable results: on any given day, it was between 9 and 12. Assuming that the people drawn to this game are not themselves a group of outliers (other than possessing lively, intelligent minds), this result suggests a surprising—at least to me—uniformity of "theory of mind" reasoning in the general population on a game such as this. In order to control for the more trivial explanation that very few people were playing the game and the pool of "100 most recent players" did not change considerably across any five consecutive days, I checked the website for another five days, this time more dispersed, a few months later. The average guesses made by the players were very similar to those before: 12, 13, 13, 13, 14 (and closer to my own guess).

The uniformity of performance among the "ordinary" people (assuming, of course, that those drawn to a game such as this are "ordinary") would make the "2/3 of the average" and other such games well-suited for identifying individuals with unusual "theory of mind" processes, perhaps including those endowed with unusual talents of various kinds.

Creativity and Intelligence

How creative is an intelligent mind? How intelligent is a creative mind? The relationship between intelligence and creativity has intrigued psychologists for decades, and research on this relationship has expanded into a whole genre, whose father was arguably Joy Paul Guilford (1897–1987). The question posed by Guilford went as follows: "Is creativity a corollary of general intelligence, or is it a separate trait which can be at variance with the general intelligence?" Guilford posited that a meaningful level of creativity requires a relatively high intelligence, but at very high levels of intelligence, this relationship breaks down. This became known as the "threshold" theory, according to which intelligence and creativity were somewhat correlated in people with an IQ below 120, but the correlation no longer held for higher IQ values. Some of the more recent research seems to provide support for this notion.[19]

Of course, any rigorous discussion of intelligence and creativity, together or separately, hinges on our ability to operationalize and quantify these constructs. In the contemporary literature, *intelligence* is usually operationalized as the intelligence quotient (IQ) measured by the most current version of the Wechsler Adult Intelligence Scale, or WAIS. How about creativity? Guilford introduced the concept of "divergent thinking" (which he contrasted with "convergent thinking"), and it became the cornerstone of creativity research and measurement. But what exactly is it? In his delightfully creative book *Creativity 101*, James Kaufman defines divergent thinking as a "response to questions with no obvious, singular answers."[20] Well . . . it sounds like an attempt to define "divergent thinking" is an exercise in divergent thinking.

So what, exactly, are we measuring? Psychologists are rightfully concerned about the "ecological validity" of their tests—the degree to which they reflect real-life cognitive demands. How about the "existential validity" of our tests— the degree to which they reflect what is important and consequential? When co-workers and acquaintances think of Johnny as being "highly intelligent," they mean "bright" or "smart"; and when they think of Bobby as being of "low intelligence," they mean "dumb" or "stupid." They have no idea what Johnny and Bobby's respective WAIS-IQ's expressed as three- (or, well . . . two-) digit numbers are, and they don't care. What they do care about is that elusive yet "I know it when I see it" quality of the individual that we refer to in everyday parlance (as distinct from psychological research or clinical reports) as "intelligence."

An implicit assumption has pervaded our culture that this elusive quality is captured by and can be quantified in a single number. The notion of "general intelligence," presumably captured in the magic IQ, has been firmly entrenched in the popular culture for decades. Numerous bureaucratic, administrative, and legal dispositions are based on this implicit assumption, and hundreds of scientific papers have been written about it. Yet the whole notion that WAIS-IQ is a meaningful measure of "Intelligence with a capital I" may have been an almost comical consequence of an accident of word choice. Had David Wechsler named his famous IQ test "The Wechsler Adult Mental Function Test," or "The New York–Bellevue Mental Function Test," or "The Happy Psychologist's Romp Test," or anything else other than "The Wechsler Adult Intelligence Test," it is very possible that none of the surplus meaning implicit in the lofty word "intelligence" would have become attached to it, and the notion of a variable capturing human "intelligence" in a single number may have never arisen. But this is precisely what happened. It has been asserted that the individual variation in intelligence defined through IQ will predict individual variation on any cognitive task.[21] However, even aside from the concern that "any" is a very big place, the fact that IQ is calculated as a derivative measure summarizing individual performance on a large number of specific tasks makes this assertion inherently circular.

What is the relationship between the WAIS-IQ, or, for that matter, of any other psychometric measure of "intelligence," and the everyday judgment passed by individuals about one another and placing them on the intuitive "bright–dumb" continuum? We don't know. In my earlier book *The New Executive Brain*,[22] I proposed an experiment designed to clarify this relationship. To the best of my knowledge, it has yet to be conducted.

Let's sketch out a modified version of this experiment here. Two demographically matched panels of lay participants, all unfamiliar with psychological theories of intelligence (no psychologists onboard!), will be assembled: "interviewers" and "interviewees" (these may be two different groups, or one group with every member performing both functions). Each "interviewer" will spend a pre-specified period of time (perhaps a few hours) with each "interviewee" in a freewheeling or semi-structured interaction. Based on this interaction, each interviewer will rate each interviewee on a multipoint "bright–dumb" (BD) scale, and an average BDQ (for "Bright–Dumb Quotient) value will be computed for each interviewee, this resulting in ranking them on the BD scale. Each interviewee will also be given the most current version of the Wechsler Adult Intelligence Test (WAIS-IV at the time of this writing)[23] or some other commonly used psychometric "intelligence" scale, and their IQs acquired in this fashion will be ranked. How well will the IQ ranking be correlated with the BDQ ranking? This is an interesting question that allows a straightforward answer, yet to be obtained. Let's table this as Experiment 1.

A similar question can be asked with respect to creativity. When we judge someone as "creative" and someone else as devoid of originality, we have no idea how they would perform on a test of "divergent thinking," and we don't particularly care. Yet, based on our assessment of the products of their labors, we have some sense of how creative different members of "creative" professions and entrepreneurs are. Scientists, artists, and entrepreneurs constantly compare themselves to their peers, as well as their peers to one another, and such peer ratings have been used in a number of creativity research projects.[24] In that spirit, Lev Landau (1908–1968), a Nobel Prize–winning Soviet theoretical physicist, among the most important ones of his generation and a colorful personality to boot, even developed a "logarithmic scale" of productivity and creativity, ranging from 0 (highest) to 5 (lowest) on which he ranked his fellow important physicists. Newton was 0; Einstein was 0.5; the founders of quantum mechanics Niels Bohr, Paul Dirac, Werner Heisenberg, and Erwin Schrodinger were each 1; and Landau himself was 2.[25]

There is no way of knowing how Landau would have performed on the divergent thinking problems commonly used in creativity research, but there are pretty good reasons to believe that he would have declined them with disdain as "too dumb to solve." At the age of 54, Landau suffered a serious head injury in a car accident and was hospitalized at the Burdenko Institute of Neurosurgery in Moscow, where I began my apprenticeship in Alexander Luria's laboratory a few years later. According to the institutional lore, as well as the memoir written by his widow, when neuropsychologists approached Landau with their tests, he chased them out of the room in a state of cold fury, evidently offended by the tests' apparent simplicity.[26] But even had it been possible to talk him into taking a few divergent thinking tests, there is no guarantee that Landau would have done well, despite being among the most brilliant theoretical physicists of his generation, held in awe by his colleagues as a near-genius. According to Keith Sawyer, a leading creativity researcher, the growing consensus among creativity researchers is that the divergent thinking tests "aren't valid measures of real-life creativity." Likewise, a meta-analysis of a large number of studies has led to the conclusion that the ability of divergent thinking tests performance in children to predict their real-life creative achievement in adulthood is quite low (correlation of 0.216); and so is that of IQ (correlation of 0.167).[27]

Let's now consider Experiment 2. Take a sample of scientists (or artists, or writers, or entrepreneurs) and have them rate one another (all members of the same field of human endeavor) anonymously on a multipoint "creative–barren" (CB) scale—hopefully putting the tribal rivalries and jealousies aside. An average of such ratings for every participant will be computed, this resulting in a CBQ (for "Creative–Barren Quotient") value. The individual CBQs will be ranked on the CB scale.

Then let's give our participants the commonly used "creativity" tests of divergent thinking (our participants will probably be more agreeable than Lev

Landau, since most of them will not be Nobel or Pulitzer Prize winners) and rank their performance on these tests. How well will the "divergent thinking" ranking be correlated with the CBQ ranking? Another interesting question that also allows a straightforward answer, yet to be obtained.

Finally, let's consider Experiment 3, which is really a version of Experiment 1 with the subjects of Experiment 2 as participants. Here the participants of Experiment 2 are the "interviewees" (for whom we already have the CBQ rankings) and the "interviewers" are members of the general public not invested or particularly interested in the area of creative pursuits in question—just people. In keeping with the Experiment 1 rules, the interviewers will rate the interviewees on the BD scale, and individual BDQ's will be computed for each interviewee. Now we will have two "existentially valid" rankings—one of intelligence and the other one of creativity—reflecting the judgment of real people in the real world and having nothing to do with either WAIS-IQ (or other psychometric measures of intelligence), or with the laboratory tests of divergent thinking commonly used in creativity research. How well will the BDQ and CBQ rankings be correlated? This is a very different way of asking the question about the relationship between intelligence and creativity, and the answer, if and when it is available, may surprise us.

A Few Worthy Tests

Since recognized geniuses are in lamentably short supply, and the availability of their brains for neuroimaging and autopsy in even shorter, much of the research on the subject of brain mechanisms of creativity and innovation has had to contend with relatively ordinary subjects performing on laboratory tests presumed to measure creativity. Numerous studies have been conducted relating individual brain differences to performance on such tests—tests of divergent thinking, generativity, and so on. One may doubt the relationship of these tests to the real thing—to Creativity with the capital "C"—and I am one of those doubters. While examining some of the psychological tests designed to measure "creativity," I often felt that the flash of effervescent spontaneity, elegance, and parsimony was sadly absent from their design. On the contrary, they often invite just the opposite: a labored, contrived slogging through with panting and heavy breathing. The "metrics" designed to rank the output of these labors are often equally artificial, inelegant, and contrived. Another big problem with "divergent thinking" tests is that they fall short of the main criterion of creativity: a combination of novelty and utility. Here is where the constructs of creativity and novelty diverge. An esoteric, bordering on the bizarre, use of a brick (an object that seems to be particularly favored in the "multiple uses" tasks) may be novel, but it is hardly useful.

Nonetheless, several studies conducted with "creativity tests" are genuinely interesting and incisive. Such studies often employ the Torrance Tests of Creative Thinking (TTCT). Designed by Ellis Paul Torrance to measure "divergent thinking," this collection of tests requires a subject to come up with as many uses as possible of an object such as—unsurprisingly—a brick; to embellish a simple design in as many ways as possible; and to solve a number of other ingenuous tasks. TTCT has been the mainstay of creativity research for over half a century.[28] It turns out that performance on this test is positively correlated with the volume of the right parietal lobe.[29]

In a different study, Rex Jung and his colleagues administered the Creative Achievement Questionnaire and three "divergent thinking" tests to a group of young subjects. When their performance was correlated with cortical thickness in various cortical regions, a distinctive pattern emerged: increased creativity was associated with *increased* cortical thickness in the angular gyrus and posterior cingulate cortex of the *right* hemisphere; and with *decreased* cortical thickness in multiple areas in the frontal, parietal, occipital, and temporal lobes of the *left* hemisphere.[30]

In a series of studies, some of which were already described in Chapter 5, Takeuchi and his colleagues at Tohoku University in Japan have demonstrated that performance on a divergent thinking test in a group of healthy young adults was positively correlated with the size of the right dorsolateral cortex as well as with the white matter integrity in the right inferior parietal lobule (an area consisting of the angular and supramarginal gyri, known to play a central role in complex cognition).[31]

So, all the admonitions against linking complex traits to specific brain structures notwithstanding, "size matters" when it comes to the right hemisphere in creativity—that is, assuming that the performance on the tests of divergent thinking and similar tests has something to do with the real thing, with consequential real-life creativity. And this, as we already argued, has been more an article of faith than an empirically demonstrated relationship.

One way of increasing our confidence in experimental findings is to look for convergence of evidence from different methodologies—in this instance, from structural and functional studies. A team of Austrian scientists studied electrophysiological correlates of "insightful problem solving" involving verbal remote associations. Because of the verbal nature of the task, a particular involvement of the left hemisphere would not have been unreasonable to expect; yet the task-dependent changes were demonstrated in the right temporal and right prefrontal regions at different stages of solving the problems.[32] In a related study, where the task was to come up with alternative uses of common objects, the more original subjects exhibited a predominantly right-hemispheric involvement (task-related alpha synchronization), while no task-related hemispheric asymmetries were noted in the less original subjects.[33] The exact nature of the right hemispheric involvement in these experiments is unclear, but it can be construed as the loosening of the frontal-lobe control over the posterior cortex of the sort described in Chapter 7.

The frontal-lobe engagement in the creative process is generally a common finding, and its interpretation is somewhat equivocal. Measuring regional cerebral blood flow (rCBF), a team of scientists from the University of Lund in Sweden found differences between high- and low-creativity subjects in a task of divergent thinking (multiple uses of—what else!—a brick); the former had significant bilateral activation in the prefrontal cortex, and the latter had only unilateral activation on the left side.[34]

A number of studies have shown that the increase in alpha frequency (8–12 Hz) is often present when subjects are engaged in divergent thinking and other "creativity" tasks.[35] To clarify the role of this increase in the creative process, a team of scientists from University of North Carolina induced alpha frequency in the frontal lobes using transcranial alternating current stimulation (tACS). As a result, the subjects' performance on the TTCT significantly improved.[36] The exact mechanisms linking alpha frequency in the frontal lobes to creativity are uncertain; they may be paradoxical, representing a diminished control by the frontal lobes over the rest of the cortex, in effect resulting in "transient hypofrontality." But then again, frontopolar activation with transcranial direct current stimulation (tDCS) improved performance on a "creative" task of analogical reasoning.[37]

It looks like some of the findings suggest frontal activation ("hyperfrontality") and others frontal deactivation ("hypofrontality"), this being consistent with the dual role of the prefrontal cortex in the creative processes described in Chapter 7. And the same nagging question remains: how much—or how little— do brief "snapshot" tests, like multiple uses of a brick, tell us about real-life consequential creativity, as opposed to frugality, sociopathy, or nothing at all?

How Bad Is Mad?
Creativity and Psychiatric Illness

Italian criminologist Cesare Lombroso (1835–1909) is best known for his controversial theory positing that propensity toward criminality is an atavistic biological trait reflected also in certain physical and physiognomic features unique to criminals. My first exposure to his theories was through my recklessly irreverent and politically incorrect ("ideologically unsound" in the Soviet vernacular of the time) mother. She used to point at the photographs of the Soviet leaders conspicuously displayed on the front pages of *Pravda*, the official daily outlet of the Communist Party of the Soviet Union and the number-one newspaper in the land, and say, "See, they all look like Lombroso types." This was part of her private but relentless campaign to inoculate her son (me) against the toxic effects of Soviet political indoctrination, never mind that at the age of ten I had no idea what she was talking about.

Lombroso's other, less well-known theory, expounded in his book *L'Uomo di Genio (The Man of Genius)*, was that artistic genius is a form of madness, a psychiatric disorder.[38] This was one of the first influential theories linking creativity to insanity. The image of a mad scientist or artist overturning the established preconceptions has titillated the imagination of the general public, film directors, and science fiction writers for generations. Many serious scientists have also been intrigued by an association between creativity and psychopathology; and this idea does have a certain heuristic appeal. It has been argued, for instance, that certain neural and cognitive traits—cognitive disinhibition, attraction to novelty, and neural hyperconnectivity among them—are the shared prerequisites of both creativity and psychopathology.[39]

Indeed, exceptional talent is by definition a departure from the norm defined as the population average. A small number of perturbations of the statistically normative neural makeup may confer advantages in certain areas, albeit perhaps at the cost of disadvantages in others; left-handedness, discussed earlier in the book, may serve as an example. But the vast majority of such perturbations probably fail to confer any advantage. Most highly creative individuals are not mad, and the vast majority of those suffering from madness are not creative in a societally meaningful way. Furthermore, there are many forms of "madness" and many forms of creativity, so any serious discussion of the relationship between the two must have some degree of specificity. Indeed, schizophrenia, bipolar disorder, epilepsy, and Tourette's syndrome have all been linked to creativity, in the eyes of both the general public and the patients themselves. I used to know a young man with Tourette's syndrome who refused medications despite his very severe tics, because he felt that his condition came with a silver lining of creativity, which he was loath to lose.

Based on historic reconstructions and biographical accounts, it has been asserted that Beethoven, Byron, Dickens, Pushkin, Schumann, and van Gogh suffered from bipolar disorder, as did Churchill and Napoleon. It has also been suggested that Julius Caesar, Mohammed, Joan of Arc, Martin Luther, Peter the Great of Russia, and the writer Fyodor Dostoyevsky suffered from epilepsy; and that the dancer Vaclav Nijinsky had schizophrenia (this has also been written about van Gogh). Some of these assertions are based on well-documented accounts, but many are conjectures based on rather questionable evidence.[40]

Then there is an "incomplete data set" issue. It is relatively easy to list a number of consequentially creative individuals afflicted with a documented or suspected psychiatric disorder, and the list may look deceptively impressive. But the association is meaningful only if examined in relationship to the total number of individuals afflicted with the disorder in question, and this ratio in turn is compared to a similar ratio calculated for the creative vs. ordinary people in the general population. At least in principle, such ratios can be calculated and compared with respect to the modern times for which epidemiological and demographic data exist and samples can be rigorously matched. But unless one is prepared to make some very loose assumptions, such estimates can hardly be calculated for the distant, or even not so distant, past.

One should also keep in mind the difference between being "creative" and being a member of a "creative profession" and not fall into the trap of this semantic conflation. Not every writer, painter, or musician is truly creative; in fact, most of them probably are not. A sample of Manhattan restaurant waiters, most of whom introduce themselves as actors, singers, or dancers (and technically they often are, but sporadically and barely part-time), would lead you to conclude that membership in a "creative profession" is often aspirational rather than actual. Depending on the selection criteria, they all may have qualified as "members of creative professions" in a research sample, even though realistically they are not. A devil's advocate may even argue that their wishful, mildly delusional self-perception is associated with psychopathology, rather than the real talent or creativity. One only wonders how these "aspirants" would fill out some of the creativity self-reports, the questionnaires sometimes used in research where subjects are asked to rate their own creative accomplishments and traits, such as the Creative Achievement Questionnaire or Gough's Adjective Check List.[41]

Nonetheless, several rigorous studies of the relationship between creativity and psychiatric disorders have been conducted. Nancy Andreasen compared the rates of mental illness in 30 creative writers and 30 matched controls and their respective first-degree relatives. Higher rates of mental illness, particularly bipolar disorder, were found in the writers and their relatives than in the control sample.[42] Kay Redfield Jamison conducted a similar study involving a group of eminent British writers and artists and came up with similar results: prevalence of mood disorder among her subjects was considerably higher than in the general population. In a similar vein, a team of scientists from Stockholm's Karolinska Institute has reported that people with bipolar disorder and their relatives, as well as the relatives of schizophrenic patients (but not schizophrenics themselves), were over-represented in the creative professions. So the pattern appears to be universal and is present across several Western societies.[43]

Both Nancy Andreasen and the Swedish team have demonstrated that the creative professions are over-represented not only in the patients, but also in their first-degree relatives, a finding that is often interpreted to mean that the underlying cognitive traits are inherited. Assuming that a relationship between creativity and psychiatric illness is real, what are the underlying biological mechanisms? Several shared genetic factors have been proposed. One of them is linked to a polymorphism (variant) of the dopamine D2 receptor gene *DRD2*, which has been implicated in schizophrenia, novelty seeking, and creativity (more about this gene in Chapter 10).[44]

Another possible association between creativity and psychosis has been proposed by the Hungarian scientist Szabolcs Keri. He reported a highly provocative finding, showing that a polymorphism of a particular gene is related to high creativity, assessed with the Creative Achievement Questionnaire and the "Just Suppose" subtest of the TTCT. A variant of the gene in question, *Neuregulin 1*, has been linked to high risk for psychosis, decreased frontal and temporal lobe activation during cognitive tasks, and reduced white matter density and structural connectivity in the anterior limb of the internal capsule—a major bundle containing the fibers connecting the frontal lobes with several subcortical structures. In short, a gene variant that predisposes one to psychosis and undermines the structure and function of the frontal lobes, probably putting the person in a permanent state—trait really—of hypofrontality, has been reported to enhance creativity. Multiple creativities to say the least![45]

"Hypers" and "Hypos" of Creativity and Madness

Assuming that certain forms of creativity and certain types of psychiatric illness (neither of the two is a monolithic construct) share certain cognitive traits and possibly even have shared causation, what are the neural mechanisms mediating these similarities? Multiple disparate and not necessarily consistent factors, or a combination thereof, may be at play.

Some of these factors may be related to the interplay between hyperfrontality and hypofrontality. As we argued in Chapter 7, the creative process is driven by the alternation between hyperfrontality that drives the deliberate, effortful preparatory stage, and hypofrontality that is necessary for the "creative spark" if the deliberate stage falls short. Hypofrontality is a prerequisite of creativity as long as it is transient and the brain's ability to switch between hyper- and hypofrontal states is intact; the nimbler is this ability, the more it benefits the creative process. In contrast, most disorders associated (folklorically, scientifically, or both) with creativity are characterized by predominant ongoing hypofrontality, and with reduced or distorted communication between the prefrontal cortex and other brain structures, where this is no longer a transient state but a relatively permanent trait. This is true for schizophrenia, affective disorder, Tourette's syndrome, and certain types of seizure disorder.[46]

In all these disorders, the balance between the two prerequisites of an efficient creative process—hyperfrontal and hypofrontal states—is distorted. The second of the two prerequisites of creativity is often overexpressed, but the first one is woefully underexpressed. Because of this imbalance on the continuum of cognitive traits, there may be a point where creative imagination and tangential loose associations (a common symptom of frontal-lobe damage and schizophrenia) are precariously close; as are the monomaniacal but adaptive perseverance necessary to propel the creative process and frankly pathological perseveration (another common symptom of frontal-lobe pathology and of certain types of seizure disorder).

Even though hypofrontality is often the predominant attribute of a disordered brain, certain fluctuations do take place. A team of Chinese neuroscientists examined patterns of consistency of the physiological activation levels over time in specific brain regions ("regional homogeneity," or ReHo for short) and found it decreased in bipolar disorder, particularly in the frontal lobes. This means that the changes in the levels of activation in the frontal lobes are subject to volatile fluctuations. Is it possible that the propensity toward fluctuation between hypo- and hyperfrontality may also facilitate creativity in bipolar disorder?[47]

Certain attributes of neural connectivity may serve as other possible factors in the intersection of creativity and psychopathology. Shelley Carson of Harvard University proposed that hyperconnectivity may be a shared factor in psychiatric illness and creativity.[48] Indeed, as we argue in Chapter 7, a certain optimal level of neural connectivity is a prerequisite for the ability to put disparate ideas together. But most biological systems operate on inverted U-curves: too little is bad, but so is too much. There may be a point on the connectivity inverted U-curve where the boundary between "just right" and "too much" is blurred, this facilitating both creativity and psychopathology. Excessive neural connectivity due to insufficient early-life pruning has been proposed as the mechanism behind certain types of autism, and it is also a risk factor for seizure disorder. Hyperconnectivity has also been described in people with certain forms of schizophrenia and their first-degree relatives.[49]

As we discussed earlier, in the healthy brain, "hyperconnected" states may arise when the posterior association cortex, particularly in the right hemisphere, escapes the control of the prefrontal cortex during hypofrontal states. But in certain forms of pathology, this condition may take the form of a permanent trait due to excessive structural connectivity—this, too, resulting in a condition functionally similar to permanent hypofrontality. And even though it may come with a silver lining, it is, on balance, not a good thing.

Creating Minds

Can creativity and talent for innovation be fostered, and if so, how? A loose question like this invites a myriad of responses, ranging from those broadly and scathingly critical of the current educational systems, to hands-on attempts at coming up with constructive alternatives. Passionate TED talks by the British educator Sir Kenneth Richardson, with titles like "Do Schools Kill Creativity?" full of witticisms and pithy declarations like "Creativity is as important today as literacy" and "If you are not prepared to be wrong, you will never come up with anything original," are examples of the former.[50]

The latter are represented by several innovative educational programs. Regardless of their theoretical bent, all such programs are premised on the assumption that a creative mind *can* be molded through properly designed educational intervention; because if they cannot be, then the failure to enhance them is understandable, and any attempt to do so is from the outset foolhardy. What would serve as definitive evidence one way or the other? Probably not an improved performance on the divergent thinking tests or progressive matrices, since we already know that the performance on these tests does not predict a real-life record of innovation. In order to be meaningful, the evidence has to be rooted in real life, and therein lies the conundrum. A really compelling study would have to be longitudinal, following and comparing the life and career trajectories of the graduates of different educational programs. And in order not to be at the mercy of idiosyncratic anecdotes, the study would have to involve a sufficiently large number of students. In effect, the project would have to be akin to one assessing the long-term effects of a new pharmaceutical product. This makes it a prohibitively tall, almost unfairly tall order.

But then again, even though no compelling evidence exists that creativity can be programmatically molded, there is no evidence to the contrary, either. So, instead of submitting to "paralysis by analysis," several teams took a leap of faith and designed such programs. Even though not yet sufficiently supported by the kind of empirical evidence outlined here, at least some of these programs are guided by reasonable scientific rationale.

Even though enhancing creativity is often the stated goal of these programs, this lofty but elusive concept is usually deconstructed into several more easily defined and targeted cognitive and metacognitive processes—mental flexibility, depth of processing, critical thinking, inhibitory control, and so on. This takes the mystique out of "creativity," but leaving mystique out of the educational process is probably a good thing. All these approaches are driven by the premise that instilling metacognitive skills is as important as, or more important than, teaching specific subject content like history or geography, and that this can be accomplished through direct instruction. Many such programs have been designed or at least attempted, covering the whole educational spectrum from the kindergarten to the university.[51] Two of them, bracketing the spectrum, are particularly interesting case studies: *Tools of the Mind* and *Minerva Schools*.

Tools of the Mind is a product of collaboration between a Russian émigré psychologist Elena Bodrova and American educator Deborah Leong.[52] Based on the theories of Lev Vygotsky (we discussed his work in the chapter on animal intelligence; it's time to invoke it where it truly belongs—human cognitive development), it has existed since 1993 and is intended for preschool and kindergarten. The concept of "mental tools" internalized from culture was central to Vygotsky's approach to cognitive development; in fact, the earliest paper he coauthored with Alexander Luria, where these ideas were formulated in an embryonic form, was titled "The Tool and the Symbol" ("*Orudiye i znak*").[53] In today's parlance, Vygotsky's "tools of the mind" roughly correspond to self-regulation, inhibitory control, and executive functions. Trained in Russia, Elena Bodrova imported some of Vygotsky's educational ideas to the United States, and together with Deborah Leong, adapted them to the local context. The approach that resulted from this effort is a combination of carefully designed social pretend-play activities aimed at the development of inhibition, self-control, and cooperation, and instruction aimed at fostering self-regulation. The children are encouraged to approach problems critically and seek multiple alternative solutions.

With any program aimed at instilling general skills, cognitive or physical alike, the challenge is one of transfer: will the improvement be limited to the tasks directly used in training, or will it extend to a broader range of tasks above and beyond those used in training? The broader the transfer, the greater the value of training; on the other hand, narrow improvement without transfer is of limited utility.

Indeed, the cognitive skills instilled by Tools of the Mind seem to generalize and transfer. When children participating in the program were compared to those enrolled in a more conventional one in their performance on tasks of executive functions that were not part of the training routines, the Tools of the Mind graduates did better. They also did better on tasks of attention and had a superior speed of mental operations. The Tools of the Mind graduates have also excelled in more traditional areas of school instruction: their reading and math skills were superior to those of the students who participated in a more traditional educational program.[54] The ultimate, and the only truly important question is how Tools of the Mind graduates will fare long-term in real life. The program has existed long enough to make a study addressing this question possible, and hopefully one is forthcoming.

Minerva Schools is where some of the Tools of the Mind kids may choose to enroll when they are ready for college. It is a university but a very unusual one, a true experiment in higher education. Founded by an entrepreneur, Ben Nelson, in 2012, for-profit and funded with venture capital, it is envisioned as a college of the future offering (at this point) several undergraduate degrees. It is unabashedly elitist but, oxymoronic as this may sound, in a good way. The selection process emphasizes aptitude and capacity for independent learning, intellectual curiosity, and a critical mind—all the attributes that the Tools of the Mind alumni may have a leg up with. Tuition is kept very low compared with most private universities, the admissions process is blind to family income and racial or ethnic background, and the student body is more international than that of most American universities. Named after the Roman goddess of wisdom (and Jupiter's daughter, to boot), Minerva Schools have a tough pedigree to live up to, and their mission is appropriately lofty: to help educate leaders of society and not just narrow experts.

Even though the two programs—Tools of the Mind and Minerva Schools—target the opposite ends of the educational spectrum (pre-kindergarten and kindergarten children vs. college age), they are both based on cognitive science and espouse similar principles. The Minerva curriculum emphasizes "deep" cognitive processing as opposed to rote memorization; leadership, effective team work, effective communication, critical thinking, and alternative solutions. The emphasis is on breaking the traditional boundaries between disciplines (damned balkanization again), developing universal cognitive tools ("habits of mind") and constructs ("foundational concepts"), and addressing "big questions" relevant across societies. Lecture format is eschewed, since, according to Minerva Schools' leaders, "Lectures are a great way to teach but a terrible way to learn," and the bulk of factual content material is acquired by the students on their own through various online sources. In the classroom (a virtual one), students are engaged in discussions and learn how the acquired knowledge can be applied. Broad exposure to the world and immersion in it is central to the educational process at Minerva. In the course of the program, the students spend time in several major cities of North and South America, Europe, and Asia. All this occurs according to a very carefully designed curriculum, and the educational process is guided by a team of accomplished faculty, two of whom are prominent cognitive neuroscientists.[55]

Tools of the Minds and Minerva Schools are among the most interesting experiments in molding the mind directly through education, and there are others. A very intelligent man (he happened to be my late, German-speaking father) liked to ask rhetorically, "How come there are so many *Wunderkinder* (wunderkinds) but so few *Wundermenschen* ("wonder-men"—his neologism)?" Perhaps with these programs' success, there is hope that the *Wunderkind*-to-*Wundermensch* conversion rate will vastly improve, and the world will be better for it.

How realistic is the whole idea of fostering the creative mind? The question is being asked by developmental psychologists, educators, policy makers, corporate gurus, and even by the military. We don't have a definitive answer to this question. But whatever the answer will ultimately be, it will not be a binary "yes or no." The answer—or rather answers—will have to be more nuanced, taking into account many types of creative accomplishments, their many degrees, and the many kinds of creative minds. We will also need better ways of defining and measuring creativity in numerous arenas of human endeavors. One thing is clear enough: the armchair deliberations and *a priori* formulations alone will not do; we must keep trying. Going beyond teaching specific content and skills and aiming to instill higher-order metacognitive "habits of the mind" is a step in the right direction, and there will be more.

The Creative Brain

A Few Worthy Brains

The notion that a gift as precious and unique as creativity can reveal itself in something as unsubtle as the gross anatomy of the brain sounds off-putting, almost profane. But this objection begins to sound hollow if one notes that the neuroscience journals are replete with publications relating individual differences in brain morphology—regional size, volume, surface area—to cognitive performance. So why not creativity? A small collection of brains exists, dispersed through various scientific institutions and museums worldwide and meticulously studied, that belonged to individuals whose place in history clearly warrants the assumption that their diseased owners were indeed endowed with a high degree of capital-C "Creativity"—for better or for worse. Here are a few.

The Genius

The creative contribution of Albert Einstein's brain requires no elaboration in this book, but its posthumous fate is a bit macabre. Upon the great scientist's death at the age of 76, his brain was autopsied and preserved by the pathologist Thomas Harvey, who kept it hidden from the public view for a number of years. It is a matter of some debate whether or not this was done with Einstein's or his family's permission. The existence of the preserved Einstein's brain became public knowledge only more than 20 years later, and its various sections ended up in the National Museum of Health and Medicine, the University Medical Center at Princeton, and the Mütter Museum of University of Pennsylvania. Several scientific investigations of Einstein's brain ensued, most of them conducted with the photographs of its slices rather than with the brain itself.

One of the better-known studies, conducted by Sandra Witelson and her colleagues at McMaster University in Canada, revealed the absence of the parietal operculum and part of the Sylvian sulcus. This unusual cortical anatomy may have resulted in the expansion of a different area, the inferior parietal lobule, which is part of the heteromodal association cortex known to be important in particularly complex cognitive processes. Was this part of the secret of Einstein's genius? Any such conjecture remains a matter of speculation.[1]

A more recent study, conducted by Dean Falk and colleagues and also based on photographs, revealed additional details that may or may not shed light on the nature of Einstein's genius, or at least of his avocations. The representation of his left hand in the motor cortex was unusually large, forming a "knob-shaped fold." This feature is commonly seen in the brains of right-handed violinists, which Einstein was, and may have only a scant, if any, relationship to his genius as a physicist. Perhaps of greater relevance to his exceptional cognitive abilities was the unusual morphology of Einstein's prefrontal cortex. It suggested both an exceptionally elaborate gyral landscape and a larger-than-usual overall surface of the prefrontal cortex. Expanded, too, were his inferior temporal-lobe areas, also known to be critical for higher-order cognition. There was also a plethora of other findings whose possible relationship to Einstein's creativity is more elusive. These include unusually large primary somatosensory and motor cortices in the left hemisphere. Einstein's inferior parietal lobule was unusually large in the left hemisphere compared to the right hemisphere; and the opposite was true for the superior parietal lobule. The overall size of Einstein's brain was, according to the authors, "unexceptional."[2]

Einstein's corpus callosum, the large white matter bundle connecting the two hemispheres, was larger than usual compared both to the older and younger controls. This was true for the entirety of the corpus callosum, but particularly so in the splenium, which provides communication between the parietal lobes in the two hemispheres.[3] Yet other findings, by Marion Diamond and colleagues at University of California, Berkeley, involve the relative number of glial cells in Einstein's brain: their ratio to neurons was unusually high in the left parietal areas.[4] One can speculate about the meaning of this finding at one's own risk, but the proliferation of glial cells in this part of the brain may be a result of its being very extensively engaged in Einstein's thought processes, which, according to his own introspection, were driven by visual and spatial imagery more than by verbal reasoning or mathematical formalisms. The peculiarities of Einstein's brain may have been a reflection—or a cause—of his particular brand of creativity.

The Revolutionary

Regardless of one's view of the past century's history, Vladimir Ilyich Ulyanov was one of its cardinal shapers. Better known to the world under his *nom de guerre* Lenin, he was the founder of the Soviet Union, who turned a utopian fantasy into political reality with a far greater international reach than that of the enfeebled Russian Empire, whose collapse he helped engineer. You don't need the Torrance Tests of Creative Thinking to assume that the man who ushered into existence a world superpower built on a political delusion possessed creativity of sorts. After his death, Lenin became an object of state-mandated and rigorously enforced quasi-religious veneration and had a "genius" status officially conferred on him by the Soviet State.

Genius or not, Vladimir Ulyanov was unquestionably a highly intelligent man and an exceptionally deft political strategist, very possibly the most consequential one of the twentieth century. He was born into an educated multiethnic family (with Russians, Swedes, and Jews among his ancestors), a descendant of minor nobility. In addition to his political activities, he was a prolific writer with an interest in, and a certain grasp of, philosophy, who referred to himself as a "journalist." While at the height of his political power and prestige, Lenin suffered a series of debilitating strokes predominantly affecting his left hemisphere, which increasingly interfered with his ability to rule the state he had ushered into existence. Following his death at the age of 53, Lenin's brain was preserved and meticulously studied by a whole team of pathologists and neurologists with the purpose of unlocking the secrets of his presumed genius. The "Lenin's brain" project laid the foundation for a whole Institute of the Brain in Moscow, which over the years expanded into one of the largest brain collections in the world. It houses the brains of the Nobel Prize–winning physiologist Ivan Pavlov; stage director Konstantin Stanislavsky, the founder of the acting school that served as the foundation of "method acting" in the United States; film director Sergei Eisenstein of *Battleship Potemkin* fame; futuristic poet Vladimir Mayakovsky; the dictator Joseph Stalin; and other true and false luminaries of the twentieth-century Russian society.

But Lenin's brain remains the collection's centerpiece. It was dissected by Oskar Vogt, a leading neuroanatomist of his time, specifically invited for this purpose from Germany. Only the right hemisphere was studied, because the left hemisphere was too ravaged by cerebrovascular disease. Multiple slices of grey and white matter were created. The reported findings included an exceptional complexity of sulcal and gyral landscape, particularly in the frontal lobes; a very high overall cortical surface area due to an unusually great amount of intrasulcal component (cortex deep within the sulci); highly pronounced transitional ("limitrophic") cortex, especially in the frontal lobe areas; particularly large heteromodal association cortical regions, especially in the frontal lobes but also in the parietal and temporal cortex; and an unusually high number of very large layer III pyramidal neurons, whose importance in complex cognition we discussed in

Chapter 4. Lenin's frontal lobes seem to be particularly endowed in terms of both their size and their connectivity—a finding almost expected in someone who distinguished himself mostly as an exceptionally effective practical organizer and leader, never mind his philosophical pretensions. As was the case with Albert Einstein, the overall size of Lenin's brain was unremarkable.[5]

The Imposter

That a creative genius's uniqueness is not necessarily reflected in the gross neuroanatomy of his or her brain was made even more apparent through a famous mix-up. Johann Carl Friedrich Gauss (1777–1855) has been lauded as the "prince of mathematics" and "the greatest mathematician since antiquity." After his death, what was thought to be the great mathematician's brain was meticulously preserved at the Institute of Ethics and History of Medicine at University Medical Center, Göttingen, and extensively studied. That was the case until Renate Schweizer, a neuroscientist at the Max Planck Institute, discovered that the much-venerated brain in fact belonged to the Göttingen physician Conrad Heinrich Fuchs. The brains were probably inadvertently switched soon after the two men's contemporaneous deaths in 1855. The two brains were similar in weight and size, and Gauss's brain revealed certain age-appropriate changes commonly seen in people his age at the time of death.[6]

The fact that it took scientists so long to discover the swap, and even that by accident, suggests that there was nothing in the brains' gross anatomy allowing one to instantly distinguish between ordinariness and genius. Indeed, both brains were morphologically unremarkable; there was nothing apparent in their gross structure distinguishing one of the greatest mathematical minds in history from a presumably intelligent but generally ordinary contemporary. Ironically, the only unusual feature found, a discontinuous ("divided") central fissure, a large fold (sulcus) separating the parietal and frontal lobes, which had been erroneously attributed to Gauss's brain before the mix-up was discovered, in fact belonged to Fuchs's brain. Therein is a cautionary note for anyone who may endeavor to discern unique biological hallmarks solely from the macroscopic morphological studies of "creative individuals'" brains. They may reveal the secret of creativity and talent; but then again, they may not. A motley variety of incidental findings—enlarged ventricles, aneurysms, pituitary adenomas, hemangiomas, calcified cysts, and small vessel disease—are unfortunately a more likely outcome than the neuroanatomical key to genius.

But how about the two brains that did belong to indisputably remarkable individuals? Albert Einstein (1879–1955) and Vladimir Lenin (1870–1924) were the products of roughly the same era, even though one outlived the other by a generation. Each man left an indelible mark on the history of the twentieth century, even though their respective marks were of very different kinds, and the nature of their respective talents was obviously very different, too. Ultimately, any attempt to relate the peculiar anatomical features of these brains to their unique minds is an exercise of uncertain outcome, speculative at best, gratuitous at worst. Yet the fact remains that the two brains had certain features in common: *they both had unusually developed frontal lobes, unusually well-developed overall cortical gyral landscapes, and a high degree of interregional connectivity, even though in Einstein's brain it was interhemispheric (corpus callosum) and in Lenin's brain, intrahemispheric (layer III pyramidal cells)*. Ultimately, however, none of these findings seems to offer the key to the extraordinariness of the two exceptional personalities' minds. Based on what we know about the brain, these findings would be expected in many highly intelligent but generally undistinguished individuals.

Connectivity of Creativity

The two worthy brains described here were both remarkable in having unusually well-developed frontal lobes. They were also remarkable by their enhanced connectivity, albeit of different kinds. Albert Einstein's brain had an unusually thick corpus callosum, particularly in the splenium, providing communication between the left and right posterior association cortices, including the parietal lobes, known to be critical for spatial reasoning. In contrast, Vladimir Lenin's brain was remarkable for an unusually large number of pyramidal cells, which with their long apical axons provide communication between the frontal lobes and diverse regions within the same hemisphere. These individual features of their brains may have been completely incidental to their owners' respective talents; or they may reflect the fact that Einstein was a man of deep contemplation and abstract thought, and Lenin was a man of dynamic action and strategic decision-making—we will never know. But this leaves open the door into the two broader questions raised in the beginning of the book and representing some of its central themes:

- What is the role of the prefrontal cortex in innovation and creativity?
- What is the role of brain connectivity in innovation and creativity?

In a way, the two questions are not entirely independent, since the frontal lobes are more richly interconnected with the rest of the brain than any other neuroanatomically distinct structure. Of the two, the first question has a longer history of being examined, particularly as it relates to the maturation of the

frontal lobes. What is the typical age at which a paradigm-changing idea or discovery is made, and how is it related to the maturation of the frontal lobes and
brain connectivity? Arne Dietrich and Narayaanan Srinivasan surveyed the
Nobel laureates in physics, chemistry, and physiology/medicine who received
the award between 1901 and 2003, and examined their ages at the time when
they first had the seminal idea that earned them the coveted prize. The conclusion, published in the paper with an ambitious title *The Optimal Age to Start a
Revolution*, was that the typical age was somewhere in the 20s and early 30s.[7] Of
course, all such estimates must be taken with a grain of salt. The only real revolutionary in this book, Vladimir Lenin, staged his successful political takeover in
1917, at the age of 47. But what is so magical about the age of the 20s to the early
30s? Dietrich and Srinivasan believe that it is the maturation of the frontal lobes.
Indeed, frontal lobes take a long time to mature, and their functional maturation
is not fully in place until sometime in the fourth decade of life.

The prospect of linking a complex cognitive trait to a single brain structure is
inherently seductive, but it is misguided and will almost certainly lead to a false
start. Beware of the "frontal idolatry" trap; of the impulse—quite pronounced in
neuropsychological literature (I may have contributed to this idolatry myself)—
to attribute everything that is uniquely human, intelligent, and complex to the
frontal lobes. The prefrontal cortex almost certainly plays a critical role in this
process, but it is far from being the only player. If we believe that the creative
process hinges on the interaction of many brain structures and is not just a product of a single "creativity brain center," then the ability of multiple, diverse brain
structures to communicate rapidly and efficiently must be at the heart of this
process, and this unavoidably brings brain connectivity into the narrative.

This, in turn, leads to the following consideration, which may strike one as
simplistically naïve, but it may very well capture an essential aspect of the "brain
mechanics" of novelty creation. If any novel idea arises to a large extent as a *de
novo* combination of the elements of previously accrued knowledge and concepts
that previously had not been integrated into coherent networks, then a highly
interconnected brain is the prerequisite for creative success. The ability of diverse
brain regions to interact and cooperate in the service of a creative act may be
the main key to their success. Furthermore, subtle individual differences in connectivity architectures may account for different cognitive styles and different
types of creativity, such as the artistic vs. the entrepreneurial. After all, the different emphases on the fronto–posterior vs. interhemispheric connectivity evident when Einstein's and Lenin's brains are compared, as well as other variations
in connectivity patterns, are likely to be present in many less exceptional individuals, who are nonetheless reasonably creative in a more "ordinary" sense and
contribute to society with meaningful innovations in various arenas—hence the

question about the relationship between individual differences in brain connectivity as a biological variable and the capacity for innovation as a cognitive trait. This is a question with two parts: (1) Are there stable individual differences in brain connectivity? (2) If such differences exist, do they have any relationship to the individual differences in cognitive traits?

A team of neuroscientists from Yale University addressed both questions using fMRI, and the answers were "yes" and "yes." When functional connectivity patterns were studied across a number of subjects, individual connectivity "fingerprints" emerged, each unique to a particular subject and stable across various cognitive tasks as well as at rest. Furthermore, the individual connectivity patterns predicted the level of performance on matrix reasoning tasks—a collection of puzzles commonly used as a proxy measure of "fluid intelligence," as well as on tasks of sustained attention. The connectivity networks involving the frontal and parietal regions proved to be the most distinctive.[8]

Before proceeding any further, how do we operationalize "brain connectivity"? Since we already crossed this bridge, let's proceed along the "simplistically naïve" line of reasoning and distinguish between the temporal and spatial aspects of connectivity. Enter small-world networks (already introduced in Chapter 7) and myelination (or myelinization, depending on which side of the Pond you learned English). The spatial aspect of connectivity, the extent to which anatomically distant circuits in the brain can interact, will be affected by the degree to which the brain possesses the "small-world" properties whose essential role in creativity was discussed in Chapter 7. The temporal aspect of connectivity, the speed with which different brain regions can communicate, will also be affected by the small-world properties; and it will be affected by the degree of long-pathway myelination as well. Let's discuss these aspects of brain connectivity separately.

Life in a Small World

We have already discussed the small-world properties that ensure that even very distant elements in a network are connected through a relatively small number of steps, and the advantages they confer on the neural net's ability to deal with cognitive complexity, in Chapter 7. However, an important question has remained unanswered so far: the question of individual differences. The capacity for innovation and creativity are highly variable traits. Some people are richly endowed with these qualities, and others are not. If the small-world properties of neural wiring have something to do with these cognitive traits, then they must also exhibit a high degree of variability across individuals. Is there any evidence to this effect? Indeed, there is. Using diffusion tensor imaging tractography, a team of neuroscientists from Beijing examined the relationship between IQ and the network properties of the brain. A clear relationship emerged between intelligence (at least as assessed with IQ testing) and the degree to which the small-world properties were expressed in the individual brains.[9]

Another way of addressing this question is by finding out whether the small-world properties of neural organization are heritable, and to what degree. This is precisely what was demonstrated by a team of neuroscientists from the Free University of Amsterdam who examined the connectivity patterns in the resting EEG (electroencephalography) of 573 twins and their siblings.[10] Both monozygotic and dizygotic twin pairs were examined and compared with their non-twin siblings. Such comparisons are particularly interesting, since they allow us to separate genetic from environmental factors responsible for the individual variability of certain traits. It turned out that the two crucial small-world properties of the brain are highly heritable and are under genetic control: the degree of both local and global interconnectedness within the brain.*

These findings are remarkable in several ways: they demonstrate a high degree of individual variability of the small-world properties, and the fact that these properties are under strong genetic control. The exact nature of the genetic basis of small-world properties is unclear at this time. Its elucidation should be the subject of future studies, and the research into the relationship between the genetic control of "small-worldness" and that of various cognitive traits should be the next natural step in understanding creativity and innovation. Since small-world properties are altered in several disorders, including ADHD, deciphering their genetic basis may help elucidate the mechanisms of these disorders as well.[11]

The Advantages of Having a Coat

Myelin, the fatty coating tissue surrounding long axonal pathways, is critical for effective communication between distant brain regions, and disrupted myelination has been implicated in several disorders, such as schizophrenia. In fact, the functional maturation of the frontal lobes to a large extent depends on the myelination of long pathways in the brain. Because of the role of the prefrontal cortex as the brain's "chief executive" or "neural orchestra conductor," its contribution to the neural orchestra is particularly dependent on its ability to communicate with distant brain regions and hence on the myelination of long pathways.

Any possible relationship between myelination and cognitive powers is particularly interesting, because myelin is a ubiquitous feature pervading practically

---

* More specifically, 46–89% of clustering coefficients (an index of local interconnectedness, or "cliquishness") and 37–62% of average path length (an index of global interconnectedness) appear to be under genetic control.

all of the brain. This brings the G-factor into the discussion. "G-factor" is essentially a speculative construct positing the existence of a single cognitive attribute that affects all (or at least most) of the individual's cognition in a uniform way and is highly variable across individuals—the proverbial "general intelligence." Some time ago, for reasons discussed in Chapter 9, an even more far-fetched assumption was made: that this speculative construct can be meaningfully measured by a test such as Wechsler Adult Intelligence Test and quantified in a single number—the WAIS IQ.

But this forces the following question: If "general intelligence" exists, what is its biological basis? As mentioned earlier, to qualify as the biological basis of "general intelligence," a certain brain attribute has to affect all of the individual's brain, or at least the structures directly involved in higher-order cognition, to a roughly equal extent. Furthermore, this attribute must remain constant through the lifespan in any individual, or change at a uniform rate across individuals, and must exhibit considerable variability across individuals. But even if the "general intelligence" construct were to be based in reality, its relationship to the three- or two-digit number called "WAIS-IQ" would be far from clear.

It is precisely the difficulties with identifying such a biological variable in the brain that caused people like myself to doubt the very existence of "general intelligence," but brain myelination may qualify as such a variable better than most (except it is not constant throughout the lifespan, as it tends to degrade past a certain age). Unlike many other genetic or epigenetic factors shaping the brain in a piecemeal regional way, the factors affecting myelin formation are more likely to impact the brain as a whole. Assuming that a G-factor, affecting the person's intelligence globally and distributed within a broad range across individuals, exists, individual differences in brain myelination is a plausible candidate root cause behind the individual variability in the G-factor.

The relationship between intelligence and brain myelination was proposed by Edward Miller in 1993.[12] Myelination is likely to be particularly important where the creation of novel ideas, content, or artistic forms is involved. As we argued earlier in the book, very few ideas or concepts are entirely new. For the most part, the creative process involves a novel juxtaposition of diverse bits and pieces of old information and concepts, which had not been connected and stored together as well-articulated neural networks before. Considered in that light, it would be surprising if the efficiency of connectivity between disparate brain regions did not play a role in the creative process. "Directed wandering," the process essential for the ability to generate novel insights and for creativity, which was discussed earlier in in the book in Chapter 7, also relies on a strong and efficient connectivity between brain structures. Remember also that the brains of the two exceptional individuals described earlier in this chapter were remarkable for an unusually thick corpus callosum providing communication between the two hemispheres, particularly splenium connecting parietal lobes in the two hemispheres; for unusually robust long ipsilateral connections; and for a very high glial cell content (oligodendroglia is important in myelin production). And it has been argued that the increase of white matter and cortical connectivity was a decisive factor in the expansion of cognitive abilities in evolution.[13]

The rate of myelination is conspicuously slow throughout development, particularly so in the human brain. It continues through the late twenties, well into the thirties, and possibly even into the forties (a process likely to be characterized by considerable individual differences).[14] In a meticulously conducted study, Daniel Miller of George Washington University, and an international team of colleagues, compared this process in the human and chimpanzee brains, and the differences were telling.[15] In both species, the myelination process extended well into ontogeny but at vastly different rates. The myelination of an infant chimpanzee's brain was already 20% of its maximal myelination seen in the adult brain, and it was almost 96% myelinated by adolescence. In contrast, the human infant's brain was less than 2% myelinated, and the adolescent brain was approximately 60% myelinated compared to the fully myelinated adult brain. Maximal myelination was reached only toward the very end of the third decade of life, past the age of 28. The process was particularly slow in the frontopolar cortex, the apex of the cognitive hierarchy, both in humans and in chimpanzees.

So it appears that the age by which myelination of the human brain reaches its peak coincides virtually to a tee with the optimal creativity age described by Dietrich and Srinivasan, and the functional maturation of the prefrontal cortex may be just one of several manifestations of this general trend. Since the wiring in the right hemisphere relies more on long myelinated pathways than that of the left hemisphere, its functional maturation is also likely to be reached at this age. And since the process of "directed wandering" particularly engages the right hemisphere, it will also benefit from effective brain myelination.

But linking the optimal creativity age to the maturation of a certain system in the brain addresses only part of the conundrum. Suppose the full development of this system—whatever it may be, myelinated pathways, the frontal lobe, the right hemisphere, all of the above, or something else—signals the beginning of the most creative life stage. What, then, signals its decline, which according to some authors accompanies later decades of life?

Again, myelination may contain at least part of the key to this riddle. Having peaked toward the end of the third decade of life, myelination of the brain begins to decline relatively rapidly, and a loss of myelinated fibers occurs, thus compromising the brain's ability to integrate diverse types of information. In a study conducted in Denmark, the total length of myelinated fibers in the brain was compared in subjects of various ages. Between the ages of 20 and 80 years, a loss of 45% of the myelinated fibers was noted, approximately 10% per decade. Considering that the peak of myelination probably occurred at an age older than 20, the aging-related slope of demyelination and long myelinated fiber loss was probably even steeper.[16] Using a novel methodology called myelin content imaging (MCI), Naftali Raz and his colleagues at Wayne State University found that, as luck would have it, aging-related myelin depletion is particularly pronounced in the pathways interconnecting higher-order cortical regions, those presumably involved in most complex cognition.[17] And because the right hemisphere is more dependent on long-pathway connectivity than the left one, the aging-related myelin depletion is likely to affect it more. This may contribute to a more rapid shrinkage of the right than the left hemisphere with aging.[18]

Studies with N-acetylaspartate (NAA) offer another window into the role of myelin in cognition. NAA is among the most ubiquitous molecules in the brain, and its concentration is commonly used as a marker of neural integrity. Concentrations of NAA have been shown to be correlated with cognitive abilities in healthy individuals[19]; and a reduction in NAA levels is correlated with cognitive decline in a number of neurological disorders.[20] NAA is highly concentrated in neurons but even more highly concentrated in myelin and in oligodendrocytes, a type of glial cells essential for the formation of myelin sheath. This suggests that the relationship between NAA concentration and cognitive performance is to a large degree a reflection of the role of myelin in cognition.[21]

It has already been noted that the capacity for innovation and creativity is characterized by a wide range of individual differences. Therefore, any biological attribute underlying these traits must also exhibit a wide range of individual differences. Does evidence of such differences exist for pathway myelination? This question can be addressed with diffusion tensor imaging (DTI), a form of MRI that examines the direction of water molecule diffusion and allows one to assess the integrity and extent of long-pathway myelination, among other variables. A less random and more constrained direction of diffusion implies greater integrity of the pathway and by extension more efficient signal transmission along it; and the degree to which diffusion is constrained is expressed in the *fractional anisotropy coefficient*.[22]

A group of neuroscientists from University of Trier in Germany used DTI to study connectivity via the corpus callosum, the major pathway bundle connecting the two hemispheres. The single most striking finding arose when the effects of handedness were examined: there was significantly less diffusion in the callosal pathways of the left-handers than of the right-handers (it remains unclear whether the finding is limited to "practicing" left-handers or could also be replicated in right-handed "converts").[23] In a limited way, this finding converges with the assertion made in Chapter 6, about the relationship between left-handedness and the propensity toward novelty-seeking and creativity. More broadly, it points to the variability in the degree of long-pathway myelination in the general population.

An even more direct evidence of a relationship between individual differences in white matter integrity and those in performance on the commonly used "creativity" tests, was reported by a team of Japanese neuroscientists. According to Takeuchi and colleagues, performance on a test of divergent thinking was positively correlated in a sample of healthy young adults with fractional anisotropy in the white matter of the frontal lobes, corpus callosum, basal ganglia, temporo-parietal areas, and the right inferior parietal lobule.[24] What is especially interesting here, is that the relationship between cognition and white matter integrity was not limited to a particular part of the brain but seems to be relatively pervasive, facilitating communication across very distant brain structures containing very different types of information.

The Advantages of Not Having a Coat

Appealing as the idea of creativity's being linked to enhanced neural connectivity may be, it is not universally supported by research. Dana Moore and colleagues studied the relationship between the size of the corpus callosum and performance on the Torrance Tests of Creative Thinking.[25] TTCT consists of many subtests. In the TTCT subtest used in the study, the participants were given shapes or lines and asked to come up with as many designs as possible that incorporated them as components.[26] This is how I handled a similar task some time ago (Figure 10.1).

Perhaps unexpectedly, the authors found a negative relationship between the size of the corpus callosum and performance on TTCT. The negative correlation was particularly evident in the splenium, the portion of the corpus callosum connecting the parietal lobes in the two hemispheres.[27] The meaning of these findings is uncertain. It may have more to do with the peculiarities of TTCT than with creativity itself, since the whole notion that this test measures real-life, consequential creativity is highly speculative and has been questioned by many people, including me. Remember, the splenium of the corpus callosum was unusually large in Albert Einstein, whose creativity is considerably less in doubt than TTCT's ability to measure it. But it may also mean that not all aspects of brain connectivity are equally important for all cognitive challenges. It may mean, for instance, that, at least for certain tasks, the capacity for generating novel content inherent in the right hemisphere may benefit from being liberated from the stifling impact of the left hemisphere.

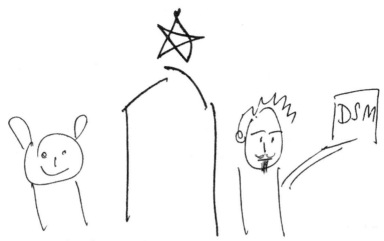

FIGURE 10.1 **Gremlin, Kremlin, Kraepelin.** The task is to embellish two vertical lines in as many ways as possible and to make up a story connecting the images. "Gremlin went to the Kremlin to have his head examined by Kraepelin." (Emil Kraepelin was one of the most important nineteenth–twentieth century psychiatrists and one of the founders of modern psychiatry.)

This interpretation would certainly agree with the findings of my Australian neuroscientist friend Allan Snyder and his colleagues from the Centre for the Mind of the University of Sydney, who studied "out-of-the-box" thinking. Using transcranial direct current stimulation (tDCS) in a group of healthy young subjects, Allan suppressed the left temporal lobe with cathodal stimulation and activated the right temporal lobe with anodal stimulation. As a result, the subjects' ability to solve the puzzles commonly used as measures of "creative thinking" and found daunting by most people—the "nine dots problem" and "matchstick arithmetic"—vastly improved.[28]

In the "nine dots problem," the task is to connect the nine dots with no more than four lines. The problem turns out to be insurmountable for most people because they make an implicit assumption that the lines must stay within the perimeter of the rectangle made of the dots, and that every dot can be crossed only once. In fact, none of these constraints is stipulated in the task, and without them, the solution becomes quite straightforward.[29] In the "matchstick arithmetic" problems, a previously formed habit (mental set) has to be overcome for the correct solution to be found. Most people find it very difficult.[30] Both problems are depicted in Figure 10.2.

The positive role of frontal connectivity in creative thinking has also been challenged. In a DTI study, Rex Jung and his colleagues found a negative relationship between fractional anisotropy (FA, a measure of white matter integrity) in

(a)

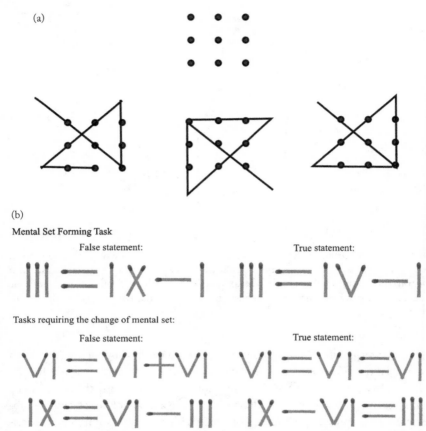

(b)

Mental Set Forming Task

False statement: True statement:

‖‖=IX−I   ‖‖=IV−I

Tasks requiring the change of mental set:

False statement: True statement:

VI=VI+VI   VI=VI=VI

IX=VI−‖‖   IX−VI=‖‖

FIGURE 10.2 **Thinking out of the box.** (A) *The nine-dots problem.* The task is to connect the nine dots with no more than four lines, without lifting the pen off the page. A few solutions are above. (B) *The matchstick arithmetic.* The task is to turn a false statement into a true one by moving only one matchstick.

Adapted from R. P. Chi and A. W. Snyder, "Facilitate Insight by Non-invasive Brain Stimulation," *PLoS One* 6 (2011): e16655.

the inferior frontal regions and performance on tests of "divergent thinking" and "openness to experience."[31] A lower frontal FA would imply reduced frontal-lobe control over the posterior cortical and subcortical structures. In a process dominated by an alternation between hyper- and hypofrontality, this would hinder the former but probably facilitate the latter. The so-called uncinate fasciculus projecting from the orbitofrontal cortex to various limbic structures, including the amygdala and insula, was particularly affected in this study. Damage to this pathway has been noted in several psychiatric conditions, such as schizophrenia and affective disorders.[32] Functionally, this pathway is closely linked to the default mode network (DMN), which was discussed in Chapter 4, and in keeping with this, is more robust in the left than right hemisphere in healthy brains but not in schizophrenia.[33] One can only speculate how disruption in the DMN may indirectly affect processes in other distributed neural networks, and possibly enhance the central executive network (CEN), known to be "anticorrelated" with DMN.

Taken together, these findings may sound like a tangle of inconsistencies. Frontal connectivity is more advantageous—frontal connectivity is less advantageous. A large corpus callosum confers an advantage—a small corpus callosum confers an advantage. A more active anterior cingulate is a good thing—a less active anterior cingulate is a good thing. How does one make sense of this sea of contradictions, aside from the concern—too deflating in its implications to be belabored here—that many of these findings have not been replicated? Ultimately, the inconsistencies between these diverse and seemingly contradictory findings may not be inconsistencies at all, but rather a reflection of the fact that the affinity for novelty and creativity may take many forms and may rely on multiple alternative brain systems. The more one immerses oneself into the brain machinery of innovation and creativity, the more one is compelled to conclude that these are not monolithic processes. As we already established, the paths to creative solutions are likely to be different in different individuals, even when they are engaged in broadly similar pursuits (think of Beethoven and Mozart, Gauss and Galois); and in the same individual engaged in different pursuits. They may be even different in the same creative individual engaged in similar pursuits at different times in his or her life, or at different stages of solving a problem. And even within any one creative pursuit, tension exists between its different components: hyperfrontality and hypofrontality; guidance by experience and its rejection, and so on. A creative mind trying to understand itself may search for consistency, elegance, and parsimony, but the neural processes underlying the object of this quest are neither consistent nor parsimonious, and neither is the overall organization of the brain. Like every product of evolution, it is a hodge-podge of layered adaptations and repurposings.

In the end, whichever way you look at it, connectivity matters. Neuroscience research of the last few decades has brought about an understanding that the brain is orders of magnitude more than a sum of its parts. Much, and perhaps even most, of its computational power arises from the rich and complex connectivity between brain regions, which we are only now beginning to fully appreciate. In order to understand the brain's intricate wiring diagram, an intense multinational effort has been launched—the Human Connectome Project. It involves a number of leading universities and combines a variety of methods: structural magnetic resonance imaging (sMRI), diffusion magnetic resonance imaging (dMRI), resting-state functional magnetic resonance imaging (rfMRI), and cognitive task functional magnetic resonance imaging (tfMRI), as well as genetic methods necessary to examine the extent and mechanisms of connectivity's heritability.[34] We will undoubtedly learn much more about the role of connectivity in cognition before long.

Are "Creativity Genes" for Real?

Is the capacity for innovation and creativity linked to certain genes? Much has been learned about the expression of numerous genes in different brain structures. Can this knowledge guide us toward the discovery of genes linked to creativity? The existence of continuities between humans and other species in the brain mechanisms of creativity helps, since it is often easier to study gene expression in the brain in animal models. But one must tread carefully. There have been many false starts attempting to find simple relationships between genes and cognition. The relationship between cognitive traits and genes is a complex one, and it defies simple one-to-one mapping. With creativity, the search is further complicated by the fact that it is a product of so many moving parts: biological, cultural, and social.

Is the gift of innovation and creativity inherited? The first to rigorously ask this question was Sir Francis Galton (1822–1911), himself a multi-talented scientist, and a cousin of Charles Darwin. Galton invented a method known as "historiometry," which he used to analyze the rates of individuals among the relatives of exceptional personalities who themselves attained a level of prominence. This work, summarized in his book *Hereditary Genius*, led him to conclude that exceptional abilities were indeed inherited.[35]

Today, the likely answer to this question is "sometimes and to some degree." A few multigenerational families of famously creative individuals exist, and they span a wide range of professions and occupations. Marie Curie, her husband Pierre Curie, and their daughter Irene Joliot-Curie were all Nobel Prize–winning physicists. Alexandre Dumas *père* (father) and Alexandre Dumas *fils* (son) were both famous writers; as were the distant cousins Lev Tolstoy, regarded as one of the greatest writers of all time, and Alexei Tolstoy, also a famous writer. Andrey Markov was a famous mathematician who founded a whole branch of mathematics of probabilistic "Markovian" processes; as was his son, also Andrey Markov, renowned for his work in mathematical logic (and one of my favorite professors at Moscow State University). George Boole's nineteenth-century work laid the foundation of twentieth-century computer science, and his great-great-grandson Geoffrey Hinton is among the contemporary pioneers of artificial intelligence. Among my late friend, author and neurologist Oliver Sacks' numerous cousins were the famous Israeli diplomat and scholar Abba Eban; the Nobel Prize–winning mathematician and economist Robert John Aumann; British stage and film director Jonathan Lynn; and the cartoonist Al Capp; not to mention the fact that Oliver's mother was one of the first female surgeons in the United Kingdom. The Sacks cluster is particularly interesting, because, unlike most other talented families, it consists of individuals of many different talents. But familial clustering does not necessarily mean heritability, since shared environmental and cultural factors, as well as role modeling, may also play a role. Furthermore, most famously creative individuals were born into unremarkable, ordinary families, and their creative talent was, to use the technical vernacular of science, "sporadic."

A more modest pursuit, the search for the genetic control over that commonly presumed precursor of creativity, novelty seeking, has a relatively long history. In some of the earliest studies, teams of Israeli and American scientists found an association between the personality trait of novelty seeking and two polymorphisms (variants) of *D4DR* gene, which controls the dopamine receptor D4, in two independent samples in Israel and in the United States.[36] These promising results prompted a substantial body of research aimed at clarifying this relationship. But when several of these studies were subject to a meta-analysis, the results we equivocal.[37]

Creativity is a more complex, multidimensional construct than novelty seeking, which makes it even less likely that it is controlled by a single gene or even a small set of genes. Nonetheless, several attempts to identify the genetic basis of creativity have been made, and they have also met with mixed success. Martin Reuter and his colleagues at Julius Liebig University in Germany examined the link between creativity and three candidate-gene polymorphisms (variants) affecting major neurotransmitter systems implicated in complex cognition: dopamine (DA), norepinephrine (NE), and serotonin (5-HT). The first gene, *COMT VAL158MET*, plays a role in the inactivation of catecholamines in the synaptic cleft and thus affects both dopaminergic and noradrenergic transmission. It has been implicated in the cognitive functions linked to the frontal lobes, such as attention and working memory, and has been a trendy research focus. The second gene, *DRD2-TAQ IA*, affects the dopamine D2 receptors already discussed in earlier chapters of this book, and is also associated with novelty seeking. The third gene, *TPH-A779C*, regulates conversion of tryptophan into serotonin. The specific polymorphisms studied were particularly efficient versions of the three respective genes, and their relationship to performance on the "inventiveness" subtests of the Berlin Intelligence Structure Test was examined in 92 healthy subjects. The latter two genes, *DRD2-TAQ IA* and *TPH-A779C*, were found to be associated with performance on the subtests of verbal and figural creativity, respectively. In contrast, *COMT* turned out to be a disappointment, showing no relationship with creativity measures used in the study. None of the three genes showed any association with the measures of intelligence, and only moderate correlation was found between the measures of creativity and intelligence used in the study, thus throwing the relationship between the two constructs and the way they are operationalized in research into further confusion.[38] The D2 receptors were linked to creativity, measured with several "divergent thinking" tests, also in a study conducted by a team from Karolinska Institute in Stockholm. They reported an inverse relationship between "creativity" scores and D2 receptor density in the thalamus, a subcortical structure consisting of a large number of nuclei closely interacting with the neocortex.[39]

The genetic basis of musical creativity was examined in several studies. Some of them reported distinct linkages between specific chromosomes and the prerequisites of musical creativity, such as absolute ("perfect") pitch. Interestingly, these linkages were somewhat different in different populations: on chromosomes 8q24.21, and to a lesser extent 7q22.3, 8q21.11, and 9p21.3 in the subjects of European ancestry; but only on chromosome 7q22.3 in the subjects of East Asian ancestry.[40] A team of Finnish neuroscientists studied the genetic basis of musical creativity, defined as self-reported musical composing, arranging, or improvisation. Self-reported arranging was found to be linked to chromosome 16, and composing to chromosome 4q22.1.[41] And a team of Israeli scientists from the Hebrew University of Jerusalem found an association between creative dance performance and *AVPR1a* and *SLC6A4* gene polymorphisms.[42]

Many more such studies aiming to link various expressions of creativity to specific genes have been published. I could continue wearing the reader down by keeping the list going, but this chapter is not intended to be an exhaustive survey of the field, and I will not attempt that here. Instead, let me offer a few general thoughts prompted by the studies. On the whole, I find the state of research into the genetic basis of creativity both elating and deflating. It is elating because each of the findings is interesting, and given their sheer volume, these findings are likely to culminate in important breakthroughs sooner or later. It is deflating because so far these breakthroughs have failed to materialize.

There may be several reasons for this. Some of the reasons are related to how creativity is defined, since the measures of creativity adopted in various studies are often arbitrary and narrow, and their relationship to real-life creativity is unproven and even questionable. As our "deconstruction" of creativity in Chapter 2 suggests, creativity is a derivative rather than a primary cognitive attribute, which depends on a number of underlying, more fundamental cognitive and neural attributes and their interaction. Furthermore, different paths to creativity may be a consequence of various combinations of these interacting attributes in varying proportions (those among my readers who are fond of oxymorons will have no trouble embracing the notion of "derivative creativity"). Notably, some of the genes controlling dopamine receptors that have been linked to creativity have also been linked to novelty seeking (either directly or inversely); and the "creative dance gene" *AVPR1*, discussed a few paragraphs earlier, has been linked to social behavior. Both novelty seeking and prosocial behavior are among the fundamental prerequisites of creativity listed in Chapter 2. Instead of a head-on quest for the genetic basis of creativity, the search for the genetic basis of such more fundamental, broad *cognitive* prerequisites of creativity may prove to be more fruitful.

Just as creativity is likely to be a derivative attribute in a *cognitive* sense, it is also likely to be derivative in a *neural* sense. We discussed several more fundamental and broad neural prerequisites of creativity earlier in this chapter and elsewhere in the book. These include a high degree of pathway myelination, high expression of small-world properties of neural network connectivity, strong frontal lobe development, strong development of the right hemisphere, a wide range of arousal states controlled by the catecholaminergic nuclei of the brain stem (ventral tegmental area and locus coeruleus), and others. Instead of a head-on quest for the genetic basis of creativity, the search for the genetic basis of such more fundamental, broad *neural* prerequisites of creativity may prove to be more fruitful.

Much has already been learned about the genetic basis of these broad properties of the brain. Several proteins have been identified as controlling myelination, including myelin-associated glycoprotein (MAG) and cyclic nucleotide 3″-phosphodiesterase (CNP).[43] Several genes asymmetrically expressed in the cerebral cortex have also been identified.[44] Earlier in this chapter, we discussed the individual differences in small-world network properties. Since evidence for their heritability exists, the search for its underlying genetic basis is another promising direction of future research. Learning more about the genetic basis of such broad neural prerequisites of creativity may go a long way toward understanding its underlying mechanisms.

The other reasons behind the failure, so far, to unravel the mysteries of creativity are related to how we frame our expectations about the genetic basis of creativity that we hope to find. As mentioned earlier, considering the complexity of the whole construct of creativity, the many paths leading to it, and the unlikelihood of a single "royal road" to creativity, it would be naïve to expect it to be linked to a single gene or enzyme, or even to a small set thereof. By way of an instructive parallel, the studies of a related construct, intelligence, with all its limitations discussed in the previous chapter, has led to the conclusion that, while highly heritable, intelligence is not linked to a single or even a small number of genetic factors. Instead, numerous genes were implicated, each exerting a small additive effect in determining the individual variation in intelligence. These findings were the result of an ambitious multicenter collaboration between British and Norwegians scientists who studied the relationship between cognitive task performance and genetic profiles in 3,511 unrelated adult subjects and 549,692 SNPs (single-nucleotide polymorphisms, molecular variations of the genetic code). They concluded that approximately 40% of individual variation in "crystallized" intelligence (overlearned knowledge) and 51% of "fluid" intelligence (capacity for solving new problems) could be accounted for through heritability, but that these differences were controlled by the combined effects of a very large, and difficult to identify, genetic factors. Longer chromosomes contributed more than the short ones to individual variability, which further supported the notion that many nucleotides were involved.[45] These findings imply that the subsets of candidate SNPs, whatever they are, may appear in multiple combinations shaping "intelligence" in a myriad of different ways, thus resulting in multiple "intelligences."

Almost certainly, the same can be presumed to be the case with the genetic basis of creativity; perhaps even to a greater degree. This further challenges the notion of "creativity" as a monolithic trait and supports the notion of "multiple creativities." The uncertain relationship between the commonly used "creativity" tests and questionnaires—those on divergent thinking and others—to real-life creativity, makes the heuristic value of studies correlating performance on such tests with various specific types of gene expression equally uncertain, and they may contribute to confusion more than to clarity. Instead of—or in addition to—this "frontal assault" trying to find direct correlations between very specific genetic factors, such as SNPs, and performance of arbitrarily selected cognitive tests (including the workhorses of "creativity research," the tests of "divergent thinking"), a more top-down, hierarchical multi-step approach may prove to be more productive, where the first step would involve looking for the genetic control over potentially relevant broad cognitive and biological attributes of the sort listed earlier. It is not unreasonable to expect that certain properties of the brain indirectly contributing to one or more "moving parts" supporting creativity may be linked to specific, identified or potentially identifiable ensembles of proteins, genes, and their expression, and it may be possible to ask questions about their identity. Instead of looking for specific candidate genes, the search for complex gene ensembles across the genome may be more fruitful, with the further expectation that different such ensembles may underlie similar cognitive properties (remember, there are many paths to creativity).

Having identified such candidate genes (or, more likely, gene ensembles), one would then explore their role in the cognitive attributes of interest, including creativity, more directly as a second step, by examining their expression in individuals characterized by different creativity types and creativity levels. An added advantage of this approach is that a wide range of mammalian (and perhaps not only mammalian) species can be used as models in identifying the candidate genes, since both the relevant broad biological attributes and their genetic control are likely to be conserved across species. Once identified, individual differences in the expression of these genetic factors can be compared in individuals having varying degrees of real-life creativity; with performance on a wide range of cognitive tests tapping "creativity" in humans, and also, appropriately operationalized, in other species.

In conclusion, consider a gardening analogy. It is probably not a very good idea to try to figure out how to "grow" a vegetable stew. A more promising proposition, by far, is to improve the ways we grow carrots, onions, potatoes, and whatever else goes into it. And those of us who will relate better to a more spirited metaphor will agree that to improve a cocktail recipe, one must identify its ingredients first. Likewise, focusing on the genetic control over the more fundamental and better defined ingredients of creativity may prove to be more productive than a head-on pursuit of the genetic control over creativity itself—at least in the near future.

Epilogue—What's Next?

Summing Up and Looking Forward

Will this book change the way the reader thinks about the nature of human creativity, and if so, how? "Creativity" is a lofty word whose meaning may seem deceptively self-evident. Yet we already learned that, contrary to such common-sense intuition, it does not correspond to a single, well-delineated phenomenon or attribute. As we argued in the previous chapter, creativity is a derivative phenomenon, a product of many cognitive attributes that rely on many brain systems working together. It may take many forms, and there are many paths to a creative product. It is a product of complex interactions between neurobiology and culture that defies a linkage to a single brain structure or simple genetic control. This is why the discussion of various components of the creative process took us on a tour through much of the human brain. A creative process by definition deals with novelty, which brings the frontal lobes and the right hemisphere into the process. It benefits from a good grasp of previously accumulated knowledge and concepts, which depends on the left hemisphere. It has to be guided by a keen sense of importance and relevance, which relies on the frontal lobes and dopamine signaling.

While guided by the sense of relevance, the creative process should not be stymied by conformity, which brings a fine-tuned anterior cingulate cortex into the picture. In order to be successful, the creative process requires an interweaving of sustained goal-directed effort guided by a hyperfrontal cortex, and a seemingly effortless insight that requires a suspension of frontal-lobe control, a state of hypofrontality. We referred to the intricate dance between these two states as "directed wandering." This, in turn, requires a nimble brainstem capable of providing a wide range of arousal states and switching between them. And in order to be able to connect disparate ideas and bits of information, the brain has to be strongly interconnected and endowed with "small-world" properties.

Ultimately, however, the fate of innovation is at the mercy of society, consisting of the multitude of not especially creative consumers who may either embrace the innovation and by so doing confer on it the recognition as "creative," or dismiss and ignore it and by so doing consign it to oblivion. The latter sad outcome may be due to the fact that the innovation was truly inconsequential, which is the fate of many attempts at innovation. But an innovation, or an idea, may also be ignored because it was so far ahead of the prevailing *Zeitgeist* of the time that the society failed to recognize its potential relevance or value. I find the second scenario particularly poignant and decided to dedicate the book to the anonymous creative individuals whose genius had not been recognized by their contemporaries and whose contributions had been ignored and forgotten because they were too far ahead of their times. Such anonymous creative spirits must have undoubtedly punctuated the history of human civilization, but we will never know their names, so dedicating a book is the least that we can do for them.

What is the future of innovation and creativity research? Obviously, it will be shaped by the future changes in the processes of innovation and creativity themselves, and anyone inclined to rely on their imperfect crystal ball in predicting the course and the numerous forms these changes will take are probably fooling themselves. Nonetheless, certain cautious predictions can be made. In making these predictions, we will pick up where we started in the beginning of the book—with the distinction between consuming innovation and generating innovation.

Consuming Innovation
"Consumer's Share"

What is the discussion of how innovation is received by the consumer doing in a book on creativity? Let us remind ourselves that a creative product is defined as a combination of novel and valuable; and the verdict of what is valuable and what is not is issued by society, not by the creative individual. Most of the time, an inquiry into the nature of creativity focuses on how new ideas, new products, or any form of innovation are *generated*; and it has been the main focus of this book as well. In comparison, it is relatively uncommon to focus on how innovation is *consumed*. But we often forget that innovation and creativity are a play with two acts: any consequential innovation is a product of somebody's creativity (Act One), which is then "consumed" by society at large (Act Two), which in turn affects future creative contributions, and the cycle continues. While focusing on the first act, we often ignore the second and forget that it is as important in propelling civilization forward as the first one.

As we discussed earlier in the book, in order for innovation to be recognized as a truly creative contribution and not just as an idiosyncratic flight of fancy, it has to resonate with society and influence it. Unless society grasps the value of an innovation and embraces it—whether it is scientific, artistic, or technological— not necessarily right away but within a reasonable period of time, the innovation will be forgotten without taking hold and leaving a mark, and we will not be talking about it today. So from the get-go, the role of the consumer is as important as that of the creator in determining the fate of a novel product, idea, or artistic form.

In his book *The Age of Insight*, Eric Kandel examined the concept of the "beholder's share" in the visual arts, implying that beholding a painting is not a passive process, but rather a process of active involvement characterized by its own cognitive demands.[1] In a broader sense, one can talk about the "consumer's share" in shaping the fate of an innovation or a creative product. Whichever course the future innovation process will take, it is likely that the cognitive challenges of the "consumer's share" will grow, and its demand for the neural processes will change both in volume and in character. The way the "consumer" responds to innovation is an integral part of the creative cycle, and it deserves close examination.

Why is this "consumer's share" an interesting subject to examine? It is interesting because, while innovations are generated by relatively few creative individuals or teams, they are consumed by thousands, millions, or even hundreds of millions. Just think about the Internet and the smartphones. First conceived by a handful of visionaries in a few rarified academic institutions and high-technology hubs, they have become pervasive worldwide and directly or indirectly touch the life of virtually every denizen of our planet.

Why is the question about how innovation is consumed more interesting today than ever before? What makes the "consumer's share" especially interesting today is the rapid acceleration of the rate at which the general public is presented with and is absorbing innovation. In the static societies of the past, innovations were few and far between. As a result, the consumers of these innovations, the proverbial masses, did not have to update their repertoire of knowledge, concepts, or skills that much. Once acquired, such a basic repertoire could carry one through life with virtually no updating at all. A human being and a generation could have lived through life without consuming much, if any, innovation. Therefore, the "consumer's share" was not a significant factor in the social dynamics of creativity and innovation.

But in a fast- and ever faster-moving society like ours, the vast masses of consumers are constantly challenged with the imperative of acquiring new skills and embracing new concepts; and the speed and scope of this process is likely to accelerate even more, at least in the foreseeable future. Following its invention in or about the fifth millennium BCE, it took centuries for the wheel to become widely adopted throughout the societies of antiquity. In contrast, it took barely a few decades for the Internet to become a universal means of communication in the end of the twentieth century.

In a dynamic society, the "consumer's share" of innovation and creativity becomes a hugely significant factor in social dynamics, whose importance has yet to be fully recognized and studied. Even though the way innovation is received by society has not been part of the traditional narrative about creativity, in an informationally dynamic society, it must become so. The demographically massive phenomenon of the changes in the rate with which innovation is introduced and propagates through society is often overlooked, but its implications for society are profound. As the rate at which the consumer masses are exposed to innovation accelerates, the demands imposed by this process on the consumers' cognition and even on their brains will change as well. What are the consequences of these changes? With our clouded crystal ball, we cannot even remotely anticipate the full scope of these consequences. Nonetheless, we will examine two of them here: how increased exposure to novelty may affect brain aging; and the unprecedented challenges posed to the consumer's brain by the advent of "virtual reality."

Brain Aging and the End of Autopilot

One intriguing possibility is that constant exposure to novelty will affect, and may have already begun to affect, the very way in which the human brain ages— and will affect it for the better. Farfetched as this idea may sound, it may help explain some of the recent changes in the incidence of dementia in society.

Against the backdrop of gloomy predictions of the catastrophically expanding dementia epidemic—an unexpected, even surprising ray of hope is seen: the rate of new dementia cases ("incidence") is declining. According to the Framingham Heart Study, this decline has been noted over the last few decades. Compared to the late 1970s through the early 1980s, the rate of new dementia cases dropped by 22% in the late 1980s to early 1990s; by 38% in the late 1990s to early 2000s; and by 44% in the late 2000s to early 2010s. During this time period, the average age at which dementia is diagnosed has increased by five years; which means that even those who succumb to it eventually are able to "hold their cognitive own" longer. Curiously, the dementia risk reduction was noted only in people with at least high-school education or higher. When the known risk factors linked to vascular illness, stroke, atrial fibrillation, and heart failure were considered, their decrease over time still could not completely explain the drop in dementia incidence.[2]

The findings were consistent with those of a few earlier studies, which showed a decline in both prevalence and the incidence of dementia in various populations. These studies went largely unnoticed because they flew in the face of the commonly made assumptions positing an increase, not a decrease, in dementia prevalence as a result of increased longevity and the demographic changes increasing the geriatric slice of the overall population pie; but here they are. A team of scientists from the Duke University Center for Demographic Studies reported a drop in the prevalence of severe cognitive impairment in the population of those 65 years old and older, from 5.7% to 2.9% between the years of 1982 and 1999.[3]

In a similar vein, according to a multicenter collaboration based on the Health and Retirement Study (HRS), the prevalence of significant cognitive impairment among those aged 70 years old and older dropped from 12.2% in 1993 to 8.7% in 2002. A more recent HRS comparison has shown that the trend continued. The prevalence of dementia among those 65 years old or older dropped from 11.6% in 2000 to 8.8% in 2012—a highly significant decline. During the same time period, the average age of dementia diagnosis went up from 80.7 to 82.4 years old—also a significant change.[4] In all these studies, education turned out to be a protective factor against dementia.

European studies reveal a similar trend. In Germany, the incidence of dementia dropped significantly between 2006/2007 and 2009/2010. At the same time, the age of onset of dementia increased significantly, so that in the 65-year-olds, remaining life free of dementia increased by an annual rate of 1.4 months in males and 1.1 months in females.[5] Similar trends were noted in the United Kingdom, the Netherlands, and Sweden.[6]

What are the causes behind these welcome but somewhat unexpected trends? Increased cerebrovascular and cardiovascular health are usually mentioned, but according to the authors of the Framingham Heart Study, these changes cannot fully explain the decline in dementia incidence. In fact, the drop in dementia rates observed in the HRS project occurred *despite* the increase in hypertension, diabetes, and obesity prevalence in the population studied, which made the findings even more puzzling. Higher education is usually mentioned as a neuroprotective factor; so is the complexity of one's adult-life occupational activities; and the concept of "cognitive reserve," a product of lifelong strenuous mental activities, is invoked.[7] The latter findings are particularly revealing, since they imply that how—and how much—one uses one's brain has an impact on that brain's health. Indeed, it has been suggested that vigorous lifelong cognitive activities not only invigorate the aging brain, but up to a point even provide a protective effect against dementia.[8]

What remained unnoticed, or at least not commented on in the scientific literature, is a concurrence between the drop in the incidence of dementia and the advent of mass-produced, and ever-changing consumer digital technologies—personal computers, cell phones and other mobile devices, and the Internet, which began to saturate developed societies from the late 1980s on. Increasingly, even the proverbial "couch potatoes" with a natural predisposition toward mental laziness and aversion to hi-tech were being drawn into the digital world and prodded by societal changes to embrace and harness these constantly evolving consumer technologies. The trend was not limited to the young, and the use of these technologies by the elderly is increasingly commonplace. The surge of new digital technologies for the masses predated the drop in the incidence of dementias by a decade or two—precisely the kind of temporal relationship that one would expect for the causal relationship between the two to be plausible.

This raises an intriguing question: Did the increasingly pervasive advent of digital consumer technologies and their relentless updating and change, forcing the consumers to embrace novelty at a rate unprecedented in the history of humanity, contribute to the drop in the incidence of dementias and to the delay of the age at which they begin to manifest themselves? Another finding of the HRS project—a finding that is both counter-intuitive and "politically incorrect"—could also be explained by the digital technology hypothesis: the risk of dementia was lower in overweight people than in those of normal weight. In contrast, the risk of dementia was elevated in the underweight people.[4] Could it be that an inverse relationship exists between the amount of time people spend in weight-reducing vigorous physical activities and the amount of time spent with digital technologies and other cognitively challenging activities? The (presumably inverse) relationship between the use of digital technologies and the risk of developing dementia in the aging population is an intriguing possibility, which can and should be examined more closely through rigorous research.

The "use it or lose it" adage of brain health has been around for so long that it often sounds like a truistic platitude, but in the age of relentless novelty, this notion takes on a new meaning. In order to exert their neuroprotective effect, cognitive activities must be challenging, varied, and novel. Yet, as we argued in the very beginning of the book, until very recently, one was able to live a happy and successful life of a respected professional without much cognitive exertion. In an informationally static environment, even a high-level professional—a physician, an engineer, or a college professor—could engage in activities perceived by an awestruck observer as dauntingly "intellectual," while being essentially on mental autopilot. The soothing protection of mental autopilot was irresistibly seductive by virtue of its being possible—using the same diagnostic techniques and prescribing the same treatments to patients, using the same equations for designing machines, and giving lectures from the same notes for years.

This was even more the case for members of less-exalted vocations. In every walk of life, reliance on mental autopilots increased with age. Barring some drastic life discontinuities—being immersed in a totally different culture, radically changing one's profession, morphing into a dolphin, or being transported to the Moon—with age, the exposure to novelty typically shrank and the reliance on set patterns expanded. But that means that, with aging, the "use it or lose it" premise was becoming increasingly hollow and gutted of its neuroprotective essence. It is not by accident that the cortical structure most critical for complex problem-solving—the prefrontal cortex—is among the first to succumb to the effects of age-related atrophy even in so-called normal aging[9]; and according to some data, the novelty-hungry right hemisphere succumbs to these effects before the left hemisphere.[8]

But in the age of novelty, reliance on mental autopilots will become increasingly untenable for every member of society, even for those not involved in the activities traditionally perceived as "intellectual." A typical member of society will be forced to "use it," one's brain, in an increasingly real, rather than perfunctory, way.

What effect will a relentless and accelerating exposure to novelty have on brain aging? Will it change the very way in which aging affects the brain, so that the prefrontal cortex and the right hemisphere will no longer be the most vulnerable targets of the aging process? Will it change the cognitive patterns and natural history of dementia? Will it forestall and delay the detrimental cognitive effects of aging and even protect against the onset of dementia? Is it possible that the declining incidence of dementia in advanced societies over the last few decades signaled the beginning of this trend, as these societies were increasingly novelty-driven, this forcing the banishment of mental autopilot? These are tantalizing possibilities, but they need to be better understood. The relationship between the culture of innovation and brain aging should become a topic of future research, with the potential for profound societal implications.

Jane Blane in a Multiverse

Saying that the novelty-driven society will be increasingly technological and that future technologies will take numerous forms is self-evident truism. It has become fashionable to lament the ills of the Internet, social media, and digital devices, and to commiserate about their alienating and "dumbing down" effects. Even had they been valid, these concerns are idle because they are not going to reverse or even slow down the advent of digital technologies; so live with it! But they are not even valid. As a species and a civilization, we have been through similar inflection points before. The advent of written language millennia ago may have triggered similar misgivings in its time, and very likely did. Reading is an inherently more solitary activity than being part of a group regaled by a wise man around a bonfire in the spirit of the oral story-telling tradition. And in some narrow, platitudinous sense, written language does have a "dumbing down" effect, because it relieves one from the need to strain one's memory and memorize a vast body of information.

Which exact forms will the advent of new technologies take? We really don't know. As history shows, even the greatest science fiction minds—Lucian of Samosata, Jules Verne, Herbert George Wells, and others—were basically off the mark trying to divine the future. But whatever trajectory it will take, the process will be non-negotiable. Even the most conservative and reluctant consumer of this deluge of innovation will not be able to dodge it, and the pressure to constantly learn new stuff will be relentless and increasingly rapid. The history of knowledge is an esoteric field that aims to catalogue the totality of knowledge across all fields of human endeavor and the rate at which it changes and expands through the history of human civilization. There has even been a book written under the ambitious title *A History of Knowledge: Past, Present, and Future*, whose author, very appropriately, was the editor of *Encyclopedia Britannica*, Charles van Doren.[10]

As a discipline, the history of knowledge has been traditionally concerned with the rate of accumulation of scientific knowledge, but an innovating (pun intended) historian of knowledge may someday undertake the challenge of quantifying the totality of knowledge and skills that an ordinary, unambitious, and unexceptional human being needed to competently navigate the environment in a given historic time. He may also undertake to calculate the rate at which this knowledge had to be updated or replaced across the historic times and plot this as a curve. Will the shape of this curve resemble the one describing Moore's law of technological development, or some other exponential curve? One can argue that it most likely will, since the impact of scientific and technical innovation on the lives of ordinary people, the enthusiastic and reluctant consumers alike, is probably broadly proportionate to the total volume of knowledge in society and the rate of its accumulation and replacement.

Among the many future wonders of the brave new world, one is likely to be particularly profound and may have an impact on the very way in which human mind—and human brain—operates. This is the advent of virtual reality and the *fusion revolution* it will eventually usher. For now, an ordinary person's exposure to virtual reality is limited or altogether absent; it is used mostly in gaming, education, professional training, physical rehabilitation, and to a very limited extent, in the movies. But a time may come in a relatively near future when virtual travel will supplant physical travel, and when streams of multisensory images may supplant verbally conveyed information, if not completely, then at least to a large extent. How will this change cognition and possibly the brain itself? What demands will it impose on the "beholder's share," the consumer's cognition? Will the world become more or less complex? Will it become more or less confusing?

As I argued in the beginning of the book, a person living a few generations from now may inhabit a world where the physical and virtual realities will be fused to a nearly complete extent, and where the laws of the virtual worlds may be constructed in multiple, perhaps even mutually contradictory ways. The multitude of "parallel universes," sometimes referred to as the "multiverse," which have so far been the exclusive domain of the more esoteric brands of quantum mechanics and science fiction, will become part of the macroscopic and generally ordinary lives. How will a typical human being navigate and reconcile them? For this question to be addressed, the "multiverse" of virtual reality and its impact on the brain will have to become the subject of neuroscientific inquiry.

A skeptical reader will do well to remember that the word "multiverse" was coined in the end of the nineteenth century by the psychologist William James, who used it in a cognitive context ("moral multiverse"), decades before it was repurposed by the physicists.[11] Counter-intuitive as this may sound, "parallel mental universes" have been part of human experience throughout the whole history of our species. The ability to evoke memories and to conjure up arbitrary images in one's head has been the source of such parallel universes. The advent of language magnified this ability many times. Language allows us to construct parallel realities that may be at loggerheads with physical reality and among themselves. Despite the potential for conflict, the parallel realities constructed through language often merge in our minds with the physical reality, and the information received through these two channels is intertwined and blended in our brain. Sometimes this fusion is seamless, to the point that the boundary between the two information streams is blurred; and sometimes it leads to a disturbing dissonance. But a healthy human being is usually able to distinguish between the actual, physical reality and the "parallel universes" constructed through imagination and language. When this ability breaks down in certain psychiatric and neurological conditions, we call the ensuing disorder "psychosis."

But the human brain's ability to handle this distinction in the future is far from assured. In hi-tech parlance, an environment where physical and virtual realities are blended is sometimes called "augmented reality." Is it possible that as the increasingly immersive virtual and augmented reality permeates our lives, the distinction between the physical and the digital will be increasingly difficult to make? What if, in certain environments and for certain purposes, the "beholder" will do better by *not* making this distinction? How will all this challenge the human mind and human brain in ways not experienced by our species, or any species for that matter, before?

The belief that human experience will be profoundly impacted by virtual reality is shared by the people best qualified to make predictions about technologies of the future. Mark Zuckerberg, the founder of Facebook, feels that the gaming applications of virtual reality are just a prelude to bigger and hopefully better things to come. And by spending two billion dollars on the acquisition of the virtual reality development company Oculus VR, he literally put his money where his mouth is. This is what Zuckerberg wrote in the release announcing the acquisition:

> Imagine enjoying a court side seat at a game, studying in a classroom of students and teachers all over the world or consulting with a doctor face-to-face—just by putting on goggles in your home. This is really a new communication platform. By feeling truly present, you can share unbounded spaces and experiences with the people in your life. Imagine sharing not just moments with your friends online, but entire experiences and adventures. . . . One day, we believe this kind of immersive, augmented reality will become a part of daily life for billions of people. . . .[12]

Other digital behemoths are in the game as well. Microsoft has launched *Project Camradre*. The project, spearheaded by Jaron Lanier, a polymath computer scientist often credited with coining the term "virtual reality," is about creating a multi-user augmented reality environment where several persons would interact with the same virtual objects or scenes.[13] A number of startups are also in the game; one of them, a company called Magic Leap, has raised more than $1 billion.

The prospect of a virtual or augmented reality–driven "cognitive multiverse" is rife with profound philosophical implications about the boundary between epistemology and ontology, and about the definition of reality itself. As mentioned in the Introduction, the questions about the relationship between that which is perceived and that which truly *is* absorbed the great minds of the past, like Immanuel Kant and Hermann von Helmholtz, and one can only imagine how they would have reacted to the brave new virtual worlds. But it is even more interesting to imagine how the minds—and the brains—of regular human beings immersed in these environments will operate and what changes in our mental makeup these changes will usher in.

The virtual reality technologies of today are still too embryonic to start exploring all the possibilities. Current research into the interaction between the brain and virtual reality revolves mostly around its applications in rehabilitation and education. Among the relatively few studies of a more basic nature examining the effects of virtual reality on the brain, the most high-profile study at the time of this writing seems to be about the hippocampal activity in rats, but this is likely to change in the very near future.[14] The mind and the brain of a person fully immersed in the virtual or augmented reality environment will become one of the subjects of intense research if we are to understand the cognitive challenges facing the consumer of digital innovation in the not-so-distant future, as well as its impact on the consumer's brain.

Creating Innovation
Minds in Context

The romance of a solitary intellectual odyssey culminating in a paradigm-shifting breakthrough is for the most part gone. To reflect the trend away from individuals and toward teams, even the term "collaborative intelligence" has been coined. It is not as if collaborative effort has not existed before. In a broad sense, even a solitary creative individual is not really solitary, since all the yesteryear giants on whose shoulders he or she stands are the implicit team members, and so are his intellectual soulmates whose ideas he supports, as well as the intellectual opponents whose ideas he is trying to debunk. Any creative process occurs within a cultural context, which by definition makes it collaborative. In his books *Group Genius* and *Explaining Creativity*,[15] Keith Sawyer provides many examples of such collaborative efforts, both vertical (drawing on earlier work) and horizontal (through interaction with contemporaries) in science, in the arts, and in business.

But even in a more direct, immediate sense, the creative process is increasingly driven by a group rather than by an individual. In science, consequential discoveries and innovations are increasingly made by teams of variable sizes and compositions. As every reader of scientific journals must have noticed, an average list of authors of a scientific paper has grown in length dramatically over the last few decades, and solitary authorship is increasingly rare. As an individual, I sometimes lament the change, because temperamentally and stylistically, a solitary intellectual pursuit has always been my preferred *modus operandi*, and I assume that there are many scientists and scholars like myself; but this regret, too, is idle, and we adapt.

As the new art forms become increasingly intertwined with technology, this collaborative trend is also likely to be on the ascendancy in the arts. This means that the effort to understand the nature of innovation and the creative process must no longer revolve exclusively or even predominantly around the creative individual; it must increasingly emphasize the studies of creative ensembles. Understanding the "do's" and "don'ts" of a successful innovation team composition is in itself a creative process, and according to the late J. Richard Hackman, a professor of social and organizational psychology at Harvard University and a leading expert on teams, not a simple one.[16]

Broad societal, cultural, and demographic changes affect the processes of innovation. The entrenched notion that the capacity for innovation comes with an age-based expiration date is being increasingly challenged.[17] Even in mathematics, which has been assumed for centuries to be exclusively the young mind's game, a careful analysis failed to establish a clear relationship between the mathematician's age and the quality and quantity of productive output.[18] Do these findings contradict some of the neuroscientific considerations expressed earlier throughout the book? No, they don't, but they do make the point that there are many paths toward a creative product, which may be complementary and reliant on different experiences and different neural attributes. They also make the point—and a crucial one—that these paths may be different in different times and in different cultural and informational contexts.

What are the implications of these differences for the optimal age composition of a creative team in different fields of innovation? It has been suggested that an effective team should include both the young members unburdened by the dated preconceptions, and the seasoned members bringing with them experience and knowledge.[19] As a general premise, this makes sense, but how it applies to different areas of creative pursuit needs to be better understood. Indeed, working this out is more than a scientific challenge; it is a sociodemographic imperative. Given the aging of developed societies, these societies simply cannot afford to not use the creative potential of the not-so-young.

Then there is gender and gender gap. The male domination of sciences and the arts is increasingly on the wane, and the trend toward gender equality will undoubtedly continue. Do systematic differences in the contributions made by the members of the two sexes to a creative team exist, and if so, what are they, and how can they be best combined into productive synergies? This line of inquiry may have a politically incorrect ring to it today, but this is so only in a culture dominated by gender inequality. Once gender equality and parity are firmly established, the questions about the complementarities in gender contributions to creative pursuits (as well as any other pursuits) can be addressed constructively and rationally, without hysteria, defensiveness, or the corrosive effects of "political correctness." In his interviews of 91 "exceptional individuals," conducted in 1990–1995, Mihaly Csikszentmihalyi was unable to reach his goal of a fifty–fifty split between sexes, since women were underrepresented in certain domains of creative endeavor. Instead, he had to settle for seventy–thirty in favor of men. One hopes that today that ratio would be much closer to parity.[20]

Creative Spirits on the Island of Gods and in Other Places

Cutting-edge scientific and technological innovation is no longer the near-monopoly of Europe and North America. In neuroscience and neuropsychology, the ascendancy of first-rate publications from China, Japan, Singapore, and other non-Western countries over the last few decades has been nothing short of spectacular, and I assume that this is the case in other fields of creative human endeavor. But while science and technology are becoming increasingly internationalized and homogenized, cultural differences still exist. It is precisely the globalization of significant creative pursuits and the emergence of international teams that make it imperative that we better understand the influence of cultural context on innovation and the creative process. Cross-cultural neuroscience is a relatively young discipline concerned with the interaction between culture and individual cognition or even between culture and the brain, and cross-cultural neuroscience of innovation is its natural future extension.[21]

True, the globalization of knowledge industries and the increasing participation in it of non-Western societies, a signature trend of the latter part of the twentieth century, was somewhat of a one-way street: the rest of the world was adopting the Western ways and mostly benefiting from them. There is absolutely no guarantee that this trend will continue in the twenty-first century; in fact there are good reasons to believe that it won't. As the historically advanced—turned backward—turned advanced again societies of Asia reclaim their place on the forefront of world stage and shed the posture of cultural submissiveness of the last few centuries, their ancient cultural traditions and traits will increasingly reassert themselves as well. And as the societies of Africa will be joining the global innovation scene, they, too, will bring with them their own traditions and traits. Yes, the world may be getting increasingly "flat," to borrow from the title of Thomas Friedman's bestseller, but the ensuing flatland will not be a mere extension on the North American prairie or the East European steppe. It will be both a blending and an amalgam of different cultural traits and personality types, and of carryovers from vastly different historical backgrounds.

As the process of modern innovation ceases to be the monopoly of the West, the innovation and creativity research must take notice and let go of the tacit assumption that whatever we learned about the innovation and creativity traits, and about cognition in general, in North America and Western Europe, automatically applies to the rest of the world. Cross-cultural science of innovation and creativity is—or at least should be—coming of age. In a globalized world, the regions that in the not so distant past could be dismissed as insignificant in terms of their consequentially creative output, will become major players, there will be many innovation hubs, and understanding both their similarities and their differences will be essential for them to interact smoothly and productively.

Cross-cultural research on creativity and innovation will become more than a merely academic pursuit. It will be a practical necessity in a "flat world."

Different cultures give rise to different cognitive styles, and these differences manifest themselves both in everyday life and in scientific and artistic pursuits. To someone like myself, whose formative years took place in Russia and the bulk of his professional career in the United States, this is not a provocative armchair proposition but a felt split-life experience. A distinct cognitive style may be a fundamental, if sometimes elusive, attribute of a culture, and I find interacting with different cognitive cultures more interesting, by far, than sampling ethnic cuisines or visiting exotic destinations. Such different, culturally shaped cognitive styles come with consequential, albeit often subtle, complementarities whose essence the clichés like "relative strengths and weaknesses" do not even remotely capture. Combined, these complementarities may result in team synergies whose collective creative powers far outstrip those of culturally homogeneous teams. I strongly believe that the influx to American universities of students and young scientists from China, India, post-Soviet countries of Europe and Asia, and other faraway places contributes to the robustness of American science and is its unique strength. Even though these young people receive their advanced education in the United States, they bring with them the cognitive styles and cognitive habits shaped by the cultural contexts of their origin, and blending them into creative teams this side of the Atlantic and Pacific results in powerful nonlinear effects. Systematic research into the nature of such culturally shaped cognitive differences and complementarities is a worthy challenge for creativity research in and of itself, with the practical potential for devising systematic methods of optimizing creative team compositions in different fields and for different purposes. Even though on the surface the idea of strategically combining individuals of different cultural backgrounds into creative ensembles has a tinge of political incorrectness, as someone with lifelong disdain for political correctness, even during my days in the old Soviet Union, I find its promise undiminished.

The relationship between the neurobiology and culture in shaping and giving direction to the creative process has been among the main themes of this book. The critical importance of this relationship is indisputable, but we don't stand a chance of truly understanding the nature of the neurobiology–culture interaction in the creative processes so long as creativity research is limited to a culturally homogeneous Western environment. In order to truly understand the nature of this interaction, we must overcome the cultural parochialism (or is it cultural hubris?) and conduct comparative creativity research in diverse cultural contexts. As every scientist knows, a variable must be manipulated in order to understand its contribution to the process in question, but so far, we have by and large failed to do so in our effort to understand the role of host culture in individual creativity.

In contrast to technological creativity, artistic creativity has never been a near-monopoly of the West; it has always blossomed in disparate corners of the world. I am writing parts of this chapter in Bali, where I have been vacationing on and off for close to 30 years. Known as "the Island of Gods," this Hindu enclave in the midst of mostly Muslim Indonesia is renowned for its seemingly inexhaustible artistic creativity—painting, woodcarving, sculpture, textile, metalwork, as well as dance and music. The old royal city of Yogyakarta on the nearby island of Java is another hub of artistic creativity with multiple forms of indigenous, highly refined cultural expression blossoming in unusual concentration.

Bali's and Yogyakarta's uniqueness has not escaped the notice of entrepreneurial types of various stripes, and numerous commercial "creativity" workshops, classes, and centers have sprung up on the island of Bali, wooing Westerners in search of new experiences. Yet my Google and PubMed searches cross-referencing "creativity" with "Bali," "Yogyakarta," or "Java" have yielded only one English-language peer-reviewed journal research publication.[22] It seems like in a self-absorbed Western-centric frame of mind, the creativity researchers have so far failed to take advantage of the opportunities offered by this natural creativity laboratory. This is a shame, because many of the paradigms commonly employed to study creativity in the West can be also implemented in the culturally different environments such as Bali and Yogyakarta. Among other questions, such research would elucidate the nature of the relationship between neurobiology and culture in the creative process and help advance the broader theme of "cross-cultural cognitive neuroscience."

The advent of "cross-cultural neuroscience" will help elucidate a wide range of questions related to creativity. We conduct our research on the relationship between the brain and the mind in a Western context, and then we take a leap of faith and assume that our findings are universal. But are they? Is the genetic control over specific forms of artistic creativity, of the sort discussed in Chapter 10, the same or different in diverse populations? Is the optimal age of creative accomplishment the same or different across cultures, for instance in Western as compared to Balinese and Javanese artists? Is the rate of brain myelination, whose relationship to creativity we discussed in Chapter 10, the same or different across cultures?

In my earlier book *The New Executive Brain*, I briefly discussed a historical puzzle. If we assume that the age of the very late 20s to mid-30s is the universal age of complete brain myelination, then we have to assume that some of the most important historical events were the products of immature brains, since some of the most influential personalities of the past embarked on their history-changing pursuits while in their late teens to early twenties. These include Pharaoh Ramses the Great of Egypt, King David of the Hebrews, Alexander the Great of Macedon, Louis XIV of France, Peter the Great of Russia; with Elizabeth I not much older, acceding to the throne and embarking on one of the longest and most consequential reigns in the history of England at the age of 25; as well as Napoleon Bonaparte, winning his first major military victory at the age of 26. Or is it perchance the case that the rates of pathway myelination, and perhaps other neurodevelopmental variables, are to some extent under the cultural control? "Cross-cultural neuroscience" will make it possible to address these and many other intriguing questions related to creativity and innovation, as well as a wide range of other questions posed by the imperative to understand the nature of humanity.

Distributed Brain Power

As the subject of social science, social and organizational psychology, research on the teams in innovation has been underway for quite some time, and a few excellent books have been published examining at an anecdotal level how the creative process benefits from being distributed among several individuals—in the arts, in hi-tech entrepreneurship, and in science.[23] But neuroscience has lagged behind. How does one move from the studies of optimal team compositions to the studies of the optimal assemblies of individual brains, of the *distributed brain power*? Neuroscience has accumulated enough knowledge to tackle this question.

In fact, the question about the optimal group constellation of individual brain traits should not sound particularly outlandish, and there have been several reasons to phrase this question very broadly and fundamentally at the evolutionary population level. In my earlier books *The Executive Brain* and *The New Executive Brain*,[24] I discussed the sex differences in the cortical connectivity architecture. In females, the interhemispheric connectivity is emphasized compared to males, the corpus callosum being thicker in the former. The female pathway architecture promotes communication between the two hemispheres. In contrast, the intrahemispheric front-back connectivity is emphasized in males compared to females, some of the longitudinal fasciculi being thicker in the former. The male pathway architecture promotes communication between the frontal lobes and the posterior cortex, particularly the parieto-temporal association cortex.

I reached these conclusions by combining the results of several earlier, disparate neuroimaging studies examining interhemispheric and intrahemispheric connectivity in separate samples, and also by considering the effects of lateralized lesions in males and females. In a recent study conducted at University of Pennsylvania, the findings of a differential emphasis on interhemispheric connectivity in females vs. intrahemispheric connectivity in males were confirmed and amplified. The Penn study is particularly compelling, since a very large sample of young subjects (428 males and 521 females aged 8–22 years old) was examined using sophisticated diffusion tensor imaging methodology.[25]

What, if any, was the evolutionary advantage for the two halves of the species to have different and complementary cortical connectivity architectures? One can speculate, as is commonly done, about how these different architectures suited the complementary roles of the Cro-Magnon males and females in their hunting and gathering pursuits, but we weren't there, and in the final analysis, this is nothing but loose talk. The really interesting question, which can be answered rigorously and without too much speculation, is whether the sex differences in cortical connectivity are unique to humans, or whether they are present in other primates and perhaps even in other non-primate mammalian species. The degree to which these sex differences in brain connectivity are universal, as opposed to being unique to humans, may shed some light on the scope and nature of their adaptive value. On the other hand, should these differences turn out to be unique to humans, this will trigger the next interesting question: are the female–male differences in brain wiring universal across cultures, or do they exhibit cultural differences? Are they sex differences or gender differences, or an admixture of the two? "Cross-cultural neuroscience" again. But ultimately, as I argue in *The New Executive Brain,* the way to find out whether mixing different connectivity architectures in the population in certain proportions confers any functional advantage on the group as a whole, and to characterize this advantage, is probably by creating computational models and computer simulations.

Left-handedness may be another case in point. If indeed the cognitive style of the left-handers is different from that of the right-handers, then what, if any, is the evolutionary advantage for the species to have this minority cognitive style emphasizing novelty-seeking represented in approximately 10% of the population (even though significant variability across cultures has been noted)? This and similar questions have been debated for some time.[26]

The answer—at least a partial one—may lie in the peculiarities of the left-handed brain. The connectivity in the left-handed brain is remarkable for a larger corpus callosum than in the right-handed brain, and less diffusion in the callosal pathways; and there may be other peculiarities, which a future comprehensive study akin to the one conducted by the University of Pennsylvania team could reveal.[27] What, if any, are the cognitive advantages for the population in endowing approximately 10% of the individual brains with these architectural features?

Then there are the hemispheric differences. As we argued earlier, the small-world network properties are more expressed in the right hemisphere than in the left hemisphere. Morphometric neuroimaging research has also shown that the allocation of cortical space is different in the two hemispheres: the territories of the lateral prefrontal cortex and inferoparietal heteromodal association cortex are larger in the right hemisphere than in the left hemisphere, and the territories of some of the modality-specific association cortex are larger in the left than in the right hemisphere.[28] What are the relative cognitive advantages of these two cortical space allocations? Are there individual differences in the degree of these hemispheric differences (there almost certainly are), and what are the functional consequences of these individual differences? Do these differences in cortical hemispheric organization relate to cognitive differences between the right- and left-handers, and if so, how? What, if any, are the implications of these differences for optimal team composition?

The way we phrased the questions both with respect to sex differences and handedness implies an approach not commonly used in neuroscience. It implies regarding cognition as a group phenomenon distributed across an ensemble of interacting individual brains (an unintended analogy with an insect colony inevitably comes to mind; but the discussion of the multiple limitations, as well as the possible heuristic value of this analogy, is way outside the scope of this book). Instead of, or rather in addition to, looking into the functional consequences of certain characteristics of individual brains, the time has come to start looking at the emergent functional properties arising in a group as a result of combining individual brains with different properties in different ways.

The idea of "group" or "population" neuroscience may sound outlandish to a neuroscientist today, but it is likely to elicit a yawn in a sociologist, political scientist, historian, or organizational psychologist, because this is how they have been developing their theories and conducting their research all along. And while the experimental methodology of "group cognitive neuroscience" will have to be worked out, computational neuroscience may find itself relatively prepared to hit the ground running; and the methodology of neural net modeling as a way of understanding individual brains can be retooled for the purpose of examining group interactions among multiple brains. Research into the behavior of interacting computational units performing together a task distributed among them has been underway for decades, and the so-called multi-agent systems have been used in a wide range of artificial intelligence applications.[29] In fact, my own first humble independent research project at University of Moscow, at the impressionable age of 19, involved examining how a collection of individually very mediocre simple devices, "low-reliability von Neumann automata" may rise to the occasion and perform a decent job once a number of them is put to work together—as a strictly paper-and-pencil enterprise before the age of computers (at least in the Soviet Union) more than 50 years ago.

Earlier in the book, the case was made that the creative process leading to consequential innovation requires an interplay between hyperfrontal and hypofrontal states. What will happen in a team where some of the individual brains exhibit hyperfrontality and hypofrontality to different degrees and in different proportions? Or where the emphasis on the interhemispheric vs intrahemispheric connectivity is represented in different proportions? Or where the small-world properties of wiring and cortical space allocations are represented in different proportions? How will these and other differences in group composition affect their ability to collectively solve a distributed cognitive task?

Suppose that actual, real-life successful creative teams are identified, and the cognitive and neuroimaging studies of each of their members conducted. What may this tell us about the optimal complementarity of several individual brains, with the total bigger than the sum of its parts? Suppose also that the activities of individual team member brains are recorded in real-time during brainstorming interactions; this is already eminently possible with portable electrophysiological (EEG), functional near-infrared spectroscopy (fNIRS) devices, and perhaps with other tools as well; and new technologies of this kind will undoubtedly appear in the future. What kinds of useful insights into the nature of group creative processes will be gained through such studies?

How are the problem-solving abilities of individual team members related to the creative output of the team? Is it perchance possible that with certain team compositions, exceptionally innovative products can be created by a team whose individual members, while being bright and competent, are basically unexceptional—something akin to aggregating the von Neumann automata in my early fledgling project? Some very interesting "whole bigger than the sum of its parts" non-linearities may emerge from such studies, guided by the concept of group cognition distributed across several individual brains. The societal ramifications of such discoveries can be enormous, since a society will no longer depend on Mother Nature to oblige by giving birth to geniuses (we still don't know how to produce or train them by fiat, and probably never will). Instead, "genius teams" will be configured out of relatively ordinary individuals whom the society will always have in ample supply. How do these distributed brainpower considerations apply to different types of innovation and to different cultural contexts?

These and myriad other questions are waiting to be addressed with the full force of cutting-edge neuroscience. To remain relevant to the changing realities of the innovation processes in society, the "neuroscience of creativity" will need to move beyond the studies of individuals into the new territory of group creativity and distributed cognition. To meet this challenge, far from being an insurmountable roadblock, the process of forging innovative paradigms and methodologies—both experimental and computational—will be rife with exciting opportunities for the new generation of cognitive neuroscientists, an unprecedented exercise in scientific creativity and daring in its own right.

The Digital Brain

If artificial intelligence (AI) is possible, then why not artificial creativity? The idea that machines can be creative has been entertained for a long time, not the least owing to the work by Allen Newell and Herbert Simon.[30] Offensive as this proposition may sound to a proponent of human exclusivity, let's be consistent. If the criterion of a creative product is a conjunction of two attributes, (1) substantial novelty and (2) significant utility, then the origins of the product shouldn't matter. Computer-generated output, judged by human experts as "creative," has been generated in music, visual arts, and in other forms of traditionally human endeavor. One of the dismissive arguments used by the doubters of artificial intelligence is that the AI devices can only do what their human designers build into them. Therefore, as the argument goes, their output is by definition derivative and therefore cannot be judged as creative. But this is a sleight-of-hand argument, since it can be equally applied to human creativity. Since even the most unorthodox creative individual is a product of his time and a beneficiary of the previously accumulated knowledge, insight, and tradition, any creative product generated by that individual, no matter how brilliant, is also in a broad sense derivative. Even though most that is derivative is not considered creative, everything that is creative is derivative, which takes the wind out of the argument.

Derivative or not, AI devices are capable of generating products judged by humans as being different and valuable. Harold Cohen, an artist, engineer, and pioneer of computer-generated art, used to refer to AARON, the painting program he designed, as his "partner." According to the artist's son Paul, "Cohen viewed AARON as his collaborator. At times during their decades-long relationship AARON was quite autonomous, responsible for the composition, coloring and other aspects of a work."[31] In a similar vein, EMI (for Experiments in Musical Intelligence) and Emily Howell, music-generating programs designed by the University of California at Santa Cruz professor David Cope, composed pieces in the styles of Beethoven, Vivaldi, and Bach, as well as other compositions judged by human listeners as beautiful. I am enjoying an opus collection by Emily Howell titled *From Darkness Light* this very moment while writing this chapter.[32] And more recently several AI music projects with evocative names like Jukedeck and Flow Machines were rapidly gaining prominence.

Can the future design of creative AI systems benefit from the human creativity neuroscience research, and have we arrived at an inflection point where the promise of such interdisciplinary interaction may hold particular promise? The answer is "maybe," which means that revving up the interaction is at least worth trying.

It is not as if an interaction between AI and neuroscience has not existed, but it has waxed and waned over the decades. From the outset, beginning with the classic work by Warren McCulloch and Walter Pitts,[33] the whole idea of AI was inspired by the analogy with the human brain. This analogy was at the heart of the formal neural nets, brain-like assemblies of basic nodes ("neurons") interconnected in multiple complex ways. As in the biological brain, complex functional properties may *emerge* in a neural net as a result of learning, without being explicitly built into its design. But at a later stage, the formal neural nets were pushed aside as the tool of AI design in favor of higher-level "symbolic" units aiming to represent more complex cognitive constructs, instead of examining the emergent properties of very large assemblies of massively interconnected small units ("neurons").[34] A more recent revival of the neural nets as a tool of modeling the brain often aims to capture the interaction between larger units, each better compared to a neural structure rather than to an individual neuron. Some of these models are informed by functional neuroanatomy, aiming to reflect the actual relationship between specific neural structures.[35] In another development, a hybrid cognitive-neural approach was adopted, sometime referred to as a "semantic neural network."[36] Here a node represents a concept rather than a neuron. Multilayered neural nets in particular, capable of "deep learning," have enjoyed a vigorous revival.

In principle, neural nets can be constructed of nodes of different molarity, from simple "neurons" to complex "concepts," "ideas," or "actions." In the latter cases, a node will itself be a shorthand for a network consisting of a lower-molarity nodes, this resulting in recursive network hierarchies. This is akin to what Joaquin Fuster proposed in his book *The Neuroscience of Freedom and Creativity,* where he refers to these higher-order representations as "cognits."[37] As a result of the shift from the neuron to the cognit as the basic unit of the model, more recent AI architectures have been informed mostly by cognitive science, while the input from brain science has been pretty scant. But much of the foundational AI work took place before neuroimaging and neurochemical studies of the creative brain had been conducted, or, at least, much of the AI design has not been informed by these studies.

Meanwhile, a lot has happened in the field of innovation and creativity research as it increasingly embraced neuroscience and employed the tools of structural and functional neuroimaging. As a result, creativity research has become relevant to AI in the way that it had not been in the past. Virtually every finding and idea related to the neurobiology of human creativity reviewed in this book, as well as many other ideas not reviewed, can be in principle translated into a feature of future AI architectures, at least the architectures that are based on neural nets. These features include some of those discussed in earlier chapters, including structural differences between the two hemispheres, relative sizes of different regions in the two hemispheres, enhanced intra- vs. interhemispheric and shallow vs. deeply indented connectivity, hyper- and hypofrontality, neurotransmitter modulation, "frontal phantoms," small-worldness, myelination, interplay between the central executive network and the default mode network, as well as many others not discussed in this book. As a result, the neuroscience of innovation and creativity is ready to be integrated with the AI the way cognitive science has been for decades. It will be for the next generation of neuroscientists and AI engineers to make this happen.

On this high note, the book had been almost written, and I was practically packing to go on vacation in Indonesia when I found out about a meeting downtown—the 2016 Annual International Conference on Biologically Inspired Cognitive Architectures, or BICA 2016 for short—precisely the kind of convergence between cognitive neuroscience and AI that I had just finished writing about, and I still had a few days before my long-awaited trip! So, at the last moment I registered and went.

The BICA meeting attracted members of some tribes very different from my own—computer scientists, mathematicians, artificial intelligence architects, experts in machine learning and informatics, electrical engineers—many of them in their twenties and thirties. They came to the meeting from more than a dozen countries from every continent, and they were all interested in the brain and cognition to varying degrees.

I was both delighted and encouraged by the convergence of interests of many of the participants and my own: delighted because the convergence turned out to be truly remarkable; and encouraged by finding out that some of my more far-out notions were shared, at least in a broad sense, by people who arrived at them from very different perspectives and backgrounds. Novelty generation and artificial creativity in neural net-like models was front and center in the talks by Lee Scheffler and Stephen Thaler, the author of *Creativity Machine R*.[38] Artificial artistic creativity was amply represented in two papers about dancing robots by a team of Italian scientists.[39] And pushing the limits of virtual reality, Eugene Borovikov and his colleagues shared their vision of a bidirectional interaction between the physical and virtual realities, this heralding an unprecedented fusion of the two. Borovikov and his team are developing virtual characters capable of crossing the boundary of their virtual world into the physical one and actively interacting with real, flesh-and-blood humans. Endowed with visual sensors, these virtual characters recognize humans and communicate with them, "enabling them to learn from intelligent beings and perhaps reason like them."[40] Even my novelty-routinization theory of hemispheric specialization (the one described earlier in the book) was, to my surprise and delight, represented at the BICA Conference, modeled by Olga Chernavskaya and her colleagues.[41] To quote Ray Kurzweil's memorable phrase, "the singularity is near," and the path toward it will be full of creative breakthroughs.

What are the many forms and directions that the creativity of the future will take? What glorious feats of creativity and innovation will the coming generations be dazzled with? In this final chapter, we tried to peer into the crystal ball, but the ball is cloudy. Ultimately, the answers to these questions are both unknown and to a large extent unknowable, since creativity by its very nature is the game of unexpected. But then again, expecting the unexpected, the very cloudiness of the crystal ball, is one of the joys of life. It is what makes life thrilling.

Chapter Notes

CHAPTER I: THE AGE OF NOVELTY

1. R. Kurzweil, *The Singularity Is Near: When Humans Transcend Biology* (New York: Penguin Books, 2006).
2. G. E. Moore, "Cramming More Components onto Integrated Circuits," *Proceedings of the IEEE* 86 (1998): 82–84.
3. S. J. Gould and N. Eldredge, "Punctuated Equilibria: The Tempo and Mode of Evolution Reconsidered," *Paleobiology* 3 (1977): 115–151.
4. P. Jenkins, *The Great and Holy War: How World War I Became a Religious Crusade*, reprint edn. (San Francisco, CA: Harper One, 2015).
5. Y. N. Harari, *Sapiens: A Brief History of Humankind,* 1st edn. (New York: Harper Collins, 2015).
6. M. Cole, K. Levitin, and A. R. Luria, *Autobiography of Alexander Luria: A Dialogue with the Making of Mind* (Mahwah, NJ: Psychology Press, 2005); A. Yanitsky, R. Van Der Veer, and M. Ferrari, *The Cambridge Handbook of Cultural-Historical Psychology* (Cambridge, UK: Cambridge University Press, 2014).
7. J. Spencer, "A Band of Tweeters," *New York Times* (November 6, 2015): A27.
8. S. Shane, "Online Embrace from ISIS, a Few Clicks Away," *New York Times* (December 9, 2015): A1 and A16.
9. I. Kant, *Critique of Pure Reason,* revised edn. (New York: Penguin Classics, 2008).
10. S. Greenfield, *2121* (London, UK: Head of Zeus, 2013).
11. J. Devinsky and S. Schachter, "Norman Geschwind's Contribution to the Understanding of Behavioral Changes in Temporal Lobe Epilepsy: The February 1974 Lecture," *Epilepsy and Behavior* 15 (2009): 417–424; J. I. Sirven, J. F. Drazkowski, and K. H. Noe, "Seizures Among Public Figures: Lessons Learned From the Epilepsy of Pope Pius IX," *Mayo Clinic Proceedings* 82 (2007): 1535–1540.

CHAPTER 2: THE NEUROMYTHOLOGY OF CREATIVITY

1. A. Dietrich and R. Kanso, "A Review of EEG, ERP, and Neuroimaging Studies of Creativity and Insight," *Psychological Bulletin* 136 (2010): 822–848.

2. E. S. Valenstein, *Great and Desperate Cures: The Rise and Decline of Psychosurgery and Other Radical Treatments for Mental Illness*, 1st edn. (New York: Basic Books, 1986).

3. E. Goldberg and L. Costa, "Hemisphere Differences in the Acquisition and Use of Descriptive Systems," *Brain and Language* 14 (1981): 144–173.

4. E. Goldberg, *The New Executive Brain* (New York: Oxford University Press, 2009).

5. L. T. Rigatelli, *Evariste Galois 1811–1832 Vita Mathematica* (Basel, Switzerland: Birkhäuser, 1996).

6. T. Hall, *Carl Friedrich Gauss* (Cambridge, MA: The MIT Press, 1970).

7. P. Melogran, *Wolfgang Amadeus Mozart: A Biography* (Chicago, IL: University of Chicago Press, 2008).

8. J. Swafford, *Beethoven: Anguish and Triumph* (New York: Houghton Mifflin Harcourt, 2014).

9. E. P. Torrance, "Growing Up Creatively Gifted: The 22-Year Longitudinal Study," *The Creative Child and Adult Quarterly* 3 (1980): 148–158; J. C. Kaufman and R. J. Sternberg, *The Cambridge Handbook of Creativity* (Cambridge, UK: Cambridge University Press, 2010).

CHAPTER 3: THE CONSERVATIVE BRAIN

1. E. Goldberg, *The Wisdom Paradox: How Your Mind Can Grow Stronger as Your Brain Grows Older* (New York: Gotham Books, 2004); E. Goldberg, *The New Executive Brain* (New York: Oxford University Press, 2009).

2. E. Goldberg, "The Gradiental Approach to Neocortical Functional Organization," *Journal of Clinical and Experimental Neuropsychology* 11 (1989): 489–517; E. Goldberg, "Associative Agnosias and the Functions of the Left Hemisphere," *Journal of Clinical and Experimental Neuropsychology* 12 (1990): 467–484; E. Goldberg and W. Barr, "Three Possible Mechanisms of Unawareness of Deficit," in *Awareness of Deficit: Theoretical and Clinical Issues*, Eds. G. Prigatano and D. Schacter (New York: Oxford University Press, 1991): 152–175.

3. H. Hecaen and M. L. Albert, *Human Neuropsychology,* Hardcover (New York: John Wiley & Sons Inc., 1978); A. Luria, *Higher Cortical Functions in Man* (New York: Basic Books, 1980); E. Goldberg, "Associative Agnosias and the Functions of the Left Hemisphere," *Journal of Clinical and Experimental Neuropsychology* 12 (1990): 467–484.

4. A. Luria, *Higher Cortical Functions in Man* (New York: Basic Books, 1980); E. Goldberg and W. Barr, "Three Possible Mechanisms of Unawareness of Deficit," in *Awareness of Deficit: Theoretical and Clinical Issues*, Eds. G. Prigatano and

D. Schacter (New York: Oxford University Press, 1991): 152–175; R. C. Leiguarda and C. D. Marsden, "Limb Apraxias: Higher-Order Disorders of Sensorimotor Integration," *Brain* 123 (2000): 860–879.

5. O. Sacks, *The Man Who Mistook His Wife for a Hat: And Other Clinical Tales* (New York: Touchstone, 1998).

6. J. Capgras and J. Reboul-Lachaux, "Illusion des 'sosies' dans un délire systématisé chronique," *Bulletin de la Société Clinique de Médicine Mentale* 2 (1923): 6–16.

7. N. Chomsky, *Language and Mind,* 3rd edn. (Cambridge, UK: Cambridge University Press, 2006); N. Chomsky, *Syntactic Structures* (Eastford, NJ: Martino Fine Books, 2015).

8. R. W. Byrne, "Human Cognitive Evolution," in *The Descent of Man: Psychological Perspectives of Hominid Evolution*, Eds. M. C. Corbalis and S. E. G. Lea (New York: Oxford University Press, 1999): 71–87.

9. N. Geschwind and W. Levitsky, "Human Brain: Left-Right Asymmetries in Temporal Speech Region," *Science* 161 (1968): 186–187; A. L. Foundas, A. Weisberg, C. A. Browning, and D. R. Weinberger, "Morphology of the Frontal Operculum: A Volumetric Magnetic Resonance Imaging Study of the Pars Triangularis," *Journal of Neuroimaging* 2001): 153–159.

10. A. Luria, *Higher Cortical Functions in Man,* 2nd edn. (New York: Basic Books, 1980); E. Goldberg, "The Gradient Approach to Neocortical Functional Organization," *Journal of Clinical and Experimental Neuropsychology* 11 (1989): 489–517.

11. A. Martin, C. L. Wiggs, L. G. Ungerleider, and J. V. Haxby, "Neural Correlates of Category-Specific Knowledge," *Nature* 379 (1996): 649–652; A. Martin, J. V. Haxby, F. M. Lalonde, C. L. Wiggs, and L. G. Ungerleider, "Discrete Cortical Regions Associated with Knowledge of Color and Knowledge of Action," *Science* 270 (1995): 102–105.

12. M. Cappelletti, F. Fregni, K. Shapiro, A. Pascual-Leone, and A. Caramazza, "Processing Nouns and Verbs in the Left Frontal Cortex: A Transcranial Magnetic Stimulation Study," *Journal of Cognitive Neuroscience* 20 (2008): 707–720.

13. S. M. Kosslyn, "Seeing and Imagining in the Cerebral Hemispheres: A Computational Approach," *Psychological Review* 94 (1987): 148–175.

14. For a comprehensive review of the subject, see: L. S. Rogers, G. Vallortigara, and R. J. Andrew, *Divided Brains: The Biology and Behaviour of Brain Asymmetries* (Cambridge, UK: Cambridge University Press, 2013).

15. Y. Yamazakia, U. Austb, L. Huberb, M. Hausmanna, and O. Güntürkün, "Lateralized Cognition: Asymmetrical and Complementary Strategies of Pigeons During Discrimination of the Human Concept," *Cognition* 104 (2007): 315–344.

16. K. Folta, B. Diekamp, and O. Güntürkün, "Asymmetrical Modes of Visual Bottom-Up and Top-Down Integration in the Thalamic Nucleus Rotundus of Pigeons," *Journal of Neuroscience* 27 (2004): 9475–9485.

17. J. W. Peirce and K. M. Kendrick, "Functional Asymmetry in Sheep Temporal Cortex," *Neuroreport* 13 (2002): 2395–2399; J. W. Peirce, A. E. Leigh, A. P. DaCosta, and K. M. Kendrick, "Human Face Recognition in Sheep: Lack of Configurational Coding and Right Hemisphere Advantage," *Behavioural Processes* 55 (2001): 13–26; J. W. Peirce, A. E. Leigh, and K. M. Kendrick, "Configurational Coding, Familiarity and the Right Hemisphere Advantage for Face Recognition in Sheep," *Neuropsychologia* 38 (2000): 475–483.

18. K. Guo, K. Meints, C. Hall, S. Hall, and D. Mills, "Left Gaze Bias in Humans, Rhesus Monkeys and Domestic Dogs," *Animal Cognition* 12 (2009): 409–418.

19. A. Ghazanfar, D. Smith-Rhorberg, and M. D. Hauser, "Role of Temporal Cues in Rhesus Monkey Vocal Recognition: Orienting Asymmetries to Reversed Calls," *Brain Behavior and Evolution* 58 (2001): 163–172; M. D. Beecher, M. R. Petersen, S. R. Zoloth, D. B. Moody, and W. C. Stebbins, "Perception of Conspecific Vocalizations by Japanese Macaques. Evidence for Selective Attention and Neural Lateralization," *Brain Behavior and Evolution* 16 (1979): 443–460; H. E. Heffner and R. S. Heffner, "Temporal Lobe Lesions and Perception of Species Specific Vocalizations by Macaques," *Science* 226 (1984): 75–76.

20. R. Hamilton and B. A. Vermeire, "Complementary Hemispheric Specialization in Monkeys," *Science* 242 (1988): 1691–1694.

21. N. Kriegeskorte, M. Mur, D. A. Ruff, R. Kiani, J. Bodurka, H. Esteky, K. Tanaka, and P. A. Bandettini, "Matching Categorical Object Representations in Inferior Temporal Cortex of Man and Monkey," *Neuron* 60 (2008): 1126–1141.

22. E. Goldberg, "The Gradiental Approach to Neocortical Functional Organization," *Journal of Clinical and Experimental Neuropsychology* 11 (1989): 489–517; E. Goldberg, "Higher Cortical Functions in Humans: The Gradiental Approach," in *Contemporary Neuropsychology and the Legacy of Luria*, Ed. E. Goldberg (Mahwah, NJ: Lawrence Erlbaum, 1990): 229–276.

23. G. Huth, S. Nishimoto, A. T. Vu, and J. L. Gallant, "A Continuous Semantic Space Describes the Representation of Thousands of Object and Action Categories Across the Human Brain," *Neuron* 76 (2012): 1210–1224.

24. G. A. Miller, "WordNet: A Lexical Database for English," *Communications of the ACM* 38 (1995): 39–41. I owe a personal debt of gratitude to the late Dr. Miller, who befriended me in the mid-1970s when I conducted research as a guest scientist at the Rockefeller University in New York City, where Miller had a lab at the time.

25. G. Huth, W. A. De Heer, T. L. Griffiths, F. E. Theunissen, and J. L. Gallant, "Natural Speech Reveals the Semantic Maps That Tile Human Cerebral Cortex," *Nature* 532 (2016): 453–458.

26. L. Miller, J. Cummings, F. Mishkin, K. Boone, F. Prince, M. Ponton, and C. Cotman, "Emergence of Artistic Talent in Frontotemporal Dementia," *Neurology* 51 (1998): 978–982.

27. W. Snyder, E. Mulcahy, J. L. Taylor, D. J. Mitchell, P. Sachdev, and S. C. Gandevia, "Savant-like Skills Exposed in Normal People by Suppressing the Left

Fronto-temporal Lobe," *Journal of Integrative Neuroscience* 2 (2003): 149–158; A. Snyder, "Explaining and Inducing Savant Skills: Privileged Access to Lower Level, Less-processed Information," *Philosophical Transactions of the Royal Society of London, B: Biological Sciences* 364 (2009): 1399–1405.

28. E. Goldberg, D. Roediger, N. E. Kucukboyaci, C. Carlson, O. Devinsky, R. Kuzniecky, E. Halgren, and T. Thesen, "Hemispheric Asymmetries of Cortical Volume in the Human Brain," *Cortex* 49 (2013): 200–210; M. Harciarek, D. Malaspina, T. Sun, and E. Goldberg, "Schizophrenia and Frontotemporal Dementia: Shared Causation?" *International Review of Psychiatry*, 25 (2013): 168–177.

29. T. Q. Wu, Z. A. Miller, B. Adhimoolam, D. D. Zackey, B. K. Khan, R. Ketelle, K. P. Ranki, and B. L. Miller, "Verbal Creativity in Semantic Variant Primary Progressive Aphasia," *Neurocase* 21 (2015): 73–78.

CHAPTER 4: THE MERMAID AND THE LEGO® MASTER (AND THE CAVE LION-MAN)

1. J. R. Hayes, "Cognitive Processes in Creativity," in *Handbook of Creativity*, Eds. J. A. Glover, R. R. Ronning, and C. R. Reynolds (New York: Plenum Press, 1989): 135–145; D. K. Simonton, "Creative Development as Acquired Expertise: Theoretical Issues and Empirical Tests," *Developmental Review* 20 (2000): 283–318.

2. M. Csikszentmihalyi, *Creativity: Flow and the Psychology of Discovery and Invention* (New York: HarperCollins, 1996).

3. For a more detailed review, see E. Goldberg, *The Executive Brain: Frontal Lobes and the Civilized Mind* (New York: Oxford University Press, 2009), and E. Goldberg, *The New Executive Brain: Frontal Lobes in a Complex World* (New York: Oxford University Press, 2009).

4. J. M. Fuster, *The Neuroscience of Freedom and Creativity: Our Predictive Brain* (Cambridge, UK: Cambridge University Press, 2013).

5. D. H. Ingvar, "Memory of the Future: An Essay on the Temporal Organization of Conscious Awareness," *Human Neurobiology* 4 (1985): 127–136.

6. N. Chomsky, *Language and Mind*, 3rd edn. (Cambridge, UK: Cambridge University Press, 2006); N. Chomsky, *Syntactic Structures* (Berlin, Germany: De Gruyter Mouton, 1957); N. Chomsky, *Aspects of the Theory of Syntax* (Cambridge, MA: MIT Press, 1965).

7. E. Goldberg and R. Bilder, "Frontal Lobes and Hierarchic Organization of Neurocognitive Control," in *Frontal Lobes Revisited*, Ed. E. Perecman (New York: IRBN, 1987): 159–187.

8. D. Everett, "Cultural Constraints on Grammar and Cognition in Pirahã," *Current Anthropology* 46 (2005): 621–646; A. Nevins, D. Pesetsky, and C. Rodrigues, "Evidence and Argumentation: A Reply to Everett," *Language* 85 (2009): 671–681.

9. Y. N. Harari, *Sapiens: A Brief History of Humankind* (New York: Harper, 2015).

10. P. Shipman, *The Invaders: How Humans and Their Dogs Drove Neanderthals to Extinction*, 3rd edn. (Cambridge, MA: Belknap Press, 2015).

11. S. L. Bressler and V. Menon, "Large-Scale Brain Networks in Cognition: Emerging Methods and Principles," *Trends in Cognitive Sciences* 14 (2010): 277–290; M. D. Fox, A. Z. Snyder, J. L. Vincent, M. Corbetta, D. C. Van Essen, and M. E. Raichle, "The Human Brain Is Intrinsically Organized Into Dynamic, Anticorrelated Functional Networks," *Proceedings of the National Academy of Sciences* 102 (2005): 9673–9678.

12. D. Mantini, M. Corbetta, G. L. Romani, G. A. Orban, and W. Vanduffel, "Evolutionarily Novel Functional Networks in the Human Brain?" *The Journal of Neuroscience* 33 (2013): 3259–3275; R. N. Spreng, W. D. Stevens, J. P. Chamberlain, A. W. Gilmore, and D. L. Schacter, "Default Network Activity, Coupled with the Frontoparietal Control Network, Supports Goal-Directed Cognition," *Neuroimage* 53 (2010): 303–317.

13. For a detailed description of the "functional system" concept, see: A. R. Luria, *Higher Cortical Functions in Man* (New York: Basic Books, 1980).

14. For a detailed discussion of the heyday of cognitive "modularity," see E. Goldberg, "The Rise and Fall of Modular Orthodoxy," *Journal of Clinical and Experimental Neuropsychology* 17 (1995): 193–208.

15. D. Wang, R. L. Buckner, and X. H. Liu, "Functional Specialization in the Human Brain Estimated by Intrinsic Hemispheric Interaction," *The Journal of Neuroscience* 34 (2014): 12341–12352.

16. A. Ardestani, W. Shen, F. Darvas, A. W. Toga, and J. M. Fuster, "Modulation of Frontoparietal Neurovascular Dynamics in Working Memory," *Journal of Cognitive Neuroscience* 28 (2016): 379–401.

17. R. L. Buckner, J. R. Andrews-Hanna, and D. L. Schacter, "The Brain's Default Network Anatomy, Function, and Relevance to Disease," *Annals of the New York Academy of Sciences* 1124 (2008): 1–38.

18. A. R. Luria, *Higher Cortical Functions in Man* (New York: Basic Books, 1980); E. Goldberg, "The Gradiental Approach to Neocortical Functional Organization," *Journal of Clinical and Experimental Neuropsychology* 11 (1989): 489–517.

19. E. Goldberg, D. Roediger, N. E. Kucukboyaci, C. Carlson, O. Devinsky, R. Kuzniecky, E. Halgren, and T. Thesen, "Hemispheric Asymmetries of Cortical Volume in the Human Brain," *Cortex* 49 (2013): 200–210.

20. D. Sridharan, D. J. Levitin, and V. Menon, "A Critical Role for the Right Fronto-insular Cortex in Switching Between Central-Executive and Default-Mode Networks," *Proceedings of the National Academy of Sciences* 105 (2008): 12569–12574; D. Sridharan, D. J. Levitin, C. H. Chafe, J. Berger, and V. Menon, "Neural Dynamics of Event Segmentation in Music: Converging Evidence for Dissociable Ventral and Dorsal Networks," *Neuron* 55 (2007): 521–532; S. L. Bressler and V. Menon, "Large-scale Brain Networks in Cognition: Emerging Methods and Principles," *Trends in Cognitive Sciences* 14 (2010): 277–290.

21. E. Goldberg, *The New Executive Brain: Frontal Lobes in a Complex World* (New York: Oxford University Press, 2009); M. Koenigs and J. Grafman, "The Functional Neuroanatomy of Depression: Distinct Roles for Ventromedial and Dorsolateral Prefrontal Cortex," *Behavioural Brain Research* 201 (2009): 239–243.

22. X. J. Chai, S. Whitfield-Gabrieli, A. K. Shinn, J. D. E. Gabrieli, A. N. Castañón, J. M. McCarthy, B. M. Cohen, and D. Öngür, "Abnormal Medial Prefrontal Cortex Resting-State Connectivity in Bipolar Disorder and Schizophrenia," *Neuropsychopharmacology* 36 (2011): 2009–2017; P. J. Hellyer, M. Shanahan, G. Scott, R. J. Wise, D. J. Sharp, and R. Leech, "The Control of Global Brain Dynamics: Opposing Actions of Frontoparietal Control and Default Mode Networks on Attention," *Journal of Neuroscience* 34 (2014): 451–461.

23. C. F. Jacobsen, "An Experimental Analysis of the Frontal Association Areas in Primates," *Journal of Nervous and Mental Disease* 82 (1935): 1–14; C. F. Jacobsen, "Studies of Cerebral Function in Primates. I. The Functions of the Frontal Association Areas in Monkeys," *Comparative Psychology Monographs* 13 (1936): 1–60.

24. J. M. Fuster and G. E. Alexander, "Delayed Response Deficit by Cryogenic Depression of Frontal Cortex," *Brain Research* 20 (1970): 85–90; J. M. Fuster, "Unit Activity in Prefrontal Cortex During Delayed-Response Performance: Neuronal Correlates of Transient Memory," *Journal of Neurophysiology* 36 (1973): 61–78; J. M. Fuster and G. E. Alexander, "Neuron Activity Related to Short-term Memory," *Science* 173 (1971): 652–654.

25. A. Baddeley, "Working Memory: Looking Back and Looking Forward," *Nature Reviews Neuroscience* 4 (2003): 829–839.

26. L. D. Selemon and P. S. Goldman-Rakic, "Common Cortical and Subcortical Targets of the Dorsolateral Prefrontal and Posterior Parietal Cortices in the Rhesus Monkey: Evidence for a Distributed Neural Network Subserving Spatially Guided Behavior," *Journal of Neuroscience* 8 (1988): 4049–4068; P. S. Goldman-Rakic, "Circuitry of the Primate Prefrontal Cortex and the Regulation of Behavior by Representational Memoir," in *Handbook of Physiology, The Nervous System, Higher Functions of the Brain*, Ed. F. Plum (Bethesda, MD: American Physiological Society, 1987): 373–417; M. L. Schwartz and P. S. Goldman-Rakic, "Prenatal Specification of Callosal Connections in Rhesus Monkey," *Journal of Comparative Neurology* 307 (1991): 144–162.

27. J. M. Fuster, *The Prefrontal Cortex,* 5th edn. (London, UK: Academic Press, 2015).

28. W. K. Kirchner, "Age Differences in Short-term Retention of Rapidly Changing Information," *Journal of Experimental Psychology* 55 (1958): 352–358; S. M. Jaeggi, M. Buschkuehl, W. J. Perrig, and B. Meier, "The Concurrent Validity of the N-back Task as a Working Memory Measure," *Memory* 18 (2010): 394–412; S. M. Jaeggi, M. Buschkuehl, J. Jonides, and W. J. Perrig, "Improving Fluid Intelligence with Training on Working Memory," *Proceedings of the National Academy of Sciences* 105 (2008): 6829–6833.

29. J. M. Fuster, *The Neuroscience of Freedom and Creativity: Our Predictive Brain* (Cambridge, UK: Cambridge University Press, 2013).

30. R. Smullyan, *Gödel's Incompleteness Theorems* (Oxford University Press, 1991).

31. J. M. Fuster, *The Prefrontal Cortex,* 5th edn. (London, UK: Academic Press, 2015).

32. A. F. T. Arnsten, C. D. Paspalas, N. J. Gamo, Y. Yang, and M. Wang, "Dynamic Network Connectivity: A New Form of Neuroplasticity," *Trends in Cognitive Sciences* 14 (2010): 365–375; A. F. T. Arnsten, M. J. Wang, and C. D. Paspalas, "Neuromodulation of Thought: Flexibilities and Vulnerabilities in Prefrontal Cortical Network Synapses," *Neuron* 76 (2012): 223–239.

33. G. N. Elston, "Cortex, Cognition and the Cell: New Insights into the Pyramidal Neuron and Prefrontal Function," *Cerebral Cortex* 13 (2003): 1124–1138.

34. E. Goldberg, *The New Executive Brain: Frontal Lobes in a Complex World* (New York: Oxford University Press, 2009).

35. P. Churchland, "Self-Representation in Nervous Systems," *Science* 296 (2002): 308–310.

36. C. Koch, *The Quest for Consciousness: A Neurobiological Approach*, 1st edn (W. H. Freeman, 2004); J. M. Fuster, *The Prefrontal Cortex,* 5th edn. (London: Academic Press, 2015); E. Goldberg, *The New Executive Brain* (New York: Oxford University Press, 2009).

37. B. J. Baars, *A Cognitive Theory of Consciousness* (Cambridge, MA: Cambridge University Press, 1988); B. J. Baars, *In the Theater of Consciousness* (New York: Oxford University Press, 1997); B. J. Baars, "The Conscious Access Hypothesis: Origins and Recent Evidence," *Trends in Cognitive Sciences* 6:1 (2002): 47–52.

38. A more neuroscientifically informed reader of this chapter may have noticed that the relationship between the parieto-temporal association cortex and prefrontal cortex portrayed here is conspicuously similar to the commonly accepted relationship between the hippocampi and the neocortex. The similarity is not coincidental. As I proposed in my earlier book *The New Executive Brain* (New York: Oxford University Press, 2009), the role of the hippocampi in facilitating the long-term representations of veridical information, representing input from the external world, is similar to the role of the prefrontal cortex in facilitating the long-term representations of internally generated, agent-centered constructs.

CHAPTER 5: IT IS ALL ABOUT SALIENCE!

1. For salience definitions, see: http://dictionary.cambridge.org/dictionary/english/salience http://www.oxforddictionaries.com/us/definition/american_english/salient

2. E. Goldberg, *The New Executive Brain: Frontal Lobes in A Complex World* (New York: Oxford University Press, 2009).

3. M. Koenigs, L. Young, R. Adolphs, D. Tranel, F. Cushman, M. Hauser, and A. Damasio, "Damage to the Prefrontal Cortex Increases Utilitarian Moral Judgements," *Nature* 446 (2007): 908–911.

4. M. Harciarek, T. Sun, D. Malaspina, and E. Goldberg, "Schizophrenia and Frontotemporal Dementia: Shared Causation?" *International Review of Psychiatry* 25 (2013): 168–177.

5. E. Goldberg, D. Roediger, N. E. Kucukboyaci, C. Carlson, O. Devinsky, R. Kuzniecky, E. Halgren, and T. Thesen, "Hemispheric Asymmetries of Cortical Volume in the Human Brain," *Cortex* 49 (2013): 200–210.

6. M. D. Fox, A. Z. Snyder, J. L. Vincent, M. Corbetta, D. C. Van Essen, and E. M. Raichle, "The Human Brain Is Intrinsically Organized into Dynamic, Anticorrelated Functional Networks," *Proceedings of the National Academy of Sciences USA* 102 (2005): 9673–9678.

7. R. L. Buckner, J. R. Andrews-Hanna, and D. L. Schacter, "The Brain's Default Network Anatomy, Function, and Relevance to Disease," *Annals of the New York Academy of Sciences* 1124 (2008): 1–38.

8. J. Smallwood, E. M. Beech, J. W. Schooler, and T. C. Handy, "Going AWOL in the Brain—Mind Wandering Reduces Cortical Analysis of the Task Environment," *Journal of Cognitive Neuroscience* 20 (2008): 458–469.

9. S. L. Bressler and V. Menon, "Large-Scale Brain Networks in Cognition: Emerging Methods and Principles," *Trends in Cognitive Sciences* 14 (2010): 277–290; D. Sridharan, D. J. Levitin, C. H. Chafe, J. Berger, and V. Menon, "Neural Dynamics of Event Segmentation in Music: Converging Evidence for Dissociable Ventral and Dorsal Networks," *Neuron* 55 (2007): 521–532.

10. N. Swanson, T. Eichele, G. Pearlson, K. Kiehl, Q. Yu, and V. D. Calhoun, "Lateral Differences in the Default Mode Network in Healthy Controls and Schizophrenic Patients," *Human Brain Mapping* 32 (2011): 654–664; D. Wang, R. L. Buckner, and X. H. Liu, "Functional Specialization in the Human Brain Estimated by Intrinsic Hemispheric Interaction," *The Journal of Neuroscience* 34 (2014): 12341–12352.

11. L. Tian, J. Wang, C. Yan, and Y. He, "Hemisphere- and Gender-related Differences in Small-World Brain Networks: A Resting-State Functional MRI Study," *NeuroImage* 54 (2011): 191–202.

12. J. D. Medaglia, T. D. Satterthwaite, T. M. Moore, K. Ruparel, R. C. Gur, R. E. Gur, and D. S. Bassett, "Flexible Traversal Through Diverse Brain States Underlies Executive Function in Normative Neurodevelopment," *Quantitative Biology* 2015: 1–14.

13. E. Goldberg, S. P. Antin, R. M. Bilder, L. J. Gerstman, J. E. Hughes, and S. Mattis, "Retrograde Amnesia: Possible Role of Mesencephalic Reticular Activation in Long-Term Memory," *Science* (1981): 1392–1394; E. Goldberg, R. M. Bilder, and J. E. O. Hughes, "Reticulo-frontal Disconnection Syndrome," *Cortex* 25 (1989): 687–695.

14. E. Goldberg, R. Bilder, S. Mattis, S. Antin and J. Hughes, "Reticulo-frontal Disconnection Syndrome," *Cortex* 25 (1989): 687–695.

15. T. Brozoski, R. M. Brown, H. E. Rosvold, and P. S. Goldman, "Cognitive Deficit Caused by Regional Depletion of Dopamine in Prefrontal Cortex of Rhesus Monkey," *Science* 205 (1979): 929–931.

16. S. M. Cox, M. J. Frank, K. Larcher, L. K. Fellows, C. A. Clark, M. Leyton, and A. Dagher, "Striatal D1 and D2 Signaling Differentially Predict Learning from Positive and Negative Outcomes," *Neuroimage* 109 (2015): 95–101.

17. K. A. Zalocusky, C. Ramakrishnan, T. N. Lerner, T. J. Davidson, B. Knutson, and K. Deisseroth, "Nucleus Accumbens D2R Cells Signal Prior Outcomes and Control Risky Decision-Making," *Nature* 531 (2016): 642–646.

18. T. W. Robbins and A. F. T. Arnsten, "The Neuropsychopharmacology of Fronto-Executive Function: Monoaminergic Modulation," *Annual Review of Neuroscience* 32 (2009): 267–287.

19. E. Goldberg, *The New Executive Brain: Frontal Lobes in a Complex World* (New York: Oxford University Press, 2009).

20. H. L. Campbell, M. E. Tivarus, A. Hillier, and D. Q. Beversdorf, "Increased Task Difficulty Results in Greater Impact of Noradrenergic Modulation of Cognitive Flexibility," *Pharmacology, Biochemistry and Behavior* 88 (2008): 222–229; S. F. Smyth and D. Q. Beversdorf, "Lack of Dopaminergic Modulation of Cognitive Flexibility," *Cognitive and Behavioral Neurology* 20 (2007): 225–229; D. Q. Beversdorf, J. D. Hughes, B. A. Lewis, and K. M. Heilman, "Noradrenergic Modulation of Cognitive Flexibility in Problem Solving," *Neuroreport* 10 (1999): 2763–2767.

21. U. Kischka, T. Kammer, S. Maier, M. Weisbrod, M. Thimm, and M. Spitzer, "Dopaminergic Modulation of Semantic Network Activation," *Neuropsychologia* 34 (1996): 1107–1113; J. S. Cios, R. F. Miller, A. Hiller, M. E. Tivarus, and D. Q. Beversdorf, "Lack of Noradrenergic Modulation of Indirect Semantic Priming," *Behavioral Neurology* 21 (2009): 137–143.

22. T. W. Robbins, "Shifting and Stopping: Fronto-striatal Substrates, Neurochemical Modulation and Clinical Implications," *Philosophical Transactions of the Royal Society of London, B: Biological Sciences* 362 (2007): 917–932; D. Q. Beversdorf, "Pharmacological Effects on Creativity," in *Neuroscience of Creativity*, Eds. O. Vartanian, A. S. Bristol, and J. C. Kaufman (Cambridge, MA: MIT Press, 2013): 151–173.

23. H. Takeuchi, Y. Taki, Y. Sassa, H. Hashizume, A. Sekiguchi, A. Fukushima, and R. Kawashima, "Regional Gray Matter Volume of Dopaminergic System Associate with Creativity: Evidence from Voxel-based Morphometry," *Neuroimage* 51 (2010): 578–585.

24. C. R. Cloninger, D. M. Svrakic, and T. R. Przybeck, "A Psychobiological Model of Temperament and Character," *Archives of General Psychiatry* 50 (1993): 975–990.

25. I. Greese and S. D. Iversen, "The Role of Forebrain Dopamine Systems in Amphetamine Induced Stereotyped Behavior in the Rat," *Psychopharmacologia* 39 (1974): 345–357; J. J. Canales and A. M. Graybiel, "A Measure of Striatal Function Predicts Motor Stereotypy," *Nature Neuroscience* 3 (2000): 377–383; E. Saka, C. Goodrich, P. Harlan, B. K. Madras, and A. M. Graybiel, "Repetitive Behaviors in Monkeys Are Linked to Specific Striatal Activation Patterns," *Journal of Neuroscience* 24 (2004): 7557–7565; O. De Manzano, S. Cervenka, A. Karabanov, L. Farde, and F. Ullén, "Thinking Outside a Less Intact Box: Thalamic Dopamine D2 Receptor Densities Are Negatively Related to Psychometric Creativity in Healthy Individuals," *PLoS One* 17 (2010): E10670.

26. K. A. Zalocusky, C. Ramakrishnan, T. N. Lerner, T. J. Davidson, B. Knutson, and K. Deisseroth, "Nucleus Accumbens D2R Cells Signal Prior Outcomes and Control Risky Decision-Making," *Nature* 531 (2016): 642–646.

27. V. D. Costa, V. L. Tran, J. Turchi, and B. B. Averbeck, "Dopamine Modulates Novelty Seeking Behavior During Decision Making," *Behavioral Neuroscience* 128 (2014): 556–566.

28. R. M. Bilder, J. Volavka, H. M. Lachman, and A. A. Grace, "The Catechol-*O*-Methyltransferase Polymorphism: Relations to the Tonic–Phasic Dopamine Hypothesis and Neuropsychiatric Phenotypes," *Neuropsychopharmacology* 29 (2004): 1943–1961.

29. S. D. Glick, D. A. Ross, and L. B. Hough, "Lateral Asymmetry of Neurotransmitters in Human Brain," *Brain Research* 234 (1982): 53–63; R. Carter, *Mapping the Mind* (London, UK: Phoenix Publishing, 2004); S. D. Glick, *Cerebral Lateralization in Non-Human Species* (Cambridge, MA: Academic Press, 1985); S. D. Glick, R. C. Meibach, R. D. Cox, and S. Maayani, "Multiple and Interrelated Functional Asymmetries in Rat Brain," *Life Sciences* 25 (1979): 395–400; S. L. Andersen and M. H. Teicher, "Sex Differences in Dopamine Receptors and Their Relevance to ADHD," *Neuroscience & Biobehavioral Reviews* 24 (2000): 137–141.

30. W. James, *Principles of Psychology* (New York: Henry Holt and Company, 1890).

31. E. Goldberg, *The Wisdom Paradox: How Your Mind Can Grow Stronger as Your Brain Grows Older* (New York: Gotham Books, 2005).

32. E. R. Kandel, *In Search of Memory: The Emergence of a New Science of Mind* (New York: W. W. Norton & Company, 2007).

33. W. Barr, E. Goldberg, J. Wasserstein, and P. Novelly, "Patterns of Retrograde Amnesia in Unilateral Temporal Lobectomies," *Neuropsychologia* 28 (1990): 243–255.

34. A. R. Luria, *The Mind of a Mnemonist: A Little Book About a Vast Memory* (Cambridge, MA: Harvard University Press, 1987).

35. J. L. McGaugh, "Making Lasting Memories: Remembering the Significant," *Proceedings of the National Academy of Sciences USA* 110 (2013): 10402–10407.

36. E. M. Hubbard and V. S. Ramachandran, "Neurocognitive Mechanisms of Synesthesia," *Neuron* 48 (2005): 509–520.

37. K. Vick, "Opiates of the Iranian People," *Washington Post Foreign Service* (September 23, 2005).

38. D. Martino, A. J. Espay, A. Fasano, and F. Morgante, *Disorders of Movement: A Guide to Diagnosis and Treatment*, 1st edn. (New York: Springer, 2016).

39. S. Varanese, B. Perfetti, S. Mason, A. Di Rocco, and E. Goldberg, "Lateralized Profiles of Frontal Lobe Dysfunction in Parkinson's Disease," Presented at the Seventh International Congress on Mental Dysfunctions and Other Non-motor Features in Parkinson's Disease and Related Disorders (Barcelona, Spain: 2010).

40. M. Jaffe, "Finding Equilibrium in Seesawing Libidos," *New York Times* (March 8, 2015): A6.

41. G. Giovannoni, J. D. O'Sullivan, K. Turner, A. J. Manson, and A. J. L. Lees, "Hedonistic Homeostatic Dysregulation in Patients with Parkinson's Disease on Dopamine Replacement Therapies," *Journal of Neurology, Neurosurgery, and Psychiatry* 68 (2000): 423–428.

42. G. Giovannoni, J. D. O'Sullivan, K. Turner, A. J. Manson, and A. J. L. Lees, "Hedonistic Homeostatic Dysregulation in Patients with Parkinson's Disease on Dopamine Replacement Therapies," *Journal of Neurology, Neurosurgery, and Psychiatry* 68 (2000): 423–428.

43. G. Rylander, "Psychoses and the Punding and Choreiform Syndromes in Addiction to Central Stimulant Drugs," *Psychiatria, Neurologia, Neurochirurgia* 75 (1972): 203–212; E. Schiorring, "Psychopathology Induced by 'Speed Drugs'," *Pharmacology, Biochemistry and Behavior* 14 (1981): 109–122; N. A. Graham, C. J. Hammond, and M. S. Gold, "Drug-Induced Compulsive Behaviors: Exceptions to the Rule," *Mayo Clinic Proceedings* 84 (2009): 846–847.

44. P. Seeman, "Parkinson's Disease Treatment May Cause Impulse-Control Disorder via Dopamine D3 Receptors," *Synapse* 69 (2015): 183–189; T. J. Moore, J. Glenmullen, and D. R. Mattison, "Reports of Pathological Gambling, Hypersexuality, and Compulsive Shopping Associated with Dopamine Receptor Agonist Drugs," *Journal of the American Medical Association: Internal Medicine* 174 (2014): 1930–1933.

45. B. Levant, "The D_3 Dopamine Receptor: Neurobiology and Potential Clinical Relevance," *Pharmacological Reviews* 49 (1997): 231–252.

46. J. Olds and P. Milner, "Positive Reinforcement Produced by Electrical Stimulation of Septal Area and Other Regions of Rat Brain," *Journal of Comparative and Physiological Psychology* 47 (1954): 419–427; D. Nakahara, N. Ozaki, Y. Miura, H. Miura, and T. Nagatsu, "Increased Dopamine and Serotonin Metabolism in Rat Nucleus Accumbens Produced by Intracranial Self-Stimulation of Medial Forebrain Bundle as Measured by in Vivo Microdialysis," *Brain Research* 495 (1989): 178–181.

47. V. Menon and D. J. Levitin, "The Rewards of Music Listening: Response and Physiological Connectivity of the Mesolimbic System," *NeuroImage* 28 (2005): 175–184; L. Aharon, N. Etcoff, D. Ariely, C. F. Chabris, E. O'Connor, and

C. Breiter, "Beautiful Faces Have Variable Reward Value: FMRI and Behavioral Evidence," *Neuron* 32 (2001): 357–551; C. F. Ferris, P. Kulkarni, J. M. Sullivan, J. A. Harder, T. L. Messenger, and M. Febo, "Pup Suckling Is More Rewarding Than Cocaine: Evidence from Functional Magnetic Resonance Imaging and Three-Dimensional Computational Analysis," *Journal of Neuroscience* 25 (2005): 149–156; M. Numan, "Motivational Systems and the Neural Circuitry of Maternal Behavior in the Rat," *Developmental Psychobiology* 49 (2007): 12–21.

48. A. J. Robison and E. J. Nestler, "Transcriptional and Epigenetic Mechanisms of Addiction," *Nature Reviews Neuroscience* 12 (2011): 623–637; E. J. Nestler, "Cellular Basis of Memory for Addiction," *Dialogues in Clinical Neuroscience* 15 (2013): 431–443.

49. V. Voon, P. O. Fernagut, J. Wickens, C. Baunez, M. Rodriguez, N. Pavon, J. L. Juncos, J. A. Obeso, and E. Bezard, "Chronic Dopaminergic Stimulation in Parkinson's Disease: From Dyskinesias to Impulse Control Disorders," *Lancet Neurology* 8 (2009): 1140–1149.

50. A. Verdejo-Garcia, R. Vilar-Lopez, M. Perez-Garcia, and E. Goldberg, "Altered Adaptive but Not Veridical Decision-Making in Substance Dependent Individuals," *Journal of the International Neuropsychological Society* 12 (2006): 90–99; A. H. Evans, R. Katzenschlager, D. Paviour, J. D. O'Sullivan, S. Appel, A. D. Lawrence, and A. J. Lees, "Punding in Parkinson's Disease: Its Relation to the Dopamine Dysregulation Syndrome," *Movement Disorders* 19 (2004): 397–405; S. S. O'Sullivan, A. H. Evans, and A. J. Lees, "Punding in Parkinson's Disease," *Practical Neurology* 2007 7 (2007): 397–399.

51. E. Goldberg, K. Podell, R. Harner, M. Lovell, and S. Riggio, "Cognitive Bias, Functional Cortical Geometry, and the Frontal Lobes: Laterality, Sex, and Handedness," *Journal of Cognitive Neuroscience* 6 (1994): 274–294.

52. S. Varanese, B. Perfetti, S. Mason, A. Di Rocco, and E. Goldberg, "Lateralized Profiles of Frontal Lobe Dysfunction in Parkinson's Disease," Presented at the Seventh International Congress on Mental Dysfunctions and Other Non-Motor Features in Parkinson's Disease and Related Disorders (Barcelona, Spain: 2010).

53. R. A. Goldstein, N. D. Volkow, "Drug Addiction and Its Underlying Neurobiological Basis: Neuroimaging Evidence for the Involvement of the Frontal Cortex," *American Journal of Psychiatry* 159 (2002): 1642–1652; A. Verdejo-Garcia, R. Vilar-Lopez, M. Perez-Garcia, and E. Goldberg, "Altered Adaptive but Not Veridical Decision-Making in Substance Dependent Individuals," *Journal of the International Neuropsychological Society* 12 (2006): 90–99.

54. A. Verdejo-Garcia, L. Clark, J. Verdejo-Roma, N. Albein-Urios, J. M. Martinez-Gonzalez, B. Gutierrez, and C. Soriano-Mas, "Neural Substrates of Cognitive Flexibility in Cocaine and Gambling Addictions," *The British Journal of Psychiatry* (2015) 207: 158–164; O. Contreras-Rodríguez, N. Albein-Urios, J. C. Perales, J. M. Martínez-Gonzalez, R. Vilar-López, M. J. Fernández-Serrano, O. Lozano-Rojas, and A. Verdejo-García, "Cocaine-Specific Neuroplasticity in the Ventral

Striatum Network Is Linked to Delay Discounting and Drug Relapse," *Addiction* 10 (2015): 1953–1962.

CHAPTER 6: THE INNOVATING BRAIN

1. For a more detailed review of biological differences between the two hemispheres across species, see: E. Goldberg, *The New Executive Brain: Frontal Lobes in a Complex World* (New York: Oxford University Press, 2009); and E. Goldberg, *The Wisdom Paradox: How Your Mind Can Grow Stronger as Your Brain Grows Older* (New York: Gotham Books, 2005).
2. E. Goldberg and L. Costa, "Hemisphere Differences in the Acquisition and Use of Descriptive Systems," *Brain and Language* 14 (1981): 144–173.
3. T. G. Bever and R. J. Chiarello, "Cerebral Dominance in Musicians and Non-musicians," *Science* 185 (1974): 537–539.
4. C. A. Marci and G. Berlucchi, "Right Visual Field Superiority for Accuracy of Recognition of Famous Faces in Normals," *Neuropsychologia* 15 (1977): 751–756.
5. A. Martin, "Automatic Activation of the Medial Temporal Lobe During Encoding: Lateralized Influences of Meaning and Novelty," *Hippocampus* 9 (1999): 62–70.
6. M. Lezak, D. B. Howieson, E. D. Bigler, and D. Tranel, *Neuropsychological Assessment*, 5th edn. (New York: Oxford University Press, 2012).
7. M. Corbetta and G. L. Shulman, "Control of Goal-Directed and Stimulus-Driven Attention in the Brain," *Nature Reviews Neuroscience* 3 (2002): 201–215; M. Corbetta, G. Patel, and G. L. Shulman, "The Reorienting System of the Human Brain: From Environment to Theory of Mind," *Neuron* 58 (2008): 306–324; B. J. Levy and A. D. Wagner, "Cognitive Control and Right Ventrolateral Prefrontal Cortex: Reflexive Reorienting, Motor Inhibition, and Action Updating," *Annals of the New York Academy of Sciences* 1224 (2011): 40–62; D. Badre and A. D. Wagner, "Left Ventrolateral Prefrontal Cortex and the Cognitive Control of Memory," *Neuropsychologia* 45 (2007): 2883–2901.
8. D. Wang, R. L. Buckner, and X. H. Liu, "Functional Specialization in the Human Brain Estimated by Intrinsic Hemispheric Interaction," *The Journal of Neuroscience* 34 (2014): 12341–12352.
9. D. Sridharan, D. J. Levitin, and V. Menon, "A Critical Role for the Right Fronto-insular Cortex in Switching Between Central-Executive and Default-Mode Networks," *Proceedings of the National Academy of Sciences* 105 (2008): 12569–12574; D. Sridharan, D. J. Levitin, C. H. Chafe, J. Berger, and V. Menon, "Neural Dynamics of Event Segmentation in Music: Converging Evidence for Dissociable Ventral and Dorsal Networks," *Neuron* 55 (2007): 521–532.
10. T. T. Chong, R. Cunnington, M. A. Williams, and J. B. Mattingley, "The Role of Selective Attention in Matching Observed and Executed Actions," *Neuropsychologia* 47 (2009): 786–795; T. T. Chong, R. Cunnington, M. A.

Williams, N. Kanwisher, and J. B. Mattingley, "fMRI Adaptation Reveals Mirror Neurons in Human Inferior Parietal Cortex," *Current Biology* 18 (2008): 1576–1580.

11. H. P. Op de Beeck, C. I. Baker, J. J. DiCarlo, and N. G. Kanwisher, "Discrimination Training Alters Object Representations in Human Extrastriate Cortex," *The Journal of Neuroscience* 26 (2006): 13025–13036.

12. M. Delazer, F. Domahs, L. Bartha, C. Brenneis, A. Lochy, T. Trieb, and T. Benke, "Learning Complex Arithmetic—An FMRI Study," *Brain Research: Cognitive Brain Research* 18 (2003): 76–88.

13. D. Sridharan, D. J. Levitin, and V. Menon," A Critical Role for the Right Fronto-insular Cortex in Switching Between Central-Executive and Default-Mode Networks," *Proceedings of the National Academy of Sciences* 105 (2008): 12569–12574.

14. S. J. Sara, C. Dyon-Laurent, and A. Hervé, "Novelty Seeking Behavior in the Rat Is Dependent upon the Integrity of the Noradrenergic System," *Brain Research: Cognitive Brain Research* 2 (1995): 181–187.

15. C. Lee, J. W. Yang, S. H. Lee, S. H. Kim, S. H. Joe, I. K. Jung, I. G. Choi, and B. J. Ham, "An Interaction Between the Norepinephrine Transporter and Monoamine Oxidase A Polymorphisms, and Novelty-seeking Personality Traits in Korean Females," *Progress in Neuro-Psychopharmacology and Biological Psychiatry* 32 (2008): 238–242.

16. R. R. I. Kruglikov, N. V. Orlova, and V. M. Getsova, "Content of Norepinephrine and Serotonin in Symmetrical Divisions of the Brain of Rats in the Norm During Learning and with the Administration of Peptides," *Neuroscience and Behavioral Physiology* 22 (1992): 128–131; S. D. Glick, D. A. Ross, and L. B. Hough, "Lateral Asymmetry of Neurotransmitters in Human Brain," *Brain Research* 234 (1982): 53–63; R. Carter, *Mapping the Mind* (London, UK: Phoenix Publishing, 2004); S. D. Glick, *Cerebral Lateralization in Non-Human Species* (Cambridge, MA: Academic Press, 1985); S. D. Glick, R. C. Meibach, R. D. Cox, and S. Maayani, "Multiple and Interrelated Functional Asymmetries in Rat Brain," *Life Sciences* 25 (1979): 395–400.

17. S. Grossberg, *Neural Networks and Natural Intelligence* (Cambridge, MA: MIT Press, 1988); R. C. O'Reilly and Y. Munakata, *Computational Explorations in Cognitive Neuroscience* (Cambridge, MA: MIT Press, 2000).

18. Y. Hakeem, C. C. Sherwood, C. J. Bonar, C. Butti, P. R. Hof and J. M. Allman, "Von Economo Neurons in the Elephant Brain," *The Anatomical Record* 292 (2009): 242–248.

19. J. M. Allman, N. A. Tetreault, A. Y. Hakeem, K. F. Manaye, K. Semendeferi, J. M. Erwin, S. Park, V. Goubert, and P. R. Hof, "The Von Economo Neurons in the Frontoinsular and Anterior Cingulate Cortex," *Annals of the New York Academy of Sciences* 1225 (2011): 59–71.

20. P. Rourke, *Nonverbal Learning Disabilities: The Syndrome and the Model*, 1st edn. (New York: The Guilford Press, 1989).

21. A. Kluger and E. Goldberg, "Comparison of VIQ/PIQ Ratios in Patients with Affective Disorders, Diffuse and Right Hemisphere Brain Disease," *Journal of Clinical and Experimental Neuropsychology* 12 (1990): 182–194.

22. C. Chiron, I. Jambaque, R. Nabbout, R. Lounes, A. Syrota and O. Dulac, "The Right Brain Hemisphere Is Dominant in Human Infants," *Brain* 120 (1997): 1057–1065.

23. E. Goldberg, *The Wisdom Paradox: How Your Mind Can Grow Stronger as Your Brain Grows Older* (New York: Gotham Books, 2005).

24. V. Llaurens, M. Raymond, and C. Faurie, "Why Are Some People Left-handed? An Evolutionary Perspective," *Philosophical Transactions of the Royal Society of London, B: Biological Sciences* 364 (2009): 881–894.

25. H. I. Kushner, "Why Are There (Almost) No Left-handers in China?" *Endeavour* 37 (2013): 71–81.

26. S. Wang and S. Aamodt, "A Vast Left-handed Conspiracy," *The Washington Post* (July 6, 2008): http://www.washingtonpost.com/wp-dyn/content/article/2008/07/03/AR2008070303202.html

27. J. Goodman, "The Wages of Sinistrality: Handedness, Brain Structure, and Human Capital Accumulation," *Journal of Economic Perspectives* 28 (2014): 193–212; C. S. Ruebeck, J. E. Harrington, Jr., and R. Moffitt, "Handedness and Earnings," *Laterality: Asymmetries of Brain Body and Cognition* 12 (2007): 101–120.

28. Goldberg, K. Podell, R. Harner, M. Lovell, and S. Riggio, "Cognitive Bias, Functional Cortical Geometry, and the Frontal Lobes: Laterality, Sex, and Handedness," *Journal of Cognitive Neuroscience* 6 (1994): 274–294.

29. R. Kumar and A. E. Lang, "Coexistence of Tics and Parkinsonism: Evidence for Non-dopaminergic Mechanisms in Tic Pathogenesis," *Neurology* 49 (1997): 1699–1701.

30. Goldberg, K. Podell, R. Harner, M. Lovell, and S. Riggio, "Cognitive Bias, Functional Cortical Geometry, and the Frontal Lobes: Laterality, Sex, and Handedness," *Journal of Cognitive Neuroscience* 6 (1994): 274–294; K. Podell, "When East Meets West: Systematizing Luria's Approach to Executive Control Assessment," in *Luria's Legacy in the 21st Century,* Eds. A. L. Christensen, E. Goldberg, and D. Bougakov (New York: Oxford University Press, 2009): 122–145.

31. S. Varanese, B. Perfetti, S. Mason, A. Di Rocco, and E. Goldberg, "Lateralized Profiles of Frontal Lobe Dysfunction in Parkinson's Disease," Presented at the Seventh International Congress on Mental Dysfunctions and Other Non-motor Features in Parkinson's Disease and Related Disorders (Barcelona, Spain: December 9–12, 2010)

32. D. M. Sheppard, J. L. Bradshaw, R. Purcell, and C. Pantelis, "Tourette's and Comorbid Syndromes: Obsessive Compulsive and Attention Deficit Hyperactivity

Disorder. A Common Etiology?" *Clinical Psychology Review* 19 (1999): 531–552; R. Rizzom, M. Gulisano, P. V. Cali, and P. Curatolo, "Tourette Syndrome and Comorbid ADHD: Current Pharmacological Treatment Options," *European Journal of Paediatric Neurology* 17 (2013): 421–428; M. Bloch, M. State, and C. Pittenger, "Recent Advances in Tourette Syndrome," *Current Opinion in Neurology* 24 (2011): 119–125; R. H. Bitsko, J. R. Holbrook, S. N. Visser, J. W. Mink, S. H. Zinner, R. M. Ghandour, and S. J. Blumberg, "A National Profile of Tourette Syndrome, 2011–2012," *Journal of Developmental & Behavioral Pediatrics* 35 (2014): 317–322; "Tourette Syndrome: Data and Statistics," *Centers for Disease Control* (2016): http://www.cdc.gov/ncbddd/tourette/data.html.

33. O. W. Sacks, "Tourette's Syndrome and Creativity," *British Medical Journal* 305 (1992): 1515–1516.

34. E. Goldberg, *"ADHD, Tourette's and the Fallacy of Fads,"* Keynote address at International Conference on Neuroethics (ICONE) (Lisbon, Portugal, April 9–10, 2015).

35. F. Lhermitte, B. Pillon, and M. Serdaru, "Human Autonomy and the Frontal Lobes. Part I: Imitation and Utilization Behavior: A Neuropsychological Study of 75 Patients," *Annals of Neurology* 19 (1986): 326–334; E. Goldberg and L. Costa, "Qualitative Indices in Neuropsychological Assessment: Extension of Luria's Approach. Executive Deficit Following Prefrontal Lesions," in *Neuropsychological Assessment in Neuropsychiatric Disorders*, Eds. K. Adams and I. Grant (New York: Oxford University Press, 2009): 48–64; E. Goldberg, *The New Executive Brain: Frontal Lobes in a Complex World* (New York: Oxford University Press, 2009).

36. This gap is now being filled by my former students and colleagues Andy Lopez-Williams and Kjell Tore Hovik, who have designed the exploratory behavior scale and are currently refining it.

37. E. Goldberg, *The New Executive Brain: Frontal Lobes in a Complex World* (New York: Oxford University Press, 2009).

38. K. T. Hovik, M. Øie, and E. Goldberg, "Inside the Triple-Decker: Tourette's Syndrome and Cerebral Hemispheres," *Executive Functions in Health and Disease*, Ed. E. Goldberg (Cambridge, MA: Academic Press, 2017).

39. R. H. Bitsko, J. R. Holbrook, S. N. Visser, J. W. Mink, S. H. Zinner, R. M. Ghandour, and S. J. Blumberg, "A National Profile of Tourette Syndrome, 2011–2012," *Journal of Developmental & Behavioral Pediatrics* 35 (2014): 317–322.

40. E. Goldberg, K. Podell, R. Harner, M. Lovell, and S. Riggio, "Cognitive Bias, Functional Cortical Geometry, and the Frontal Lobes: Laterality, Sex, and Handedness," *Journal of Cognitive Neuroscience* 6 (1994): 274–294.

41. S. C. Cohen, J. M. Mulqueen, E. Ferracioli-Oda, Z. D. Stuckelman, C. G. Coughlin, J. F. Leckman, and M. H. Bloch, "Meta-Analysis: Risk of Tics Associated with Psychostimulant Use in Randomized, Placebo-Controlled Trials," *Journal of the American Academy of Child and Adolescent Psychiatry* 54 (2015): 728–736.

CHAPTER 7: DIRECTED WANDERING AND
THE INEFFABLE CREATIVE SPARK

1. B. Ghiselin, *The Creative Process: Reflections on the Invention in the Arts and Sciences*, 1st edn. (Oakland, CA: University of California Press, 1985).

2. D. T. Campbell, "Blind Variation and Selective Retentions in Creative Thought as in Other Knowledge Processes," *Psychological Review*, 67 (1960): 380–400; R. E. Jung, B. S. Mead, J. Carrasco, and R. A. Flores, "The Structure of Creative Cognition in the Human Brain," *Frontiers in Human Neuroscience* 7 (2013): 330.

3. H. A. Simon, *The Sciences of the Artificial*, 3rd edn. (Cambridge, MA: MIT Press, 1996): 194.

4. A. Dietrich, "Transient Hypofrontality as a Mechanism for the Psychological Effects of Exercise," *Psychiatry Research* 145 (2006): 79–83.

5. A video of the Sanghyang Jaran dance was made by my Balinese friends' son Ida Bagus Yogi Iswara Bawa, whom I asked to come along: https://youtu.be/g_nAG-NrLjiM. For more detailed discussion of transient hypofrontality in altered states of consciousness, see A. Dietrich, "Functional Neuroanatomy of Altered States of Consciousness: The Transient Hypofrontality Hypothesis," *Consciousness and Cognition* 12 (2003): 231–256.

6. M. L. Grillon, C. Oppenheim, G. Varoquaux, F. Charbonneau, A. D. Devauchelle, M. O. Krebs, F. Baylé, B. Thirion, and C. Huron, "Hyperfrontality and Hypoconnectivity During Refreshing in Schizophrenia," *Psychiatry Research* 211 (2013): 226–233.

7. A. Hampshire, A. Macdonald, and A. M. Owen, "Hypoconnectivity and Hyperfrontality in Retired American Football Players," *Scientific Reports* 3 (2013): 2972.

8. F. X. Vollenweider, K. L. Leenders, C. Scharfetter, P. Maguire, O. Stadelmann, and J. Angst, "Positron Emission Tomography and Fluorodeoxyglucose Studies of Metabolic Hyperfrontality and Psychopathology in the Psilocybin Model of Psychosis," *Neuropsychopharmacology* 16 (1997): 357–372; C. Dackis and C. O'Brien, "Neurobiology of Addiction: Treatment and Public Policy Ramifications," *Nature Neuroscience* 8 (2005): 1431–1436.

9. D. R. Weinberger and K. F. Berman, "Speculation on the Meaning of Cerebral Metabolic Hypofrontality in Schizophrenia," *Schizophrenia Bulletin* 14 (1988): 157–168; R. A. Renes, M. Vink, A. Van Der Weiden, M. Prikken, M. G. Koevoets, R. S. Kahn, H. Aarts, and N. E. Van Haren, "Impaired Frontal Processing During Agency Inferences in Schizophrenia," *Psychiatry Research* 248 (2016): 134–141; D. Senkowski and J. Gallinat, "Dysfunctional Prefrontal Gamma-band Oscillations Reflect Working Memory and Other Cognitive Deficits in Schizophrenia," *Biological Psychiatry* 77 (2015): 1010–1019; H. Tomioka, B. Yamagata, S. Kawasaki, S. Pu, A. Iwanami, J. Hirano, K. Nakagome, and M. Mimura, "A Longitudinal Functional Neuroimaging Study in Medication-naïve Depression After Antidepressant Treatment," *PLoS One* 10

(2015): E0120828; C. T. Li, T. P. Su, S. J. Wang, P. C. Tu, and J. C. Hsieh, "Prefrontal Glucose Metabolism in Medication-Resistant Major Depression," *British Journal of Psychiatry* 206 (2015): 316–323; M. E. Vélez-Hernández, E. Padilla, F. Gonzalez-Lima, and C. A. Jiménez-Rivera, "Cocaine Reduces Cytochrome Oxidase Activity in the Prefrontal Cortex and Modifies Its Functional Connectivity with Brainstem Nuclei," *Brain Research* 1542 (2014): 56–69.

10. A. Dietrich, "Functional Neuroanatomy of Altered States of Consciousness: The Transient Hypofrontality Hypothesis," *Consciousness and Cognition* 12 (2003): 231–256; A. Dietrich, "The Cognitive Neuroscience of Creativity," *Psychonomic Bulletin & Review* 11 (2004): 1011–1026.

11. K. M. Heilman, S. E. Nadeau, and D. O. Beversdorf, "Creative Innovation: Possible Brain Mechanisms," *Neurocase* 9 (2003): 369–379; K. M. Heilman, "Possible Brain Mechanisms of Creativity," *Archives of Clinical Neuropsychology* 31 (2016): 285–296.

12. A. Kaufman Et Al, "The Neurobiological Foundation of Creative Cognition," in *The Cambridge Handbook of Creativity*, Eds. J. C. Kaufman and R. J. Sternberg (Cambridge, UK: Cambridge University Press, 2010): 216–232.

13. G. B. Chand, M. Dhamala, "Interactions Among the Brain Default-Mode, Salience, and Central-Executive Networks During Perceptual Decision-Making of Moving Dots," *Brain Connectivity* 6 (2016): 249–254.

14. E. Goldberg & L. Costa, "Qualitative Indices in Neuropsychological Assessment: Extension of Luria's Approach. Executive Deficit Following Prefrontal Lesions." In K. Adams & I. Grant (Eds.), *Neuropsychological Assessment in Neuropsychiatric Disorders* (New York: Oxford University Press, 1986): 48–64.

15. E. Goldberg, K. Podell, R. Harner, M. Lovell, and S. Riggio, "Cognitive Bias, Functional Cortical Geometry, and the Frontal Lobes: Laterality, Sex, and Handedness," *Journal of Cognitive Neuroscience* 6 (1994): 274–294; E. Goldberg and K. Podell, "Reciprocal Lateralization of Frontal Lobe Functions," *Archives of General Psychiatry* 52 (1995): 159–160; E. Goldberg and K. Podell, "Lateralization in the Frontal Lobes: Searching the Right (and Left) Way," *Biological Psychiatry* 38 (1995): 569–571; K. Podell, M. Lovell, M. Zimmerman, and E. Goldberg, "The Cognitive Bias Task and Lateralized Frontal Lobe Functions in Males," *Journal of Neuropsychiatry and Clinical Neuroscience* 7 (1995): 491–501.

16. S. Varanese, B. Perfetti, S. Mason, A. Di Rocco, and E. Goldberg, "Lateralized Profiles of Frontal Lobe Dysfunction in Parkinson's Disease," Presented at the Seventh International Congress On Mental Dysfunctions and Other Non-motor Features in Parkinson's Disease and Related Disorders (Barcelona, Spain: December 9–12, 2010); K. T. Hovik, M. Øie, and E. Goldberg, "Inside the Triple-Decker: Tourette's Syndrome and Cerebral Hemispheres," *Executive Functions in Health and Disease*, Ed. E. Goldberg (Cambridge, MA: Academic Press, 2017).

17. J. D. Watts and S. H. Strogatz, "Collective Dynamics of 'Small-World' Networks," *Nature* 393 (1998): 440–442.

18. O. Sporns and G. Tononi, "Classes of Network Connectivity and Dynamics," *Complexity* 7 (2002): 28–38.

19. O. Sporns, G. Tononi, and G. M. Edelman, "Theoretical Neuroanatomy: Relating Anatomical and Functional Connectivity in Graphs and Cortical Connection Matrices," *Cerebral Cortex* 10 (2000): 127–141.

20. L. Tian, J. Wang, C. Yan, and Y. He, "Hemisphere and Gender Related Differences in Small-World Brain Networks: A Resting-State Functional MRI Study," *NeuroImage* 54 (2011): 191–202; Y. Iturria-Medina, A. Perez Fernandez, D. M. Morris, E. J. Canales-Rodriguez, H. A. Haroon, L. Garcia Penton, M. Augath, L. Galan Garcia, N. Logothetis, G. J. Parker, and L. Melie-Garcia, "Brain Hemispheric Structural Efficiency and Interconnectivity Rightward Asymmetry in Human and Nonhuman Primates," *Cerebral Cortex* 21 (2011): 56–67; J. Semmes, "Hemispheric Specialization: A Possible Clue to Mechanism," *Neuropsychologia* 6 (1968): 11–26; M. Daianu, N. Jahanshad, E. L. Dennis, A. W. Toga, K. L. McMahon, G. I. De Zubicaray, N. G. Martin, M. J. Wright, I. B. Hickie, and P. M. Thompson, "Left Versus Right Hemisphere Differences in Brain Connectivity: 4-Tesla HARDI Tractography in 569 Twins," *Proceedings of the IEEE International Symposium on Biomedical Imaging* 9 (2012): 526–529.

21. C. D. Good, I. S. Johnsrude, J. Ashburner, R. N. Henson, K. J. Friston, and R. S. Frackowiak, "A Voxel-based Morphometric Study of Ageing in 465 Normal Adult Human Brains," *Neuroimage* 14 (2001): 21–36; J. Pujol, A. Lopez-Sala, J. Deus, N. Cardoner, N. Sebastian-Galles, G. Conesa, and A. Capdevilla, "The Lateral Asymmetry of the Human Brain Studied by Volumetric Magnetic Resonance Imaging," *Neuroimage* 17 (2002): 670–679; R. C. Gur, I. K. Packer, J. P. Hungerbuhler, M. Reivich, W. D. Obrist, W. S. Amarnek, and H. A. Sackeim, "Differences in the Distribution of Gray and White Matter in Human Cerebral Hemispheres," *Science* 207 (1980): 1226–1228.

22. H. Poincaré, "The Mathematical Creation." In *The Creative Process: Reflections on Inventions in the Arts and Sciences*, Ed. B. Chiselin (Oxnard, CA: Transformational Book Circle, 1986).

23. B. Ghiselin, *The Creative Process: Reflections on the Invention in the Arts and Sciences*, 1st edn. (Oakland, CA: University of California Press, 1985).

24. N. Marupaka and A. A. Minai, "Connectivity and Creativity in Semantic Neural Networks." *Neural Networks (IJCNN)* (International Joint Conference on Neural Networks, July 31–August 5, 2011).

25. J. Hadamard, *The Mathematician's Mind: The Psychology of Invention in the Mathematical Field* (Princeton, NJ: Princeton University Press, 1945): 142–143.

26. B. Ghiselin, *The Creative Process: Reflections on the Invention in the Arts and Sciences*, 1st edn. (Oakland, CA: University of California Press, 1985), 60.

27. A. Luria, *Higher Cortical Functions in Man*, 2nd edn. (New York: Springer, 1980); A. Luria, *The Working Brain: An Introduction to Neuropsychology* (New York: Basic Books, 1976); J. M. Fuster, *The Neuroscience of Freedom and Creativity: Our Predictive Brain* (Cambridge, UK: Cambridge University Press, 2013): 176.

CHAPTER 8: IS THE BABOON CREATIVE?

1. F. De Waal, *Are We Smart Enough to Know How Smart Animals Are?* 1st edn. (New York: W. W. Norton & Company, 2016).

2. J. Grainger, S. Dufau, M. Montant, J. C. Ziegler, and J. Fagot, "Orthographic Processing in Baboons (*Papio Papio*)," *Science* 336 (2012): 245–248.

3. J. Fagot and J. Vauclair, "Video-Task Assessment of Stimulus Novelty Effects on Hemispheric Lateralization in Baboons (*Papio Papio*)," *Journal of Comparative Psychology* 108 (1994): 156–163; J. Grainger, S. Dufau, M. Montant, J. C. Ziegler, and J. Fagot, "Orthographic Processing in Baboons (*Papio Papio*)," *Science* 336 (2012): 245–248.

4. P. F. MacNeilage, L. J. Rogers, and G. Vallortigara, "Origins of the Left and Right Brain," *Scientific American* 301 (2009): 60–67.

5. S. Klur, C. Muller, A. Pereira de Vasconcelos, T. Ballard, J. Lopez, R. Galani, U. Certa, and J. C. Cassel, "Hippocampal-dependent Spatial Memory Functions Might Be Lateralized in Rats: An Approach Combining Gene Expression Profiling and Reversible Inactivation," *Hippocampus* 19 (2009): 800–816.

6. K. W. Pryor, R. Haag, and J. O'Reilly, "The Creative Porpoise: Training for Novel Behavior," *Journal of the Experimental Analysis of Behavior* 12 (1969): 653–661.

7. K. W. Pryor, R. Haag, and J. O'Reilly, "The Creative Porpoise: Training for Novel Behavior," *Journal of the Experimental Analysis of Behavior* 12 (1969): 661.

8. A. Kilian, L. Von Fersen, and O. Güntürkün, "Left Hemispheric Advantage for Numerical Abilities in the Bottlenose Dolphin," *Behavioral Processes* 68 (2005): 179–184.

9. M. Sakai, T. Hishii, S. Takeda, and S. Koshima, "Laterality of Flipper Rubbing Behaviour in Wild Bottlenose Dolphins (*Tursiops Aduncus*): Caused by Asymmetry of Eye Use?" *Behavioural Brain Research* 170 (2006): 204–210.

10. C. Blois-Heulin, M. Crével, M. Böye, and A. Lemasson, "Visual Laterality in Dolphins: Importance of the Familiarity of Stimuli," *BMC Neuroscience* 13 (2012): 9; M. Siniscalchi, S. Dimatteo, A. M. Pepe, R. Sasso, and A. Quaranta, "Visual Lateralization in Wild Striped Dolphins (*Stenella Coeruleoalba*) in Response to Stimuli with Different Degrees of Familiarity," *PLoS One* 7 (2012): E30001.

11. J. Ackerman, *The Genius of Birds* (New York: Penguin Press, 2016).

12. M. O'Hara, A. M. Auersperg, T. Bugnyar, and L. Huber, "Inference by Exclusion in Goffin Cockatoos (*Cacatua Goffini*)," *PLoS One* 10 (2015): E0134894;

A. M. Auersperg, N. Oswald, M. Domanegg, G. K. Gajdon, and T. Bugnyar, "Unrewarded Object Combinations in Captive Parrots," *Animal Behavior and Cognition* 1 (2014): 470–488; A. M. Auersperg, A. Kacelnik, and A. M. Von Bayern, "Explorative Learning and Functional Inferences on a Five-step Means-Means-End Problem in Goffin's Cockatoos (*Cacatua Goffini*)," *PLoS One* 8 (2013): E68979.

13. E. D. Jarvis, O. Güntürkün, L. Bruce, A. Csillag, H. Karten, W. Kuenzel, L. Medina, G. Paxinos, D. J. Perkel, T. Shimizu, G. Striedter, J. M. Wild, G. F. Ball, J. Dugas-Ford, S. E. Durand, G. E. Hough, S. Husband, L. Kubikova, D. W. Lee, C. V. Mello, A. Powers, C. Siang, T. V. Smulders, K. Wada, S. A. White, K. Yamamoto, J. Yu, A. Reiner, A. B. Butler, and The Avian Brain Nomenclature Consortium, "Avian Brains and a New Understanding of Vertebrate Brain Evolution," *Nature Reviews Neuroscience* 6 (2005): 151–159.

14. M. Magat and C. Brown, "Laterality Enhances Cognition in Australian Parrots," *Proceedings in Biological Sciences* 276 (2009): 4155–4162; J. N. Daisley, G. Vallortigara, and L. Regolin, "Logic in an Asymmetrical (Social) Brain: Transitive Inference in the Young Domestic Chick," *Society of Neuroscience* 5 (2010): 309–319.

15. J. Verhaal, J. A. Kirsch, I. Vlachos, M. Manns, and O. Güntürkün, "Lateralized Reward-Related Visual Discrimination in the Avian Entopallium," *European Journal of Neuroscience* 35 (2012): 1337–1343.

16. B. A. Bell, M. L. Phan, and D. S. Vicario, "Neural Responses in Songbird Forebrain Reflect Learning Rates, Acquired Salience and Stimulus Novelty After Auditory Discrimination Training," *Journal of Neurophysiology* 113 (2015): 1480–1492.

17. J. J. Templeton, D. J. Mountjoy, S. R. Pryke, and S. C. Griffith, "In the Eye of the Beholder: Visual Mate Choice Lateralization in a Polymorphic Songbird," *Biology Letters* 8 (2012): 924–927; J. J. Templeton, B. G. McCracken, M. Sher, and D. J. Mountjoy, "An Eye for Beauty: Lateralized Visual Stimulation of Courtship Behavior and Mate Preferences in Male Zebra Finches, *Taeniopygia Guttata*," *Behavioral Processes* 102 (2014): 33–39.

18. S. Moorman, S. M. Gobes, M. Kuijpers, A. Kerkhofs, M. A. Zandbergen, and J. J. Bolhuis, "Human-like Brain Hemispheric Dominance in Birdsong Learning," *Proceedings of the National Academy of Sciences USA* 109 (2012): 12782–12787.

19. S. C. Tsoi, U. V. Aiya, K. D. Wasner, M. L. Phan, C. L. Pytte, and D. S. Vicario, "Hemispheric Asymmetry in New Neurons in Adulthood Is Associated with Vocal Learning and Auditory Memory," *PLoS One* 9 (2014): E108929.

20. L. J. Rogers and G. Vallortigara, "From Antenna to Antenna: Lateral Shift of Olfactory Memory in Honeybees," *PLoS One* 3 (2008): E2340; E. Frasnelli, "Brain and Behavioral Lateralization in Invertebrates," *Frontiers in Psychology* 4 (2013): 939.

21. E. Frasnelli, "Brain and Behavioral Lateralization in Invertebrates," *Frontiers in Psychology* 4 (2013): 939.

22. L. S. Vygotsky, *The Psychology of Art* (Cambridge, MA: MIT Press, 1974).

23. L. S. Vygotsky, *Thought and Language,* revised and expanded edn. (Cambridge, MA: MIT Press, 2012); L. S. Vygotsky, *Mind in Society: The Development of Higher Cognitive Processes,* revised edn. (Cambridge, MA: Harvard University Press, 1978); J. V. Wertsch, *Vygotsky and the Social Formation of Mind* (Cambridge, MA: Harvard University Press, 1985).

24. F. G. Patterson, "The Gestures of a Gorilla: Language Acquisition in Another Pongid," *Brain and Language* 5 (1978): 72–97; V. A. Haviland, H. E. L. Prins, B. McBride, and D. Walrath, *Cultural Anthropology: The Human Challenge,* 15th edn. (Wadsworth Publishing, 2016).

25. S. Savage-Rumbaugh and R. Lewin, *Kanzi: The Ape at the Brink of the Human Mind* (Hoboken, NJ: Wiley, 1994); W. M. Fields, P. Segerdahl, and S. Savage-Rumbaugh, "The Material Practices of Ape Language Research," in *The Cambridge Handbook of Sociocultural Psychology,* Eds. J. Valsinar and A. Rosa (Cambridge, UK: Cambridge University Press, 2007): 164–186.

26. F. Warneken and A. G. Rosati, "Cognitive Capacities for Cooking in Chimpanzees," *Proceedings of the Royal Society B B* 282 (2015): 20150229.

27. I. M. Pepperberg, "In Search of King Solomon's Ring: Cognitive and Communicative Studies of Grey Parrots (*Psittacus Erithacus*)," *Brain, Behavior and Evolution* 59 (2002): 54–67; I. M. Pepperberg and S. Carey, "Grey Parrot Number Acquisition: The Inference of Cardinal Value from Ordinal Position on the Numeral List," *Cognition* 125 (2012): 219–232.

28. K. N. Laland and B. G. Galef, Eds., *The Question of Animal Culture* (Cambridge, MA: Harvard University Press, 2009).

29. A. Whiten, J. Goodall, W. C. McGrew, T. Nishida, V. Reynolds, Y. Sugiyama, C. E. G. Tutin, R. W. Wrangham, and C. Boesch, "Cultures in Chimpanzees," *Nature* 399 (1999): 682–685.

30. J. Terkel, "Cultural Transmission of Feeding Behavior in the Black Rat (*Rattus Rattus*)," in *Social Learning in Animals: The Roots of Culture,* Eds. C. M. Heyes and B. G. Galef (San Diego, CA: Academic Press, 1996): 17–48.

31. C. A. Toft and T. F. Wright, *Parrots of the Wild: A Natural History of the World's Most Captivating Birds* (Berkeley, CA: University of California Press, 2015).

32. C. M. Johnson, "Distributed Primate Cognition: A Review," *Animal Cognition* 4 (2001): 167–183; W. M. Fields, P. Segerdahl, and S. Savage-Rumbaugh, "The Material Practices of Ape Language Research," in *The Cambridge Handbook of Sociocultural Psychology,* Eds. J. Valsinar and A. Rosa (Cambridge, UK: Cambridge University Press, 2007): 164–186.

33. E. Pennisi, "The Power of Personality," *Science* 352 (2016): 644–647.

34. V. A. Haviland, H. E. L. Prins, B. McBride, and D. Walrath, *Cultural Anthropology: The Human Challenge,* 15th edn. (Belmont, CA: Wadsworth Publishing, 2016).

CHAPTER 9: THE CREATIVE MIND

1. Arrian, *The Campaigns of Alexander* (New York: Penguin Group, 1971): 105; Plutarch, *Life of Alexander* (New York: The Modern Library, 2004): 19.
2. B. Hayes, "Gauss's Day of Reckoning," *American Scientist* 94 (2006): 200.
3. P. Hermann, M. Smith, and K. L. Alexander, "Horrified Passengers Witnessed Brutal July 4 Slaying Aboard Metro Car," *The Washington Post* (July 7, 2015): https://www.washingtonpost.com/local/crime/victim-in-metro-slaying-stabbed-repeatedly-during-robbery-on-train/2015/07/07/8dd09132-249b-11e5-b72c-2b7d516e1e0e_story.html.
4. S. E. Asch, "Studies of Independence and Conformity: I. A Minority of One Against a Unanimous Majority," *Psychological Monographs: General and Applied* 70 (1956): 1–70.
5. S. Gächter and J. Schultz, "Intrinsic Honesty and the Prevalence of Rule Violations Across Societies," *Nature* 531 (2016): 496–499.
6. A. Strandburg-Peshkin, D. R. Farine, I. D. Couzin, and M. C. Crofoot, "Shared Decision-making Drives Collective Movement in Wild Baboons," *Science* 348 (2015): 1358–1361.
7. C. S. Carter, T. S. Braver, D. M. Barch, M. M. Botvinick, D. Noll, and J. D. Cohen, "Anterior Cingulate Cortex, Error Detection, and the Online Monitoring of Performance," *Science* 280 (1998): 747–749.
8. B. Slotnick, "Disturbances of Maternal Behavior in the Rat Following Lesions of the Cingulate Cortex," *Behaviour* 29 (1967): 204–235.
9. K. A. Hadland, M. F. S. Rushworth, D. Gaffan, and R. E. Passingham, "The Effect of Cingulate Lesions on Social Behaviour and Emotion," *Neuropsychologia* 41 (2003): 919–931.
10. C. F. Zink and A. Meyer-Lindenberg, "Human Neuroimaging of Oxytocin and Vasopressin in Social Cognition," *Hormones and Behavior* 61 (2012): 400–409; C. F. Zink, J. L. Stein, L. Kempf, S. Hakimi, and A. Meyer-Lindenberg, "Vasopressin Modulates Medial Prefrontal Cortex-Amygdala Circuitry During Emotion Processing in Humans," *Journal of Neuroscience* 30 (2010): 7017–7022.
11. V. Klucharev, K. Hytönen, M. Rijpkema, A. Smidts, and G. Fernández, "Reinforcement Learning Signal Predicts Social Conformity," *Neuron* 61 (2009): 140–151.
12. V. Klucharev, M. A. M. Moniek, A. Smidts, and G. Fernandez, "Downregulation of the Posterior Medial Frontal Cortex Prevents Social Conformity," *Journal of Neuroscience* 31 (2011): 11934–11940.
13. E. Goldberg, D. Roediger, N. E. Kucukboyaci, C. Carlson, O. Devinsky, R. Kuzniecky, E. Halgren, and T. Thesen, "Hemispheric Asymmetries of Cortical Volume in the Human Brain," *Cortex* 49 (2013): 200–210.
14. C. Fajardo, M. I. Escobar, E. Buriticá, G. Arteaga, J. Umbarila, M. F. Casanova, and H. Pimienta, "Von Economo Neurons Are Present in the Dorsolateral

(Dysgranular) Prefrontal Cortex of Humans," *Neuroscience Letters* 435 (2008): 215–218.

15. J. M. Allman, N. A. Tetreault, A. Y. Hakeem, K. F. Manaye, K. Semendeferi, J. M. Erwin, S. Park, V. Goubert, and P. R. Hof, "The Von Economo Neurons in the Frontoinsular and Anterior Cingulate Cortex," *Annals of the New York Academy of Sciences* 1225 (2011): 59–71.

16. A. F. Santillo, C. Nilsson, and E. Englund, "Von Economo Neurones Are Selectively Targeted in Frontotemporal Dementia," *Neuropathology and Applied Neurobiology* 39 (2013): 572–579.

17. G. Boole, *An Investigation of the Laws of Thought* (Amherst, MA: Prometheus Books, 2003).

18. J. M. Osborne and A. Rubinstein, *A Course in Game Theory* (Cambridge, MA: MIT Press, 1994). At the time of this writing, the "2/3 of the average" game's website was http://twothirdsofaverage.creativitygames.net/.

19. J. P. Guilford, *The Nature of Human Intelligence* (New York: McGraw-Hill, 1967); E. Jauk, M. Benedek, B. Dunst, and A. C. Neubauer, "The Relationship Between Intelligence and Creativity: New Support for the Threshold Hypothesis by Means of Empirical Breakpoint Detection," *Intelligence* 41 (2013): 212–221.

20. J. C. Kaufman, *Creativity 101* (New York: Springer Publishing Company, 2009).

21. J. B. Carroll, *Human Cognitive Abilities: A Survey of Factor Analytic Studies* (Cambridge, UK: Cambridge University Press, 1993).

22. E. Goldberg, *The New Executive Brain: Frontal Lobes in a Complex World* (New York: Oxford University Press, 2009).

23. A. S. Kaufman, *IQ Testing 101* (New York: Springer Publishing, 2009).; also see:http://www.pearsonclinical.com/psychology/products/100000392/wechsler-adult-intelligence-scalefourth-edition-wais-iv.html accessed April 24, 2017.

24. R. K. Sawyer, *Explaining Creativity: The Science of Human Innovation* (New York: Oxford University Press, 2012); M. Csikszentmihalyi, *Creativity: Flow and the Psychology of Discovery and Invention* (New York: Harper Collins, 1996).

25. T. Hey, *Einstein's Mirror* (Cambridge, UK: Cambridge University Press, 1997): 1.

26. K. Landau-Drobantseva, *Academician Landau: How We Lived. A Memoir*, in Russian (Moscow: Zakharov Press, 1999).

27. R. K. Sawyer, *Explaining Creativity: The Science of Human Innovation*, 2nd edn. (New York: Oxford University Press, 2012); K. H. Kim, "Meta-analyses of the Relationship of Creative Achievement to Both IQ and Divergent Thinking Tests Scores," *Journal of Creative Behavior* 42 (2008): 106–130.

28. E. P. Torrance, *Torrance Tests of Creative Thinking* (Bensenville, IL: Scholastic Testing Service, 1966).

29. D. A. Gansler, D. W. Moore, T. M. Susmaras, M. W. Jerram, J. Sousa, and K. M. Heilman, "Cortical Morphology of Visual Creativity," *Neuropsychologia* 49 (2011): 2527–2532.

30. R. E. Jung, J. M. Segall, J. H. Bockholt, R. A. Flores, S. W. Smith, R. S. Chavez, and R. J. Haier, "Neuroanatomy of Creativity," *Human Brain Mapping* 31 (2010): 398–409.

31. H. Takeuchi, Y. Taki, Y. Sassa, H. Hashizume, A. Sekiguchi, A. Fukushima, and R. Kawshima, "Regional Gray Matter Volume of Dopaminergic System Associated with Creativity: Evidence from Voxel-based Morphometry," *Neuroimage* 51 (2010): 578–585; H. Takeuchi, Y. Taki, Y. Sassa, H. Hashizume, A. Sekiguchi, A. Fukushima, and R. Kawishima, "White Matter Structures Associated with Creativity: Evidence from Diffusion Tensor Imaging," *Neuroimage* 51 (2010): 11–18.

32. S. Sandkühler and J. Bhattacharya, "Deconstructing Insight: EEG Correlates of Insightful Problem Solving," *PLoS One* 3 (2008): E1459.

33. A. Fink, R. H. Grabner, M. Benedek, G. Reishofer, V. Hauswirth, M. Fally, C. Neuper, F. Ebner, and A. C. Neubauer, "The Creative Brain: Investigation of Brain Activity During Creative Problem Solving by Means of EEG and FMRI," *Human Brain Mapping* 30 (2009): 734–748.

34. I. Carlsson, P. E. Wendt, and J. Risberg, "On the Neurobiology of Creativity: Differences in Frontal Activity Between High and Low Creative Subjects," *Neuropsychologia* 38 (2000): 873–875.

35. A. Fink and M. Benedek, "EEG Alpha Power and Creative Ideation," *Neuroscience and Biobehavioral Reviews* 44 (2014): 111–123.

36. C. Lustenberger, M. R. Boyle, A. A. Foulser, J. M. Mellin, and F. Fröhlich, "Functional Role of Frontal Alpha Oscillations in Creativity," *Cortex* 67 (2015): 74–82.

37. A. E. Green, K. A. Spiegel, E. J. Giangrande, A. B. Weinberger, N. M. Gallagher, and P. E. Turkeltaub, "Thinking Cap Plus Thinking Zap: TDCS of Frontopolar Cortex Improves Creative Analogical Reasoning and Facilitates Conscious Augmentation of State Creativity in Verb Generation," *Cerebral Cortex* (2016): Bhw080.

38. C. Lombroso, *The Man of Genius*, reprint of translated edition of the original 1889 book (North Charleston, SC: CreateSpace Independent Publishing Platform, 2015).

39. S. H. Carson, "Creativity and Psychopathology: A Shared Vulnerability Model," *Canadian Journal of Psychiatry* 56 2011: 144–153; A. Fink, M. Benedek, H. F. Unterrainer, I. Papousek, and E. M. Weiss, "Creativity and Psychopathology: Are There Similar Mental Processes Involved in Creativity and in Psychosis-proneness?" *Frontiers in Psychology* 5 (2014).

40. For a more detailed review, see my earlier book: E. Goldberg, *The Wisdom Paradox: How Your Mind Can Grow Stronger As Your Brain Grows Older* (New York: Gotham, 2005).

41. S. H. Carson, J. B. Peterson, and D. M. Higgins, "Reliability, Validity, and Factor Structure of the Creative Achievement Questionnaire," *Creative Research Journal*

17 (2005): 37–50; H. G. Gough, "A Creative Personality Scale for the Adjective Check List," *Journal of Personality and Social Psychology* 37 (1979): 1398–1405.

42. N. Andreasen, "Creativity and Mental Illness: Prevalence Rates in Writers and Their First-degree Relatives," *American Journal of Psychiatry* 144 (1987): 1288–1292.

43. S. Kyaga, P. Lichtenstein, M. Boman, C. Hultman, N. Långström, and M. Landén, "Creativity and Mental Disorder: Family Study of 300,000 People with Severe Mental Disorder," *British Journal of Psychiatry* 199 (2011): 373–379; K. R. Jamison, "Mood Disorders and Patterns of Creativity in British Writers and Artists," *Psychiatry* 52 (1989): 125–134.

44. V. E. Golimbet, M. G. Aksenova, V. V. Nosikov, V. A. Orlova, and V. G. Kaleda, "Analysis of the Linkage of the Taq1A and Taq1B Loci of the Dopamine D2 Receptor Gene with Schizophrenia in Patients and Their Siblings," *Neuroscience and Behavioral Physiology* 33 (2003): 223–225.

45. S. Keri, "Genes for Psychosis and Creativity. A Promoter Polymorphism of the Neuregulin 1 Gene Is Related to Creativity in People with High Intellectual Achievement," *Psychological Science* 20 (2009): 1070–1073; J. Hall, H. C. Whalley, D. E. Job, B. J. Baig, A. M. McIntosh, K. L. Evans, P. A. Thomson, D. J. Porteous, D. G. Cunningham-Owens, E. C. Johnstone, and S. M. Lawrie, "A Neuregulin 1 Variant Associated with Abnormal Cortical Function and Psychotic Symptoms," *Nature Neuroscience* 9 (2006): 1477–1478; A. M. McIntosh, T. W. Moorhead, D. Job, G. K. Lymer, S. Muñoz Maniega, J. McKirdy, J. E. Sussmann, B. J. Baig, M. E. Bastin, D. Porteous, K. L. Evans, E. C. Johnstone, S. M. Lawrie, and J. Hall, "The Effects of a Neuregulin 1 Variant on White Matter Density and Integrity," *Molecular Psychiatry* 13 (2008): 1054–1059; B. Barbot, M. Tan, and E. L. Grigorenko, "The Genetics of Creativity: The Generative and Receptive Sides of the Creativity Equation," in *Neuroscience of Creativity*, Eds. O Vartanian, A. S. Ristol, and J. C. Kaufman (Cambridge, MA: MIT Press, 2013): 72–93.

46. J. A. Pratt, C. Winchester, A. Egerton, S. M. Cochran, and B. J. Morris, "Modelling Prefrontal Cortex Deficits in Schizophrenia: Implications for Treatment," *British Journal of Pharmacology* 153 (2008): 465–470; C. E. Bearden, K. M. Hoffman, and T. D. Cannon, "The Neuropsychology and Neuroanatomy of Bipolar Affective Disorder: A Critical Review," *Bipolar Disorders* 3 (2001): 106–150; A. Anticevic, M. S. Brumbaugh, A. M. Winkler, L. E. Lombardo, J. Barrett, P. R. Corlett, H. Kober, J. Gruber, G. Repovs, M. W. Cole, J. H. Krystal, G. D. Pearlson, and D. C. Glahn, "Global Prefrontal and Fronto-Amygdala Dysconnectivity in Bipolar I Disorder with Psychosis History," *Biological Psychiatry* 73 (2013): 565–573; Y. I. Sheline, J. L. Price, Z. Yan, and M. A. Mintun, "Resting-State Functional MRI in Depression Unmasks Increased Connectivity Between Networks Via the Dorsal Nexus," *Proceedings of the National Academy of Sciences* 107 (2010): 11020–11025.

47. Q. Xiao, Y. Zhong, D. Lu, W. Gao, Q. Jiao, G. Lu, and L. Su, "Altered Regional Homogeneity in Pediatric Bipolar Disorder During Manic State: A Resting-State FMRI Study," *PLoS ONE* 8 (2013): E57978.

48. S. Carson, "Creativity and Psychopathology," in *Neuroscience of Creativity*, Eds. O. Vartanian, A. S. Bristol, and J. C. Kaufman (Cambridge, MA: MIT Press, 2013).

49. S. Whitfield-Gabrieli, H. W. Thermenos, S. Milanovic, M. T. Tsuang, S. V. Faraone, R. W. McCarley, M. E. Shenton, A. I. Green, A. Nieto-Castanon, P. la Violette, J. Wojcik, J. D. E. Gabrieli, and L. J. Seidman, "Hyperactivity and Hyperconnectivity of the Default Network in Schizophrenia and in First-degree Relatives of Persons with Schizophrenia," *Proceedings of the National Academy of Sciences USA* 106 (2009): 1279–1284.

50. See link for TED Talk on the effects of school on creativity: www.ted.com/talks/ ken_robinson_says_schools_kill_creativity?language=en.

51. For a comprehensive review of such programs, see: R. L. DeHaan, "Teaching Creativity and Inventive Problem Solving in Science," *NCBE Life Sciences Education* 8 (2009): 172–181.

52. For a detailed program description, visit: E. Bodrova and D. J. Leong, *Tools of the Mind: The Vygotskian Approach to Early Childhood Education*, 2nd edn. (New York: Pearson, 2006); also see: http://toolsofthemind.org.

53. R. Van der Veer and J. Valsiner, Eds., *The Vygotsky Reader*, 1st edn. (Hoboken, NJ: Wiley-Blackwell, 1994); more on the strange fate of this paper in E. Goldberg, *The Wisdom Paradox: How Your Mind Can Grow Stronger as Your Brain Grows Older* (New York: Gotham Books, 2005); and in E. Goldberg, "Thank You for Sharing This Fascinating Material—Very Interesting," *Dubna Psychological Journal* 5 (2012): 118–120.

54. A. Diamond, W. S. Barnett, J. Thomas, and S. Munro, "Preschool Program Improves Cognitive Control," *Science* 318 (2007): 1387–1388; A. Diamond and K. Lee, "Interventions Shown to Aid Executive Function Development in Children 4–12 Years Old," *Science* 333 (2011): 959–964; C. Blair and C. C. Raver, "Closing the Achievement Gap Through Modification of Neurocognitive and Neuroendocrine Function: Results from a Cluster Randomized Controlled Trial of an Innovative Approach to the Education of Children in Kindergarten," *PLoS One* 9 (2014): E112393.

55. See links for more on Minerva Schools: www.minerva.kgi.edu; www.youtube. com/watch?v=5-NRAgo_y1I.

CHAPTER 10: THE CREATIVE BRAIN

1. S. F. Witelson, D. L. Kigar, and T. Harvey, "The Exceptional Brain of Albert Einstein," *The Lancet* 353 (1999): 2149–2153.

2. D. Falk, F. E. Lepore, and A. Noe, "DOI the Cerebral Cortex of Albert Einstein: A Description and Preliminary Analysis of Unpublished Photographs," *Brain* (2012): 1304–1327.

3. W. Men, D. Falk, T. Sun, W. Chen, J. Li, D. Yin, L. Zang, and M. Fan, "The Corpus Callosum of Albert Einstein's Brain: Another Clue to His High Intelligence?" *Brain* 137 (2013): 1–8.

4. M. C. Diamond, A. B. Scheibe, G. M. Murphy, and T. Harvey, "On the Brain of A Scientist: Albert Einstein," *Experimental Neurology* 88 (1985): 198–204.

5. O. S. Adrianov, I. N. Bogolepova, S. M. Blinkov, L. A. Kukuev, "The Study of V. I. Lenin's Brain," [article in Russian] *Uspekhi Fiziologicheskikh Nauk* 24 (1993): 40–52.

6. See link for more on Gauss's brain: https://www.mpg.de/7589532/Carl_Friedrich_Gauss_brain; R. Schweizer, A. Wittmann, J. Frahm, "A Rare Anatomical Variation Newly Identifies the Brains of C. F. Gauss and C. H. Fuchs in a Collection at the University of Gottingen," *Brain* 137 (2013): 1–2.

7. A. Dietrich and N. Srinivasan, "The Optimal Age to Start a Revolution," *The Journal of Creative Behavior* 41 (2007): 54–74.

8. E. S. Finn, X. Shen, D. Scheinost, M. D. Rosenberg, J. Huang, M. M. Chun, X. Papademetris, and R. T. Constable, "Functional Connectome Fingerprinting: Identifying Individuals Using Patterns of Brain Connectivity," *Nature Neuroscience* 18 (2015): 1664–1671; M. D. Rosenberg, E. S. Finn, D. Scheinost, X. Papademetris, X. Shen, R. T. Constable, and M. M. Chun, "A Neuromarker of Sustained Attention from Whole-Brain Functional Connectivity," *Nature Neuroscience* 19 (2016): 165–171.

9. Y. Li, Y. Liu, J. Li, W. Qin, K. Li, C. Yu, and T. Jiang, "Brain Anatomical Network and Intelligence," *PLoS Computational Biology* 5 (2009): E1000395.

10. D. J. Smit, C. J. Stam, D. Posthuma, D. I. Boomsma, and E. J. De Geus, "Heritability of "Small-World" Networks in the Brain: A Graph Theoretical Analysis of Resting-State EEG Functional Connectivity," *Human Brain Mapping* 29 (2008): 1368–1378.

11. L. Wang, C. Zhu, Y. He, Y. Zang, Q. J. Cao, H. Zhang, Q. Zhong, and Y. Wang, "Altered Small-World Brain Functional Networks in Children with Attention-Deficit/Hyperactivity Disorder," *Human Brain Mapping* 30 (2009): 638–649.

12. E. M. Miller, "Intelligence and Brain Myelination: A Hypothesis," *Personality and Individual Differences* 17 (1994): 803–832.

13. J. M. Fuster, *The Neuroscience of Freedom and Creativity: Our Predictive Brain* (Cambridge, UK: Cambridge University Press, 2013): 176.

14. E. R. Sowell, B. S. Peterson, P. M. Thompson, S. E. Welcome, A. L. Henkenius, and A. W. Toga, "Mapping Cortical Change Across the Human Life Span," *Nature Neuroscience* 6 (2003): 309–315; F. I. M. Craik and E. Bialystok, "Cognition Through the Lifespan; Mechanisms of Change," *Trends in Cognitive Sciences* 10 (2006): 131–138.

15. D. J. Millera, T. Dukaa, C. D. Stimpson, S. J. Schapiro, W. B. Baze, M. J. McArthur, A. J. Fobbs, A. M. M. Sousa, N. Sestan, D. E. Wildman, L. Lipovich, C. W. Kuzawa, P. R. Hof, and C. C. Sherwood, "Prolonged Myelination in

Human Neocortical Evolution," *Proceedings of the National Academy of Sciences* 109 (2012): 116480–16485.

16. L. Marner, J. R. Nyengaard, Y. Tang, and B. Pakkenberg, "Marked Loss of Myelinated Nerve Fibers in the Human Brain with Age," *Journal of Comparative Neurology* 462 (2003): 144–152.

17. N. Raz, K. M. Rodrigue, and E. M. Haacke, "Brain Aging and Its Modifiers: Insights from in Vivo Neuromorphometry and Susceptibility Weighted Imaging," *Annals of the New York Academy of Sciences* 1097 (2007): 84–93.

18. E. Goldberg, *The Wisdom Paradox: How Your Mind Can Grow Stronger as Your Brain Grows Older* (New York: Gotham Books, 2005).

19. M. J. Valenzuela, P. S. Sachdev, W. Wen, R. Shnier, H. Brodaty, and D. Gillies, "Dual Voxel Proton Magnetic Resonance Spectroscopy in the Healthy Elderly: Subcortical-Frontal Axonal N-Acetylaspartate Levels Are Correlated with Fluid Cognitive Abilities Independent of Structural Brain Changes," *Neuroimage* 12 (2000): 747–756.

20. K. Kantarci, C. R. Jack, Y. C. Xu, N. G. Campeau, P. C. O'Brien, G. E. Smith, R. J. Ivnik, B. F. Boeve, E. Kokmen, E. G. Tangalos, and R. C. Petersen, "Regional Metabolic Patterns in Mild Cognitive Impairment and Alzheimer's: A 1H MRS Study," *Neurology* 55 (2000): 210–217; S. H. Patel, M. Inglese, G. Glosser, D. L. Kolson, R. I. Grossman, and O. Gonen, "Whole-Brain N-acetylaspartate Level and Cognitive Performance in HIV Infection," *AJNR: American Journal of Neuroradiology* 24 (2003): 1587–1591.

21. K. Nordengen, C. Heuser, J. E. Rinholm, R. Matalon, and V. Gundersen, "Localisation of N-acetylaspartate in Oligodendrocytes/Myelin," *Brain Structure and Function* 220 (2015): 899–917.

22. A. L. Alexander, J. E. Lee, M. Lazar, and A. S. Field, "Diffusion Tensor Imaging of the Brain," *Neurotherapeutics* 4 (2007): 316–329.

23. R. Westerhausen, C. Walter, F. Kreuder, R. A. Wittling, E. Schweiger, and W. Wittling, "The Influence of Handedness and Gender on the Microstructure of the Human Corpus Callosum: A Diffusion-Tensor Magnetic Resonance Imaging Study," *Neuroscience Letters* 351 (2003): 99–102; R. Westerhausen, F. Kreuder, S. Dos Santos Sequeira, C. Walter, W. Woerner, R. A. Wittling, E. Schweiger, and W. Wittling, "Effects of Handedness and Gender on Macro- and Microstructure of the Corpus Callosum and Its Subregions: A Combined High-Resolution and Diffusion-Tensor MRI Study," *Cognitive Brain Research* 21 (2004): 418–426.

24. H. Takeuchi, Y. Taki, Y. Sassa, H. Hashizume, A. Sekiguchi, A. Fukushima, and R. Kawashima, "White Matter Structures Associated with Creativity: Evidence from Diffusion Tensor Imaging," *Neuroimage* 51 (2010): 11–18.

25. D. W. Moore, R. A. Bhadelia, R. L. Billings, C. Fulwiler, K. M. Heilman, K. M. J. Rood, and D. A. Gansler, "Hemispheric Connectivity and the Visual–Spatial Divergent-Thinking Component of Creativity," *Brain and Cognition* 70 (2009): 267–272.

26. E. P. Torrance, *Torrance Tests of Creative Thinking* (Bensenville, IL: Scholastic Testing Service, 1966).

27. D. A. Gansler, D. W. Moore, T. M. Susmaras, M. W. Jerram, J. Sousa, and K. M. Heilman, "Cortical Morphology of Visual Creativity," *Neuropsychologia* 49 (2011): 2527–2532.

28. R. P. Chi and A. W. Snyder, "Facilitate Insight by Non-invasive Brain Stimulation," *PLoS One* 6 (2011): E16655; R. P. Chi and A. W. Snyder, "Brain Stimulation Enables the Solution of an Inherently Difficult Problem," *Neuroscience Letters* 515 (2012): 121–124.

29. J. Travers, *The Puzzle-Mine: Puzzles Collected from the Works of the Late Henry Ernest Dudeney* (Nashville, TN: Thomas Nelson, 1951).

30. M. Ollinger, G. Jones, and G. Knoblich, "Investigating the Effect of Mental Set on Insight Problem Solving," *Experimental Psychology* 55 (2008): 269–282.

31. R. E. Jung, R. Grazioplene, A. Caprihan, R. S. Chavez, and R. J. Haier, "White Matter Integrity, Creativity, and Psychopathology: Disentangling Constructs with Diffusion Tensor Imaging," *PLoS One* 5 (2010): E9818.

32. T. Kawashima, M. Nakamura, S. Bouix, M. Kubicki, D. F. Salisbury, C. F. Westin, R. W. McCarley, and M. E. Shenton, "Uncinate Fasciculus Abnormalities in Recent Onset Schizophrenia and Affective Psychosis: A Diffusion Tensor Imaging Study," *Schizophrenia Research* 110 (2009): 119–126.

33. S. Rodrigo, O. Naggara, C. Oppenheim, N. Golestani, C. Poupon, Y. Cointepas, J. F. Mangin, D. Le Bihan, and J. F. Meder, "Human Subinsular Asymmetry Studied by Diffusion Tensor Imaging and Fiber Tracking," *American Journal of Neuroradiology* 28 (2007): 1526–1531; H. J. Park, C. F. Westin, M. Kubicki, S. E. Maier, M. Niznikiewicz, A. Baer, M. Frumin, R. Kikinis, F. A. Jolesz, R. W. McCarley, and M. E. Shenton, "White Matter Hemisphere Asymmetries in Healthy Subjects and in Schizophrenia: A Diffusion Tensor MRI Study," *NeuroImage* 23 (2004): 213–223.

34. D. C. Van Essen, S. M. Smith, D. M. Barch, T. E. J. Behrens, E. Yacoub, K. Ugurbil, and for the WU-Minn HCP Consortium, "The WU-Minn Human Connectome Project: An Overview," *Neuroimage* 80 (2013): 62–79.

35. F. Galton, *Hereditary Genius* (London: Macmillan, 1869).

36. R. P. Ebstein, O. Novick, R. Umansky, B. Priel, Y. Osher, D. Blaine, E. R. Bennett, L. Nemanov, M. Katz, and R. H. Belmaker, "Dopamine D4 Receptor (D4DR) Exon III Polymorphism Associated with the Human Personality Trait of Novelty Seeking," *Nature Genetics* 12 (1996): 78–80; J. Benjamin, L. Li, C. Patterson, B. D. Greenberg, D. L. Murphy, and D. H. Hamer, "Population and Familial Association Between the D4 Dopamine Receptor Gene and Measures of Novelty Seeking," *Nature Genetics* 12 (1996): 81–84.

37. M. R. Munafò, B. Yalcin, S. A. Willis-Owen, and J. Flint, "Association of the Dopamine D4 Receptor (*DRD4*) Gene and Approach-Related Personality Traits: Meta-Analysis and New Data," *Biological Psychiatry* 63 (2008): 197–206.

38. M. Reuter, S. Roth, K. Holve, and J. Hennig, "Identification of First Candidate Genes for Creativity: A Pilot Study," *Brain Research* 1069 (2006): 190–197.

39. O. Manzano, S. Cervenka, A. Karabanov, L. Farde, and F. Ullen, "Thinking Outside a Less Intact Box: Thalamic Dopamine D2 Receptor Densities Are Negatively Related to Psychometric Creativity in Healthy Individuals," *PLoS One* 17 (2010).

40. E. Theusch, A. Basu, and J. Gitschier, "Genome-wide Study of Families with Absolute Pitch Reveals Linkage to 8q24.21 and Locus Heterogeneity," *American Journal of Human Genetics* 85(1) (2009): 112–119.

41. J. Oikkonen, T. Kuusi, P. Peltonen, P. Raijas, L. Ukkola-Vuoti, K. Karma, P. Onkamo, and I. Järvelä, "Creative Activities in Music—A Genome-Wide Linkage Analysis," *PLoS One* 24 (2016): 11(2).

42. R. Bachner-Melman, C. Dina, A. Zohar, N. Constantini, E. Lerer, S. Hoch, S. Sella, L. Nemanov, I. Gritsenko, P. Lichtenberg, R. Granot, and R. Ebstein, "*AVPR1A* and *SLC6A4* Gene Polymorphisms Are Associated with Creative Dance Performance," *PLoS Genetics* 1(3) (2005): E42.

43. D. J. Miller, T. Duka, C. D. Stimpson, S. J. Schapiro, W. B. Baze, M. J. McArthur, A. J. Fobbs, A. M. M. Sousa, N. Sestand, D. E. Wildman, L. Lipovich, C. W. Kuzawa, P. R. Hof, and C. C. Sherwood, "Prolonged Myelination in Human Neocortical Evolution," *Proceedings of the National Academy of Sciences* 109 (2012): 116480–16485.

44. T. Sun, R. V. Collura, M. Ruvolo, and C. A. Walsh, "Genomic and Evolutionary Analyses of Asymmetrically Expressed Genes in Human Fetal Left and Right Cerebral Cortex," *Cerebral Cortex* 16 (2006): I118–i125; T. Sun, C. Patoine, A. Abu-Khalil, J. Visvader, E. Sum, T. J. Cherry, S. H. Orkin, D. H. Geschwind, and C. A. Walsh, "Early Asymmetry of Gene Transcription Between Embryonic Human Left and Right Cerebral Cortex," *Science* 308 (2005): 1794–1798; T. Sun and C. A. Walsh, "Molecular Approaches to Brain Asymmetry and Handedness," *Nature Reviews Neuroscience* 7 (2006): 655–662.

45. G. Davies, A. Tenesa, A. Payton, J. Yang, S. E. Harris, D. Liewald, X. Ke, S. Le Hellard, A. Christoforou, M. Luciano, K. McGhee, L. Lopez, A. J. Gow, J. Corley, P. Redmond, H. C. Fox, P. Haggarty, L. J. Whalley, G. McNeill, M. E. Goddard, T. Espeseth, A. J. Lundervold, Ivar Reinvang, A. Pickles, V. M. Steen, W. Ollier, D. J. Porteous, M. Horan, J. M. Starr, N. Pendleton, P. M. Visscher, and I. J. Deary, "Genome-wide Association Studies Establish That Human Intelligence Is Highly Heritable and Polygenic," *Molecular Psychiatry* 16 (2011): 996–1005.

CHAPTER 11: EPILOGUE—WHAT'S NEXT?

1. E. Kandel, *The Age of Insight: The Quest to Understand the Unconscious in Art, Mind, and Brain, from Vienna 1900 to the Present* (New York: Random House, 2012).

2. C. L. Satizabal, A. S. Beiser, V. Chouraki, G. Chêne, C. Dufouil, and S. Seshadri, "Incidence of Dementia over Three Decades in the Framingham Heart Study," *New England Journal of Medicine* 374 (2016): 523–532.

3. K. C. Manton, X. L. Gu, and S. V. Ukraintseva, "Declining Prevalence of Dementia in the U.S. Elderly Population," *Advances in Gerontology* 16 (2005): 30–37.

4. K. M. Langa, E. B. Larson, J. H. Karlawish, D. M. Cutler, M. U. Kabeto, S. Y. Kim, and A. B. Rosen, "Trends in the Prevalence and Mortality of Cognitive Impairment in the United States: Is There Evidence of a Compression of Cognitive Morbidity?" *Alzheimer's and Dementia* 4 (2008): 134–144; K. M. Langa, E. B. Larson, E. M. Crimmins, J. D. Faul, D. A. Levine, M. U. Kabeto, and D. R. Weir, "A Comparison of the Prevalence of Dementia in the United States in 2000 and 2012," *JAMA Internal Medicine*, 177 (2017): 51–58.

5. G. Doblhammer, A. Fink, S. Zylla, and F. Willekens, "Compression or Expansion of Dementia in Germany? An Observational Study of Short-term Trends in Incidence and Death Rates of Dementia Between 2006/07 and 2009/10 Based on German Health Insurance Data," *Alzheimer's Research and Therapy* 7 (2015): 66.

6. K. M. Langa, "Is the Risk of Alzheimer's Disease and Dementia Declining?" *Alzheimer's Research and Therapy* 7 (2015): 34; C. Qiu, E. Von Strauss, L. Bäckman, L. B. Winblad, and L. Fratiglioni, "Twenty-Year Changes in Dementia Occurrence Suggest Decreasing Incidence in Central Stockholm, Sweden," *Neurology* 80 (2013): 1888–1994.

7. L. Fratiglioni and H. X. Wang, "Brain Reserve Hypothesis in Dementia," *Journal of Alzheimer's Disease* 12 (2007): 11–22.

8. E. Goldberg, *The Wisdom Paradox: How Your Mind Can Grow Stronger as Your Brain Grows Older* (New York: Gotham Books, 2005).

9. N. Raz, F. Gunning-Dixon, D. Head, K. M. Rodrigue, A. Williamson, and J. D. Acker, "Aging, Sexual Dimorphism, and Hemispheric Asymmetry of the Cerebral Cortex: Replicability of Regional Differences in Volume," *Neurobiology of Aging* 25 (2004): 377–396; N. Raz, P. Ghisletta, K. M. Rodrigue, K. M. Kennedy, and U. Lindenberger, "Trajectories of Brain Aging in Middle-Aged and Older Adults: Regional and Individual Differences," *NeuroImage* 51 (2010): 501–511.

10. C. Van Doren, *A History of Knowledge: Past, Present, and Future*, reissue edn. (New York: Ballantine Books, 1992).

11. W. James, *Is Life Worth Living?* reprint edn. (North Charleston, SC: CreateSpace, 2015).

12. See linked post written by Mark Zuckerberg on Facebook's acquisition of Oculus VR: www.facebook.com/zuck/posts/10101319050523971.

13. W. Knight, "Microsoft Researchers Are Working on Multi-Person Virtual Reality," *MIT Technology Review* (October 12, 2015): https://www.technologyreview.com/s/542341/microsoft-researchers-are-working-on-multi-person-virtual-realit/

14. Z. M. Aghajan, L. Acharya, J. J. Moore, J. D. Cushman, C. Vuong, and M. R. Mehta, "Impaired Spatial Selectivity and Intact Phase Precession in Two-Dimensional Virtual Reality," *Nature Neuroscience* 18 (2015): 121–128.

15. K. Sawyer, *Group Genius: The Creative Power of Collaboration* (New York: Basic Books, 2008); K. Sawyer, *Explaining Creativity: The Science of Human Innovation*, 2nd edn. (New York: Oxford University Press, 2012).

16. J. R. Hackman, *Collaborative Intelligence: Using Teams to Solve Hard Problems* (San Francisco, CA: Berrett-Koehler Publishers, 2011); D. Markova and A. McArthur, *Collaborative Intelligence: Thinking with People Who Think Differently* (New York: Spiegel & Grau, 2015); D. Contu, "Why Teams Don't Work," *Harvard Business Review* 5 (2009).

17. S. Cole, "Age and Scientific Performance," *American Journal of Sociology* 84 (1979): 958–977.

18. N. Stern, "Age and Achievement in Mathematics: A Case-study in the Sociology of Science," *Social Studies of Science* 8 (1978): 127–140.

19. See link for SAP's use of mixed-age teams: https://news.sap.com/young-old-powerful-combination/.

20. M. Csikszentmihalyi, *Creativity: The Psychology of Discovery and Invention*, reprint edn. (New York: Harper Perennial, 2013).

21. J. Y. Chiao, "Cultural Neuroscience: A Once and Future Discipline," *Progress in Brain Research* 178, (2009): 287–304; C. L. Fincher, R. Thornhill, D. R. Murray, and M. Schaller, "Pathogen Prevalence Predicts Human Cross-Cultural Variability in Individualism/Collectivism," *Proceedings of the Royal Society: B* 275 (2008): 1279–1285; R. B. Adams, N. O. Rule, R. G. Franklin, E. Wang, M. T. Stevenson, S. Toshikawa, M. Nomura, W. Sato, K. Kveraga, and N. Ambady, "Cross-Cultural Reading the Mind in the Eyes: An FMRI Investigation," *Journal of Cognitive Neuroscience* 22 (2010): 97–108; E. Goldberg, "Foreword," in *Embodiment and Cultural Differences*, Eds. B. M. Pirani and T. S. Smith (Cambridge, UK: Cambridge Scientific Publishers, 2016).

22. R. Gaines, and D. Price-Williams, "Dreams and Imaginative Processes in American and Balinese Artists," *Psychiatric Journal of the University of Ottawa* 15 (1990): 107–110.

23. J. W. Shenk, *Powers of Two: How Relationships Drive Creativity*, reprint edn. (New York: Eamon Dolan/Mariner Books, 2015).

24. E. Goldberg, *The Executive Brain: Frontal Lobes and the Civilized World* (New York: Oxford University Press, 2001; paperback 2002); E. Goldberg, *The New Executive Brain: Frontal Lobes in a Complex World* (New York: Oxford University Press, 2009).

25. M. Ingalhalikar, A. Smith, D. Parker, T. D. Satterthwaite, M. A. Elliott, K. Ruparel, H. Hakonarson, R. E. Gur, R. C. Gur, and R. Verma, "Sex Differences in the Structural Connectome of the Human Brain," *Proceedings of the National Academy of Sciences USA* 111 (2014): 823–828.

26. V. Llaurens, M. Raymond, and C. Faurie, "Why Are Some People Left-Handed? An Evolutionary Perspective," *Philosophical Transactions of the Royal Society of London, B: Biological Sciences* 364 (2009): 881–894.

27. S. F. Witelson, "The Brain Connection: The Corpus Callosum Is Larger in Left-Handers," *Science* 229 (1985): 665–668; Q. Gao, J. Wang, C. Yu, and H. Chen, "Effect of Handedness on Brain Activity Patterns and Effective Connectivity Network During the Semantic Task of Chinese Characters," *Scientific Reports* 5 (2015): 18262; R. Westerhausen, C. Walter, F. Kreuder, R. A. Wittling, E. Schweiger, and W. Wittling, "The Influence of Handedness and Gender on the Microstructure of the Human Corpus Callosum: A Diffusion-Tensor Magnetic Resonance Imaging Study," *Neuroscience Letters* 351 (2003): 99–102; R. Westerhausen, R. F. Kreuder, S. Dos Santos Sequeira, C. Walter, W. Woerner, R. A. Wittling, E. Schweiger, and W. Wittling, "Effects of Handedness and Gender on Macro- and Microstructure of the Corpus Callosum and Its Subregions: A Combined High-Resolution and Diffusion-Tensor MRI Study," *Cognitive Brain Research* 21 (2004): 418–426.

28. E. Goldberg, D. Roediger, N. E. Kucukboyaci, C. Carlson, O. Devinsky, R. Kuzniecky, E. Halgren, and T. Thesen, "Hemispheric Asymmetries of Cortical Volume in the Human Brain," *Cortex* 49 (2013): 200–210.

29. M. Wooldridge, *An Introduction to MultiAgent Systems* (New York: John Wiley & Sons, 2002).

30. H. A. Simon, *The Sciences of the Artificial*, 3rd edn. (Cambridge, MA: MIT Press, 1996); A. Newell, J. C. Shaw, and H. A. Simon, "The Process of Creative Thinking," in *Contemporary Approaches to Creative Thinking*, Eds. H. E. Gruber, G. Terrell, and M. Wertheimer (New York: Atherton, 1962): 63–119.

31. From Harold Cohen obituary, posted on http://www.aaronshome.com/ where information about Harold Cohen and paintings by AARON can also be found.

32. You can find some of the Emily Howell compositions on www.youtube.com.

33. W. McCulloch and W. Pitts, "A Logical Calculus of Ideas Immanent in Nervous Activity," *Bulletin of Mathematical Biophysics* 5 (1943): 115–133.

34. M. Minsky and S. Papert, *Perceptrons: An Introduction to Computational Geometry* (Cambridge, MA: MIT Press, 1969).

35. For a comprehensive review, see D. S. Levine, "Neural Network Models of Human Executive Function and Decision Making," in *Executive Functions in Health and Disease*, Ed. E. Goldberg (Cambridge, MA: Academic Press, 2017).

36. N. Marupaka and A. A. Minai, "Connectivity and Creativity in Semantic Neural Networks," *Neural Networks (IJCNN)* (International Joint Conference on Neural Networks, July 31–August 5, 2011).

37. J. M. Fuster, *The Neuroscience of Freedom and Creativity: Our Predictive Brain* (Cambridge, UK: Cambridge University Press, 2013).

38. L. Scheffler, "Which Features Matter How Much When?" Presentation at BICA 2016; S. Thaler, "Pattern Turnover Within Synaptically Perturbed Neural Systems,"

Presentation at BICA 2016; S. Thaler, "Creativity Machine Paradigm," in E. G. Carayannis (Ed.), *Encyclopedia of Creativity, Innovation and Entrepreneurship* (New York: Springer, 2013): 447–456.

39. A. Manfre', A. Augello, I. Infantino, G. Pilato, and F. Vella, "Exploiting Interactive Genetic Algorithms for Creative Humanoid Dancing," Presentation at BICA 2016; A. Augello, I. Infantino, A. Manfre', G. Pilato, and F. Vella, "Analyzing and Discussing Primary Creative Traits of a Robotic Artist," Presentation at BICA 2016; www.facebook.com/CRSSLAB

40. E. Borovikov, I. Zavorin, and S. Yershov, "On Virtual Characters That Can See," Presentation at BICA 2016.

41. O. Chernavskaya, D. Chernavskii, V. Karp, A. Nikitin, and D. Schepetov, "An Architecture of Thinking System Within the Dynamic Theory of Information," BICA 12 (2015): 144–154; O. Chernavskaya, D. Chernavskii, and Y. Rozhylo, "A Hypothesis on the Nature of "Aesthetic" Emotions and the Concept of "Masterpiece," Presentation at BICA 2016.

Index

Note: Figures are indicated by an italic *f* following the page number.